Eye Movement Research:
Physiological and Psychological Aspects

Eye Movement Research

Physiological and Psychological Aspects

edited by

Gerd Lüer, Uta Lass, Josephine Shallo-Hoffmann
University of Göttingen

C. J. Hogrefe
Toronto · Lewiston, NY · Göttingen · Zürich

Fourth European Conference on Eye movements, Volume 2

Library of Congress Cataloging-in-Publication Data

Eye movement research : physiological and psychological aspects / Gerd Lüer, Uta Lass, and Josephine Shallo-Hoffmann, editors
p. cm.

1. Eye—Movements. 2. Eye—Movements—Psychological aspects.
I. Lüer, Gerd, 1938– . II. Lass, Uta, 1949– III. Shallo-Hoffmann, Josephine, 1946– .
[DNLM: 1. Eye Movements. WW 400 E968]
QP477.5.E92 1988 612'.846 – dc19 88-16032

Canadian Cataloguing in Publication Data

Main entry and under title:

Eye movement research

Bibliography: p.
Includes index.

1. Eye—Movements—Research. 2. Eye—Movements—Psychological aspects—Research. I. Lüer, Gerd, 1938– . II. Lass, Uta, 1949– . III. Shallo-Hoffmann, Josephine, 1946– .

QP477.5.E937 1988 612'.846 C88-094112-X

P.O. Box 51
Lewiston, NY 14092

12–14 Bruce Park Ave.
Toronto, Ontario M4P 2S3

Printed in Germany

ISBN 0-88937-020-6 Hogrefe Toronto · Lewiston, NY · Göttingen · Zürich
ISBN 3-8017-0288-X Hogrefe Göttingen · Zürich · Toronto · Lewiston, NY

PREFACE

This second volume on eye movement research stems from the Fourth European Conference on Eye Movements (ECEM 4) held on September 21-24, 1987, in Göttingen, Federal Republic of Germany. While Volume 1 appeared at the beginning of the congress and includes abstracts of all contributions to the ECEM 4, this book is a selection of 18 articles published at full length. It is not a report of findings presented at the congress; rather, these 18 articles have been written at the request of the editors and reach far beyond the congress reports. One can think of the works presented here as the fully detailed result which has grown out of the ECEM 4 meeting.

Selecting papers for a collected work is never without problems. It is thus possible that some very good papers presented at ECEM 4 are not to be found here. Although several experts served as our advisors for the selection of the current articles, it is clear that not all of the fine contributions could be accepted for publication. The editors alone carry the responsibility for any error in this selection. However, we would like to take this opportunity to note that we felt these 18 articles to be particularly noteworthy among very many other good ones.

A book with many contributors is only possible with the help of many persons. Firstly, we would like to thank all the authors who made their texts available to us. The deadline pressure which we had to set as well as our many critical comments were surely occasionally uncomfortable. We are grateful for the understanding, cooperation, and, most importantly, good will of everyone concerned.

Further, we would like to thank our many colleagues for their competent advice and reviews concerning the selection of articles. They were certainly helpful with the decisions for the final manuscript.

For financial reasons the entire manuscript was prepared so that it could be simply reproduced. Thus, along with the actual editorial work, we were responsible for the layout and printed format of the book. Ms. Waltraut Fähmel prepared the final manuscript as well as took care of all correspondence with the authors. She was supported by Ms. Angelika Weber and Ms. Barbara Becker. We are indebted to them for their ever precise and very dependable assistance.

Each manuscript was additionally proofread for stylistic and orthographic accuracy. For this, we thank above all Ms. Freya Tiederle, and Dr. Christina Jones. We were also supported by Ms. Gabriele Reimann, who improved or re-drew unsuitable figures for final print.

As in Volume 1, Mr. Michael Ulrich was responsible for the entire computer word processing and printing of the manuscript. For his patience, cooperation and ability to hold the deadline we are especially thankful.

As with Volume 1, collaboration with the publishing company C.J. Hogrefe was exceptionally effective. For this, we also would like to express our gratefulness and recognition.

Göttingen, July 1988

Gerd Lüer, Uta Lass, and Josephine Shallo-Hoffmann

CONTENTS

1
Introduction

INTRODUCTION

GERD LÜER[1], UTA LASS[1], AND
JOSEPHINE SHALLO-HOFFMANN[2]

[1] Institut für Psychologie,
[2] Abteilung Strabologie und Neuroophthalmologie,
Georg-August-Universität Göttingen

The title of this book holds a two-fold meaning: firstly, the subject of discourse is the phenomenon of eye movements in correlation to various aspects of neurophysiology and perception; secondly, the reader finds a collection of intentionally interdisciplinary contributions concerning eye movements which stresses the influence of visual perception and its related processes. It was the intention of the editors to prove that such a multidisciplinary approach is fruitful.

Although many questions concerning methodological criteria for the comparability and standardization of eye movement measurements are far from satisfactorily answered, the entire area has progressed long past a simple methodology concerned with applied research. Especially in the last few years has it become more apparent that the study of eye movements as they relate to more complex recognition and decision processes contribute very basically to questions of visual perception. The contributions in this book show the intensity with which current research in this area has tackled such problems.

The volume is organized into five central sections, focusing on main topics of interest in this research field. Often the discourse achieves a remarkable refinement in solving the problem and therefore demonstrating some totally new results. However, since these are specific issues, they cannot be thought of as representative of the whole field. The present book is a mirror of the times and thus a cross-section of the research areas currently being explored.

Before we further elaborate on the outline and structure of the present volume, we would like to ask a general question: What is actually so fascinating about the research of human eye movement? We see it, above all, in the many different facets of the answers that can be given. This can best be described by focusing on a few basic themes. The breadth of the area of eye movement research extends from fundamental neurophysiology to the understanding of reading processes. Basic knowledge of the mechanisms and functional processes of eye movement allow not only for the exact characterization of the speed and precision of visual perceptive abilities, but also for higher order processing. Reading research is a good example of this. From the precise measurement of movement and duration around points of fixation, it becomes possible to interpret more complex cognitive processes such as attention or decision making. This implies that whole new results can be won through precise functional eye movement analysis. Further, new knowledge can be gained from the "indicator function" that these basal mechanisms of visual perception apparently have. Through the choice of the contributions published here the editors have attempted to exemplify the breadth and diversity which is possible and necessary for a description of eye movement function.

The discussion begins with the article from Otto D. Creutzfeldt. He provides an overview of the actual state of knowledge in this area from the perspective of a neurophysiologist. The fact that so many regions of the brain participate in the control and direction of eye movement allows for the testing of hypotheses concerning the relationship between eye movement and cortical functions. Just as cortical oculomotoric controls and perceptions are connected with each other, so is it possible to demonstrate that regions of the brain which are active in direct control of eye movements are also necessary for cognitive abilities. Creutzfeldt develops a model of perception as an active process from these neurophysiological findings.

A historical view of eye movement research is given in the article by Dieter Heller. In impressive examples he proves that the research of this area began long before the beginnings of experimental psychology. Important scientific ideas are traced back to the Middle Ages and even into ancient times. The author also theorizes on the methods of measuring and the criteria for gathering valid data. This review makes clear that the development of methods of measurement strongly influenced the course of research.

The third chapter includes six articles on smooth pursuit and saccadic eye movements. Reinhart Jürgens, Anselm W. Kornhuber, and Wolfgang Becker describe discontinuous and non-linear processes concerned in human smooth pursuit. Detailed experimental results indicate a conceptual mechanism for prediction of smooth pursuit strategies.

Lo Bour investigates the mutual interaction of human smooth pursuit and saccadic eye movements. It is his aim to achieve more insight into the initiation of saccades when both saccadic and pursuit systems are simultaneously activated. Jan A.M. van Gisbergen, Arend C. Smit, and Rob J.W. Berg explore the dynamic characteristics of saccades and report on experiments in which the dynamics-latency relation of a saccade could be studied. The results are interpreted in terms of Becker and Jürgens' saccadic system model. In a further contribution, Heiner Deubel, John Findlay, Arthur Jacobs, and David Brogan describe results from two different experimental approaches; the authors explore the effect of visual background structure on target-elicited saccades.

Roberto Schmid and Daniela Zambarbieri present a general theory on sensorimotor control. Vestibular nystagmus, for which a mathematical model is introduced, is understood here as a manifestation of a strategy of eye-head coordination. In the last article in this section, Hessel Franssen and Dirk Frederik Stegeman investigate the influence of the cerebral cortex, thalamus, or superior colliculus in saccadic decision and averaging processes through the study of patients with lesions in these areas.

The fourth section includes six papers on reading process. Marcel A. Just and Patricia A. Carpenter discuss the topics of reading and spatial cognition and review the progress of research in this area over the last ten years. Aside from reporting research data, they present two basic themes to which eye movement research has contributed substantially: theories on the organization of thought and individual differences in the way people think.

Joel Pynte, Alan Kennedy, Wayne S. Murray, and Pierre Courrieu discuss the problem of the assimilation of ambiguous sentences. They compared total re-reading times and pattern of reinspection following spatialised presentation of sentences in order to address issues in eye movement control.

Eye movement control during reading is the focus of the article written by George W. McConkie, N. Roderic Underwood, Gary S. Wolverton, and David Zola. They use data on various patterns of response that occur when readers encounter erroneous letters at different locations in their visual field. Marc Brysbaert and Géry d'Ydewalle investigate whether the two visual hemifields are sharply separated from each other or not. Further, they contemplate the possible contribution of collosal connections between hemispheres and review the literature in this area as well as present new findings.

The paper from Arthur M. Jacobs and Ariane Lévy-Schoen treats information processing during a single eye fixation. The authors demonstrate that a model with independent assimilation processes for centrally and peripherally presented information best describes the data from four experiments. Françoise Vitu and J. Kevin O'Regan show that the eye's first fixation position in a word is the probable source of variation for the various observable fixation durations. With incorporation of reading rhythm and parafoveal preprocessing as factors of normal reading, the phenomenon of optimal viewing position during normal reading is described.

The last chapter contains articles dealing with perception and cognition. The section begins with Rudolf Groner's paper on eye movements and attention processes. His overview of experimental results leads to the conclusion that both eye movement and attention processes are connected with each other but controlled by different systems. Using a computerized method of the classical slit view paradigm Kazuo Koga, Tatsuro Makino, Katsuaki Sakata, and Nobuko Takahashi show how the perception of the velocity of a moving object is influenced by pursuit eye movements. Their results indicate the importance of the role of eye movements, especially smooth pursuit eye movements, on absolute velocity perception. Werner Krause's interest lies in the acquisition and use of cognitive structures. His discussion and experimental findings incorporate data on eye movements in ordering problems in order to verify the symbol-distance effects.

Calvin F. Nodine, Harold L. Kundel, James D. Polikoff, and Lawrence L. Toto report on the importance of fixation clusters in visual search processing. The study involves the measurement of eye movements when radiologists search x-ray images for lung tumors. According to their findings, the number of fixations per cluster seems to be a more sensitive measure than fixation duration as an indication of information processing of the visual scene.

Finally, to facilitate working with the text, subject and author indexes are found at the end of the book. A list of the contributors' addresses is also included.

2
Basic Neurophysiological Description of Eye Movements

CORTICAL MECHANISMS OF EYE MOVEMENTS IN RELATION TO PERCEPTION AND COGNITIVE PROCESSES

OTTO D. CREUTZFELDT

Abteilung Neurobiologie,
Max-Planck-Institut für Biophysikalische Chemie,
Göttingen

INTRODUCTION

When the organizers had invited a sensory neurophysiologist to address this conference on eye movements, they probably had expected a synthetic view which might bring together the two aspects of visual physiology: the one which is essentially concerned with the anatomical and physiological representation of the retina and of visual stimuli in the brain, and the other concentrating on the involvement of various brain areas in eye movement control. The first aspect has dominated visual physiology during the last 25-30 years leading to a model, in which the visual world is layed out across the brain as on maps, in which either the spatial dimensions of visual stimuli or specific aspects of the visual information are faithfully and orderly represented (Creutzfeldt, 1983, 1985). Without going into the details of this model at this point, the question arises how this distributed information is recombined into a single, meaningful concept of the visual world. Is meaning, in fact, represented in feature maps of the highest order and abstraction?

Visuomotor physiologists are, on the other hand, faced with the fact that eye movements are controlled and can be elicited from many parts of the brain and that many areas of the cortex are involved in the same or different aspects of eye movements. The question which arises here is that of the command structure which activates either this or that forebrain system, and of the agent or agency which selects objects in the visual environment as goals for directing the gaze (or the fovea) towards them.

While the first line of reasoning cannot avoid to use concepts of perception and cognition for interpreting its data, the second cannot help to invoke such concepts as attention, decision or free will (*voluntary* eye movements). This becomes evident when studying some of the most recent reviews on the organization of cortical control of eye movements (see, for example, Andersen, 1987; Fischer, 1987, Heilmann et al., 1987; Robinson, 1981). These are, of course, psychological concepts and they are essentially based on an introspective analysis of cognitive and action processes, and it appears that they cannot do without a hierarchic organization.

Both, the cognitive and the action hierarchy must be symmetrical, however. They must meet at a highest level (H. Jackson, 1897, in 1932 p. 422), where the final evaluation and analysis of the perceptual details are supposed to be combined to an idea and from where the commands for appropriate action should be distributed to the various executive levels of the brain. We will ask, in the following, whether the anatomo-functional organization of the brain does in fact support such a symmetrical hierarchic model or whether we are lead by neurophysiology to consider different models. Can neurophysiology, in fact, suggest a straightforward and coherent model without refering and reverting to psychological concepts?

Cortical Control of Eye Movements

Saccadic eye movements can be elicited by electrical stimulation from many areas of the cerebral cortex (Figure 1). This has been demonstrated more than half a century ago on monkeys by Oscar and Cecile Vogt (1919, 1926) and on humans by Otfrid Foerster (1936). These areas include purely sensory areas such as the primary area 17 and the prestriate visual cortex (areas 18 and 19), precentral motor area such as the classical frontal eye field (Area 8) and the supplementary motor area (SMA, Area 6 aß), in which a supplementary eye field has recently been delineated (Schlag & Schlag-Rey, 1987), as well as the parietal (Area 7) and the temporal association cortex (Areas 21/22). These results have been essentially confirmed by recent stimulation mapping of the different eye movement related areas of the cerebral cortex. These more recent stimulation experiments (Wagmann, 1964; Schiller et al., 1979; Keating et al., 1982; Bruce & Goldberg, 1984; Goldberg et al., 1986; Mitz & Wise, 1987; Schlag & Schlag-Rey, 1987) have, in addition, revealed that the thresholds for eliciting saccades from these different areas may vary considerably and may also depend on the state of the animal. The lowest threshold regions are somewhat more restricted than suggested by the older experiments with less controlled stimulus parameters.

However, the fact that eye movements can be elicited from such a large part of the cortex concurs with the observation that eye movement related activity of single neurons can be recorded in all of these areas, except maybe for the temporal association cortex in which no saccade related activities have yet been reported to my knowledge. We shall return later to some details of eye movement related activities in these different areas. At this point, we only want to note that none of the areas from where saccadic eye movements can be elicited is it *per se* necessary for such eye movements as can be concluded from lesion experiments in animals and from clinical observation in man.

Thus, bilateral ablation of the frontal eye fields does not even eliminate purposeful, goal directed eye movements as Schiller et al. (1979) have shown,

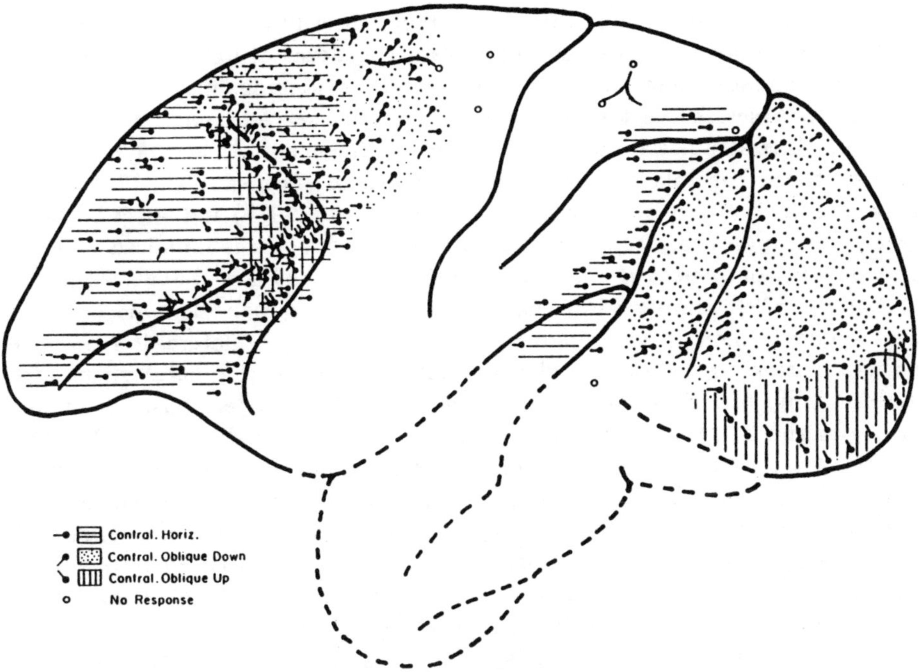

Fig. 1: Cortical map of eye movement responses to electrical stimulation of the alert, cervically transected monkey *M. mulatta* obtained by Wagman (1964). Locations of responses are indicated with *solid points*. The *lines* originating from the points indicate the direction of the eye movement. All responses were towards the contralateral side. Source: Wagman, 1964. Reprinted with permission of Harper & Row Publishers.

nor does bilateral ablation of the supplementary frontal eye field make them disappear completely (Guitto et al., 1985; Foerster, 1936; Schiller et al., 1987). Thus, neither lesion, electrical stimulation experiments nor, as we will see later, electrophysiological recordings suggest any clear and simple hierarchy of the cortical organization of eye movement control. Only lesion of area 17 eliminates goal directed eye movements almost completely because after lesion of this area, visual goals are not anymore identified and represented in the cortex. However, even after area 17-lesion, gaze shifts towards visual targets can still be observed under specific experimental conditions, a phenomenon termed blind sight (Pöppel et al., 1973; Weiskrantz et al., 1974).

On the other hand, the quality and extent of the functional deficits caused by the various lesions varies considerably. The devastating effect of area 17 lesion was already mentioned. Even optokinetic nystagmus maybe suppressed after bilateral lesions. After parietal cortex lesions, saccadic eye movements to the contralateral side are slowed down, and the latencies for eliciting eye movements into the contralateral hemifield are increased (Posner et al., 1984; Stein, 1978; Lynch, 1980). Visual search is impeded (Latto, 1978) and, after bilateral lesion, tracking of fast but not of slowly moving targets is impaired and the slow pursuit component of optokinetic nystagmus is also slowed down (Lynch & McLaren, 1979). Similar effects have been observed in man. The most prominent syndrome here is, of course, Balints syndrome after bilateral lesion of the parietal cortex which consists of what Balint called psychic paralysis of gaze with inability to look at an object in the far visual periphery, visually guided ataxia of the hand and difficulty in spatial attention (Balint, 1909; Holmes, 1919). After unilateral lesion of one parietal lobe, (especially of lobe which is not the speech dominant hemisphere since it is then not confounded with more prominent and more devastating symptomes of cognition and language), the syndrome of visual neglect is observed which has been so impressively documented by the self-portraits of the painter Räderscheidt following a right parietal infarction, collected and published by Richard Jung (1974). It thus appears, and most authors nowaday agree, that the parietal lobe is involved in mechanisms necessary for visual attention, for focussed attention in general, as well as for assessing and evaluating spatial relations between objects in the environment relative to ones own body and for appropriate visuo-motor coordination (Hyvärinen, 1982; Mountcastle, 1976, 1981).

This does not mean, however, that the parietal cortex is sufficient for such mechanisms. Clearly, other regions of the visual cortex are also involved in visual attention and also necessary for it. Furthermore, as first observed as far back as 1895 by Bianchi, visual neglect is also observed after frontal eye field lesion, although only temporarily (Foerster, 1936), but to such an extent that unilateral lesion of the frontal eye field in monkeys may be indistinguishable from an heminanopsia (Latto & Cowey, 1971). The often claimed hierarchic organization from the supplementary motor area to the motor cortex, in our case, from the supplementary to the prearcuate frontal eye field, has also not been confirmed in recent studies. The fact is that eye movements can still be elicited from the supplementary eye field after lesion of the prearcuate eye field, and spontaneous eye movements do not disappear after supplementary eye field lesions although they may be reduced. There is even a very important functional difference between the two areas in that presaccadic activation of neurons is seen in the arcuate frontal eye field only before purposeful, goal directed saccades, but not before spontaneous saccades in the dark (Goldberg & Bushnell, 1981; Goldberg & Bruce, 1986; Bizzi, 1968). Supplementary eye field neurons, on the other hand, also discharge during or before spontaneous saccades in the dark (Schlag & Schlag-Rey, 1985, 1987).

At this point then, *it appears that the various cortical regions, which are involved in eye movement control, are not so much working in series but rather in parallel.* Before dealing with this conclusion in further detail, however, let us have a short look at the apparatus through which these apparently parallel cortical mechanisms exert their control of eye movements.

The Interface for Coordination of Eye Movement Commands in the Mesencephalon

This apparatus is located in the upper brainstem. Its task is to distribute activities to the motoneurons in the various oculomotor nuclei so that the 12 eye muscles, 6 for each eye including the levator palpebrae, contract in a coordinated manner for producing conjugate saccades to the desired position, convergence movements, gaze fixation on an object or for following a moving object in pursuit These tasks have to be made independent of the position of the head and body.

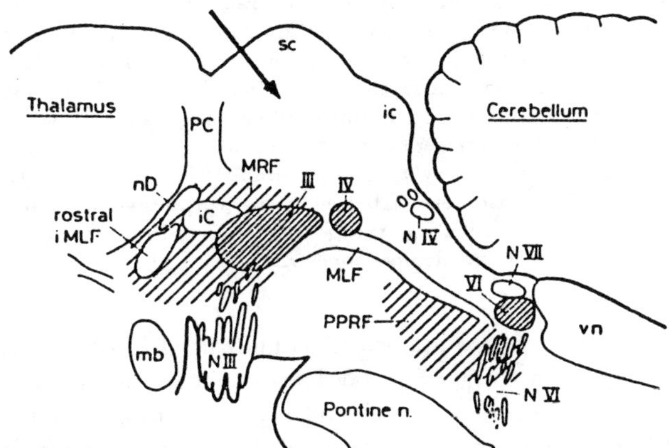

Fig. 2: Parasagittal cut through the brainstem of a rhesus monkey. The IIIrd nucleus supplies medial rectus, inferior rectus, and inferior oblique muscle ipsilaterally, the superior rectus contralaterally, and the levator palpebrae bilaterally. Trochlear fibers from the IVth nucleus cross within the brainstem; abducens fibers from the VIth nucleus are all ipsilateral. The paramedian pontine reticular formation (PPRF) and the rostral mesencephalon (MRF) are immediate premotor areas for horizontal and vertical gaze respectively. The arrow indicates the stereotaxic vertical plane. Source: Henn, Büttner-Ennever, & Hepp, 1982a. Reprinted with permission of Springer-Verlag.

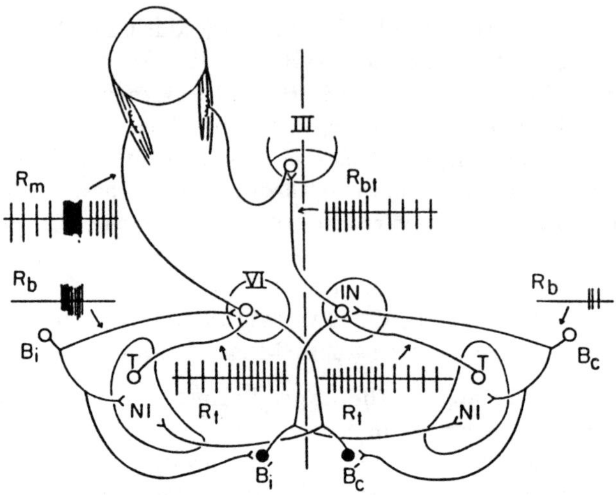

Fig 3: Push-pull arrangement by which burst cells create saccades. Ipsilateral burst cells (Bi) discharge at high rates (Rb) during leftward saccades. They excite ipsilateral abducens motoneurons in abducens nucleus (VI) and relay an inhibitory burst through Bi, located in ipsilateral rostral medulla, to burst tonic, internuclear neurons (IN) in contralateral VI, which fire at rate Rbt. This inhibitory burst silences contralateral IN cells and ipsilateral medial rectus montoneurons in oculomotor nucleus (III) during the saccade. Burst rate (Rm) in the lateral rectus motoneuron is the difference between rates Rb of Bi and that of contralateral inhibitory cells B'c relayed from contralateral burst cells Bc. Neural integrator (NI) must be formed by a pair of reciprocally acting circuits in the paramedian pontine reticular formation with midline symmetry. They are represented by tonic cells (T) and must also be stepped up or down (discharge rates Rt) by the push - pull action of burst cells to produce the final pulse - step Rm (Or pause - step Rbt) in agonist (or antagonist) motoneurons. *Closed circles*, inhibitory cells; *open circles*, excitatory cells. Source: Robinson, 1981. Reprinted with permission of the American Physiological Society.

The general layout of this apparatus is known, although a complete understanding of many, even some essential details is still missing (Henn et al., 1982 a,b). The coordination of motoneuronal activity for the different eye muscles is achieved by inter- and intranuclear connections involving synergistic excitation and antagonistic reciprocal inhibition, with the axons and axon collaterals running predominantly in the medial longitudinal fascicle which thus becomes a predominant anatomical structure for this coordination. The commands for eye movements are distributed to the motor nuclei from two major structures. One is in the *rostral reticular formation*, which delivers commands for vertical eye movements, and the more caudally located paramedian pontine reticular formation which is responsible for horizontal eye movements (Figure 2).

Cortical efferents, even from the premotor frontal eye field, do not have direct access to the motoneurons of the oculomotor nuclei. *All cortical com-*

mands have to go through the interface of oculomotor control within the upper brainstem. Within these supranuclear mesencephalic regions, functional subregions can be distinguished in that neurons responsible for certain aspects of eye movements in the horizontal or vertical domain, as e.g. upwards or downwards movements, are clustered (Henn & Cohen, 1976; Hepp & Henn, 1983). In this way, the gaze directions are roughly layed out in the supranuclear premotor regions of the reticular formation in a topographical manner like on a keyboard. Within these direction domaines various types of neurons are found. For example, those which are essentially responsible for saccade initiation by sending short bursts of activity into the motoneuronal pool (medium lead bursts), but which are tonically active during gaze fixation; others which appear to discharge earlier (long lead bursts) and again others that are inhibited (pause neurons), possibly opening the gate for burst discharges (Figure 3). These various types of neurones with activation and inhibition at various times preceding the saccades, also constitute a mechanism for the transformation of spatial vectors of directing the gaze into temporal sequences of neuronal activations within the various motoneuron pools concerned. How this is done and along which paths is still an open question although several models are proposed (Robinson, 1981). Activities from the vestibular nuclei also enter into this inter-, intra- and supranuclear oculomotor interface, which provide for correction signals from the vestibular system (vestibulo-ocular reflexes) and from the neck muscles (neck reflexes) as well as from the flocculus of the cerebellum, for controlling the continuity of pursuit eye movements (Precht, 1975). Visual input for these control signals arrives directly through subcortical visual afferents via the pretectum and the accessory optic tract which signal retinal slip of an image (Hoffmann, 1982; Precht, 1982).

This beautifully designed mesencepho-cerebellar system guarantees for fixation, pursuit and saccades in the desired manner independent of disturbances from head and body positions, object or body movements etc. It is, of course, only a visuo-motor reflex system, but it is at the same time, the interface into which the different forebrain structures send their neuronal commands and where these are distributed to produce the appropriate voluntary eye movements according to the purposes demanded by the forebrain. These commands do not only entail more or less activity for shifting the gaze into one or the other direction, but also must engage or disengage the automatic subroutines for fixation, pursuit, vestibular-ocular and neck reflexes. How this is done in detail, is still a riddle, as far as I understand the experts in this field. We know, however, that during evolution, this subcortical control system is increasingly controlled by the forebrain. Thus, in reptiles, fish, birds and even lower mammals, eye movements are under control of the vestibular and neck reflexes, while primates and especially humans can readily disengage these controls. And we also know, at least, some of the pathways and of the command signals which

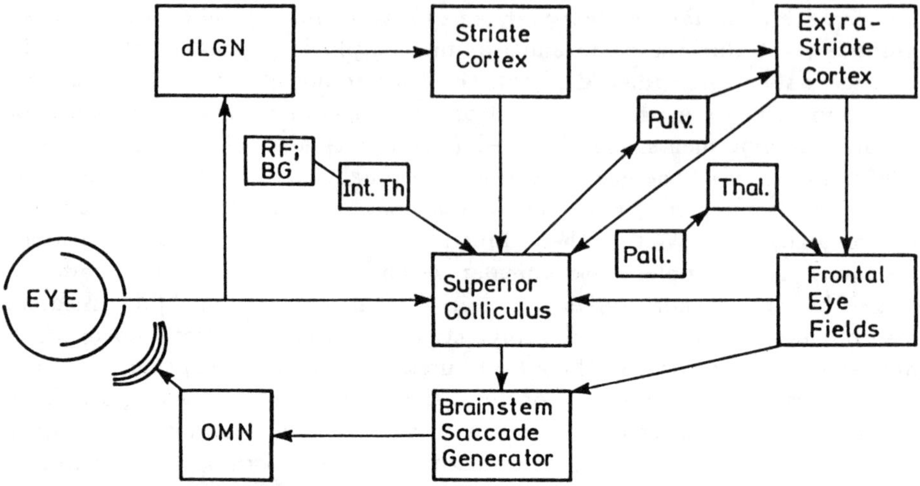

Fig. 4: Anatomical connections between the frontal eye fields and other brain structures participating in the initiation of saccadic eye movements. The frontal eye fields receive visual information via a cortico-cortical route originating in the striate cortex and directly from the thalamus. Several cortical areas, including the frontal eye fields, project to the superior colliculus, which receives a direct retinal projection as well. The brainstem's saccade generator, located in the para-pontine reticular formation (PPRF), receives a projection from the colliculus and an independent input from the frontal eye fields and other cortical areas. This model is minimal, and primarily serves to explain how the frontal eye fields can effect saccades without the colliculus, whereas striate and extrastriate cortical areas cannot. Many additional structures could be included and structures that are included could be elaborated. Abbreviation: dLGN=dorsal lateral geniculate nucleus; OMN=Oculomotor nuclei; RF=reticular formation; Int.Th.= intralaminar nuclei of the thalamus; Pulv=pulvinar; Pall=Pallidum. Source: Bruce & Goldberg, 1984, with some additions. Used with permission of Elsevier Science Publishers B.V., Amsterdam.

are transmitted from the forebrain into this mesencephalic oculomotor interface and shall discuss them in the following section.

Pathways from the Cortex to the Supranuclear Coordination System for Eye Movements

There are, at least, three access lines from the forebrain to the mesencephalic interface: (1) through the superior colliculi, (2) via a bypass directly or indirectly into the mesencephalic supranuclear, premotor regions and (3) through the pontine nuclei, from where the signals are transmitted to the cerebellum and hence back via the vestibular nucleus into the medial longitudinal fascicle. The superior colliculus receives afferent signals from virtually the whole neocortex as well as from the retina (see Wurtz & Albano, 1980). The visual field is layed out here topographically, across the surface of the superior colliculi, and electrical stimulation at a point of that map representing a certain region of the visual field will also elicit a saccadic eye movement into that region (Straschill & Rieger, 1973; Sparks et al., 1976; Schiller, 1984). Thus, visual receptive space as well as visuomotor space are layed out across the same map, and the input from the visual cortex and from the retina are in register (Goldberg & Wurtz, 1972 a,b). In primates, though apparently not in cats, the visual receptive fields and response properties of neurons in the superior colliculus are independent of the visual cortex (Schiller et al., 1974; Schiller, 1984).

This may be the pathway through which target directed saccades can still be elicited by visual stimuli after visual cortical lesion (blind sight), and also for the express saccades, i.e. for saccades with very short response times which have been described by Fischer and his colleagues (Fischer, 1986, 1987). Express saccades and gaze movement towards a goal in blind sight may then represent straightforward retino-colliculo-oculomotor reflexes bypassing the cortex and thus the neuronal substrates for detailed visual analysis, decision making and attention as suggested also by their elimination after collicular ablation (Schiller et al., 1987). However, spatial attention still appears to have an influence on express saccades, as is indicated by their more frequent appearance after appropriate cueing.

The superior colliculus is a layered structure (Figure 5A). Neurons in the superficial layers are predominantly visually responsive and receptive fields in the superficial layer are small (1° or so), while with increasing depth they may increase to 10° (Sparks et al., 1976; Goldberg & Wurtz, 1972 a; Schiller, 1984). Their visual responsiveness to a spot of light may be enhanced if the animal is trained to look at this new target, and it may increase further during the course of the learning (Goldberg & Wurtz, 1972b). However, activations are not regularly seen before spontaneous saccades. This changes drastically when the recording electrode enters the deeper layers (Mohler & Wurtz, 1976; Sparks et al., 1977). Here cells discharge in short bursts preceding saccades by 50-150 ms, no matter whether the saccades are made in the dark or light, or to selected targets (Figure 5B). The timing and duration of these presaccadic bursts varies between neurons and with depth, but this has not been systematically studied. Again, the retinotopic space (or the visual field) is layed out topographically, but instead of representing the place of a stimulus, neurons now represent the target of a saccadic eye movement. They have movement direction fields instead of receptive fields. The movement fields of neurons in the deep layer of the superior colliculi are in close topographic and retinotopic register with the receptive fields of superficial neurons.

We have mentioned already the afferent input to the superficial layers of the superior colliculi from the retina and the striate as well as the prestriate visual cortex, and we might complete this list by adding inputs from the frontal eye field and the pretectum. In fact, the superior colliculi are the only output

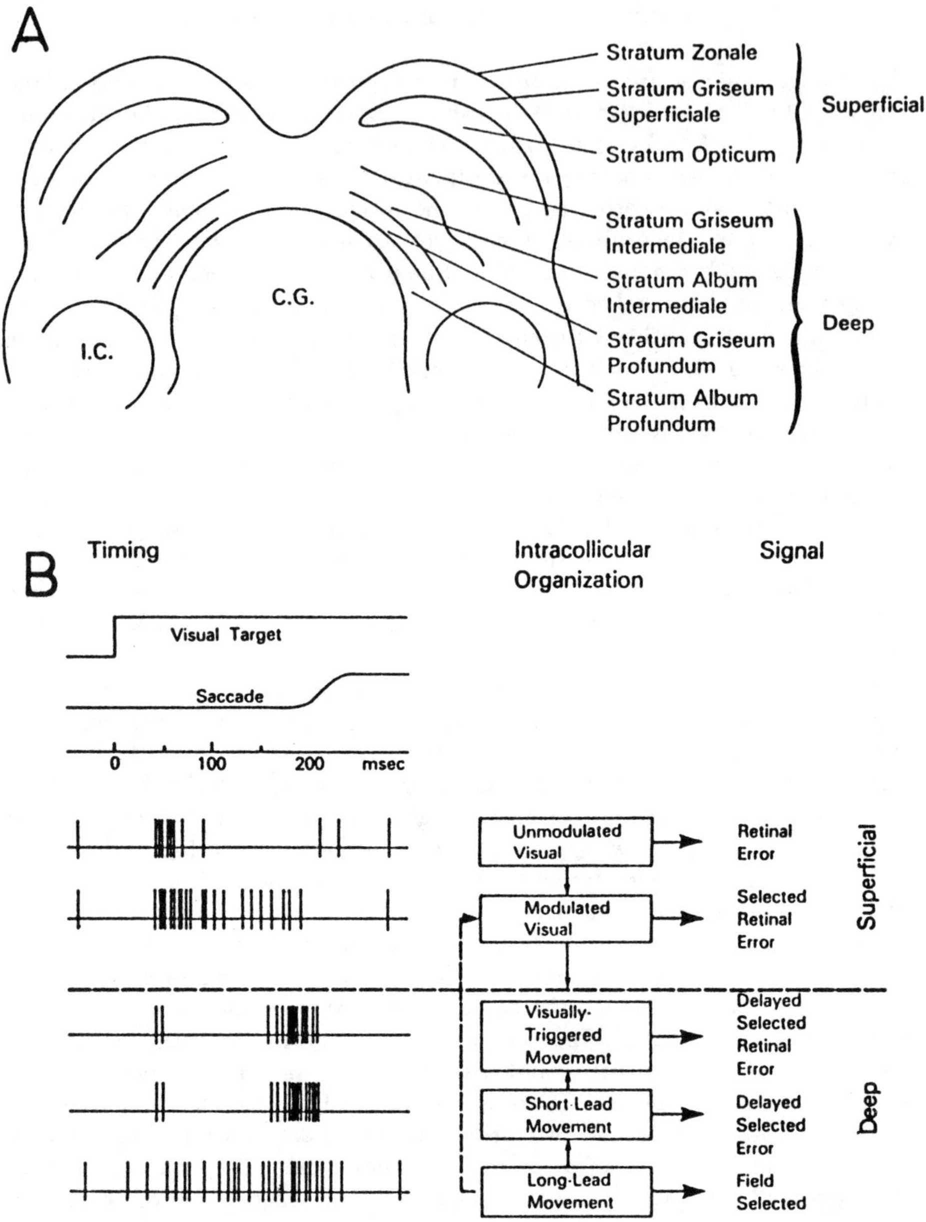

Fig. 5 A: Alternating fiber and cell layers of monkey superior colliculus. A drawing of a coronal section through the colliculus is shown. The seven layers indicated on the right are divided into three layers designated as the superficial division and four layers designated as the deep division. I.C., inferior colliculus; C.G., central gray. **B**: Temporal sequence of cell discharge in monkey superior colliculus (timing, left), hypothetical intracollicular organization based on this sequence (middle), and possible signal conveyed by each of these elements (right). Source: Wurtz & Albano, 1980. Reproduced with permission from the Annual Review of Neuroscience, Vol. 3, Copyright 1980 by Annual Review Inc.

structure for oculomotor commands from the striate cortex: after collicular lesion, electrical stimulation of area 17 will not elicit eye movements (Schiller et al., 1974; Schiller, 1984). The input to the deep layers is, however, much more diverse. Not only efferents from the whole neocortex reaching from the visual to the frontal cortex are arriving here, (to some extent in different layers), but inputs can also be traced from various afferent sensory systems of spinal and mesencephalic origin, from pontine nuclei, and also from midbrain structures with more general modulating actions such as the locus coeruleus or the raphe nuclei (see the list of afferent and efferent connections of the superior colliculi in Wurtz & Albano, 1980). The same applies to the output organization in that the superficial layers send efferents back into the prestriate visual cortex via the inferior pulvinar, while the deep layers provide a major input to our mesencephalic oculomotor interface, the supranuclear structures in the reticular formation, into other motor and premotor brainstem nuclei such as the facial nucleus or the nucleus reticularis pontis which is an important structure for extrapyramidal motor control. An upward stream goes into various specific and non-specific thalamic nuclei, such as, the suprageniculate nucleus, the intralaminar nuclei as well as to the gate controlling, inhibitory nucleus reticularis thalami.

In addition to the direct afferents from the cortex, deep collicular activity can also be controlled from the cortex through a bypass via the basal ganglia (Figure 6 A). As we know, the whole cortex projects into the basal ganglia (caudate nucleus and pallidum) in a coarse topographic manner. Output from the basal ganglia goes, inter alias, into the pars reticulata of the substantia nigra and from there into the deep layers of the superior colliculi. This output is an inhibitory one, using gamma-amino-butyric acid (GABA as transmitter). Wurtz and Hikosako (1986) have found that this inhibitory activity of neurones in the pars reticulata stops before and during the pre- and perisaccadic burst activity of the deep collicular units (Figure 6 B).

Due to these various inputs, the superior colliculus is more than a simple relay of oculomotor corticofugal activity. Outputs from the various areas are weighted against each other and the correct innervation pattern for an intended target of an eye movement may also be worked out here in this multilayered structure, in which inputs from the various cortical regions are staggered on top of each other. Electrical stimulation, for example, at a point in the supplementary frontal eye field or the intralaminar thalamus does not only determine the direction of an eye movement, but also takes into account the position of the eye at the moment of stimulation and corrects for this so that the same intended position is reached (Schlag & Schlag-Rey, 1987). We may conjecture that this correction does, in fact, take place in the superior colliculus.

Considering this intricate structure, connectivity and functional layout of the superior colliculi, it is indeed disappointing to see that removal of this structure

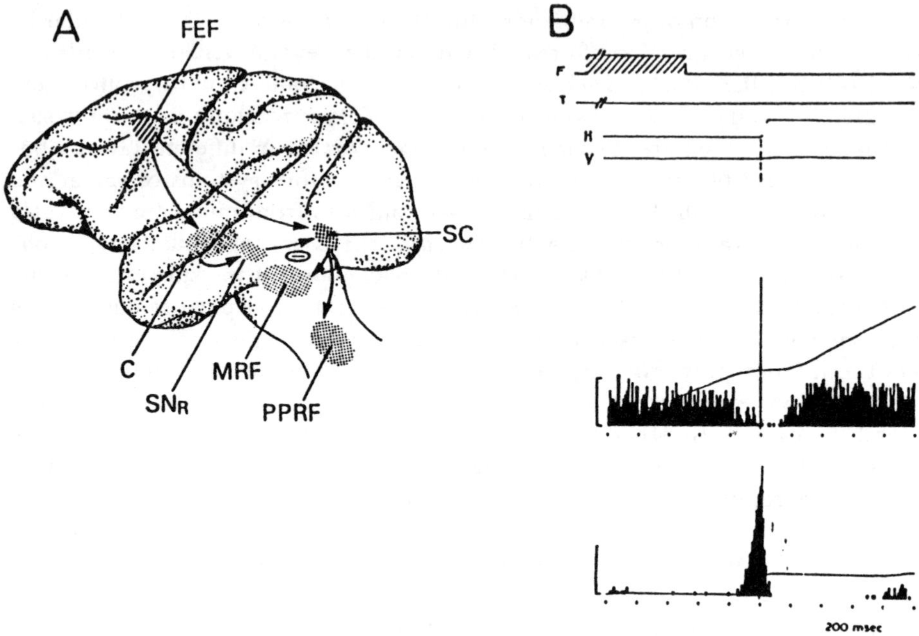

Fig. 6 A: Location of the Substantia nigra, pars reticularis (SNr) in the pathway for the initiation of saccadic eye movements. SNr is one of the two most prominent inputs to the superior colliculus (SC), the other being from the frontal eye field (FEF). SNr receives input via the caudate (C) from frontal cortex including the frontal eye field. The SNr action on the SC is probably inhibitory, as indicated by the minus sign. MRF and PPRF, mesencephalic and prepontine reticular formation. **B**: Comparison of the discharge rate of a substantia nigra cell (top) with that of a superior colliculus cells (bottom) made as the monkey made saccades to a remembered visual target. The superior colliculus cell was recorded at the point in the superior colliculus where the substantia nigra cell could be antidromically activated by stimulation of the superior colliculus. The superior colliculus cell was one that discharged before saccades made under any condition. Source: Wurtz & Hikosaka, 1986. Reprinted with permission of Elsevier Science Publishers B.V., Amsterdam.

does not wipe out voluntary eye movements completely. Target directed eye movements are still possible after such an operation, and also spontaneous eye movements do not disappear although they are less frequent (Pasik et al., 1966; Bender, 1980; Schiller et al., 1980, 1987; see Wurtz & Albano, 1960). Also, saccades are not so accurate, their latency is increased and they are slower. These deficits are more severe, however, when collicular function is disrupted acutely. e.g. by injection of an inhibitory drug (Wurtz & Hikosaka, 1986). It is clear from such acute and chronic ablation studies, which are also supported by observations on human patients (Bender, 1980; Kommerell,

1986), that cortical regions must have access to the mesencephalic supranuclear oculomotor structures through another route. The exact access route is not yet known, but it is a good guess that a thalamo-mesencephalic pathway, possibly through the intralaminar nuclei, maybe involved (see Figure 4). Recording of eye movement related activity in the intralaminar nuclei as well as rather precise stimulation effects from this region support this assumption (Schlag & Schlag-Rey, 1984). Yet, the extracollicular cortico-mesencephalic pathway is, one has to admit it, unknown. Its function is less precise, although, the stronger effects during and immediately after a functional lesion as compared to the minor effects after prolonged lesions, indicate that under normal conditions the cortico-collicular routes play the major role. One must take into account, that due to its widespread efferents into the motor system, the superior colliculus does not only serve as transmitter of visuo-motor activity, but also has more widespread functions for visuo-motor and even for multimodal sensory-motor orientation.

Cortical Control of Eye Movements: Active Perception

Here we are now, back to the cortex, which uses and controls this mesencephalic machinery. It uses it because an integral part of visual perception is active exploration of the visual environment with the fovea. Thus, for visual analysis, a continuous shift of gaze is necessary and the percept is, in fact, a recomposition of these temporally disrupted, successive and variable projections and representations of a visual scene in the various striate and prestriate visual areas. A stable and unified percept is comparable to a deconvolution of the variable representations in the retinotopic and feature sensitive maps over the temporally dispersed track of eye movements. Therefore, it is not suprising that eye movement related activity is not only seen in so-called oculomotor regions, and that neurons in oculomotor fields such as the frontal eye field but also have visual receptive fields (see Bruce & Goldberg, 1984, 1985). On the other hand, once an object of interest has been identified, it needs to be fixated and pursued not to lose it out of sight in spite of object and subject motion. Thus, the exploration program has to be suppressed, the fixation and pursuit program has to be engaged, and gaze attracting stimuli in the peripheral visual field have to be suppressed. We say, attention has to be concentrated onto the point of fixation or, *vice versa*, fixation has to be locked to the field of attention.

For further exploration of details, perception has to be switched from the preattentive to the attentive mode, as Julesz (1985) puts it, which involves detailed comparison of adjacent structures or textures and to complement these borders to a Gestalt. This involves local and global screening of a visual scene. During reading and writing, finally, progressive eye movements are controlled by the semantic identification of one fixation frame after the other, or by the whole progress of mental comprehension.

Let us now look at some cortical regions, whose neuronal activity is related to one or several aspects of visual behavior and perception. In the *parietal association cortex*, Mountcastle and Hyvärinen and their colleagues have found neurones, which are active during fixation and pursuit, and others which are active during and before saccades (for details see Hyvärinen, 1982; Andersen, 1987). Pursuit, fixation and saccade neurons are clustered in small patches, but mixed in the same areas and to some extent even with neurons activated in connection with arm movements. It was tempting to assign to these neurons the function of command neurons (Mountcastle, 1976), commands from the highest level, so to say, in the terminology of Hughling Jackson. It turned out, however, that these neurones were also visually excitable, and the visual receptive fields and the motion fields of individual neurons coincide to some extent (Robinson et al., 1978; Mountcastle, 1981). Thus, fixation and pursuit neurons should have receptive fields in the foveal and parafoveal region of the visual field, while saccade related neurones should have more peripherally located receptive fields. Unfortunately, exact data on this are not available to my knowledge. Furthermore, one might postulate that pursuit and saccade related neurones should feed into different functional subdivisions of the supranuclear occulomotor interface related to the pursuit and the saccade mode, respectively. This has not been investigated either, however.

In any case, these parietal neurons are both visual and motor. In addition, it turned out that their responses to visual stimuli may be enhanced if the subject, a monkey, is asked to pay attention to a peripheral stimulus located within the motion and receptive field, no matter whether he moves his eyes towards it or not (Lynch et al., 1977; Bushnell et al., 1981; Goldberg & Bruce, 1985; Andersen, 1987) . This enhancement effect thus indicates that localized attention is also represented by activation of these neurons, and this maybe the most important aspect of their function. It would fit with the observation that a parietal lesion produces contralateral visual neglect.

Such enhancement effects have also been discovered under various behavioral conditions, in the *prelunate visual association area V4* (Fischer & Boch, 1981; Haenny & Schiller, 1988; Moran & Desimone, 1985; see also Fischer, 1987) a visual area which is considered otherwise mainly to be an area involved in various aspects of visual perception (for further detail see Tanaka et al., 1986). Such attention related activations do not mean, however, that such neurons or such regions select the stimulus for attention, but only that attention may make these neurons more sensitive to visual stimuli in that part of the visual field. These parietal and prestriate regions may, therefore, be necessary for the expression of attentive processes, which finally lead to appropriate eye movements - as pathology shows -, but they are not sufficient. An additional function of the parietal cortex must also be the change from one mode of vision (or oculomotor program) to another, as the "fixing of gaze" after parietal lesions indicates: the subject has difficulty to disengage his/her gaze from fixation and to jump to another target (Holmes & Horrax, 1919; Cogan, 1965; Balint, 1905; for further references see Hyvärinen, 1982).

Attention related activations are also found in the *dorsal prelunate area*, (DP). Also here, neurons with eye movement related activities are mixed with those which are only or predominantly activated by the specific behavioral attention to a visual object (Li, Tanaka, & Creutzfeldt, in preparation). Such neurons may even not be visually excitable, but are visually excited only after the eye movement is terminated. These neurons in DP do not respond in connection with spontaneous eye movements in the dark or without a task, but only when a fixation task is on or when the visual environment is actively and attentively explored. The appearance of a behaviorally significant object (or person) in the field of gaze may significantly enhance their activity even without further change of predominant gaze direction (Figure 7). Thus, the attentive fixation or visual exploration of the object is represented by the activity of such neurones, but these neurons are not themselves evaluating the behavioral significance of the object as their activation occurs only after termination of the saccade indicates. The behavioral significance is represented by their activation, however. In this sense the prestriate areas and their neurons are necessary for object recognition, as was demonstrated recently by lesion studies of the prelunate visual association cortex in primates (Heywood & Cowey, 1987) and from clinical experience (see Creutzfeldt, 1983). They are not sufficient for object recognition, however, and the activities of other areas also have to be added (Tanaka et al., 1986).

When looking at an object, whether exploring it or just looking at it, as in the experimental situation which Yarbus (1967) has used, our gaze jumps around (although, introspectively, we say it wanders around) with about 2-3 saccades every second. It does the same, actually, if our mind ponders around (and we may ask whether our thought processes aren't similarly jumpy at a similar rhythm?). These continuous saccades are not randomly spread across the object, but stop at resting points of the picture or object. These resting points are regions where contours cross, and the trajectories of saccadic eye movements preferentially run along contours if they exist in the picture. If the picture contains objects with fine details which constitute a Gestalt, say an animal or a man, the gaze returns more frequently to it. When looking at a face, eyes, mouth angles, the tip of the nose are preferential resting points. Monkeys appear to explore similarly as humans though with a somewhat shorter gaze fixation period (see Wurtz et al., 1982 and own observations).

The points of actual fixation and the gaze paths (contours) are only represented in sufficient spatial detail in area 17, i.e. in the *primary visual cortex*.

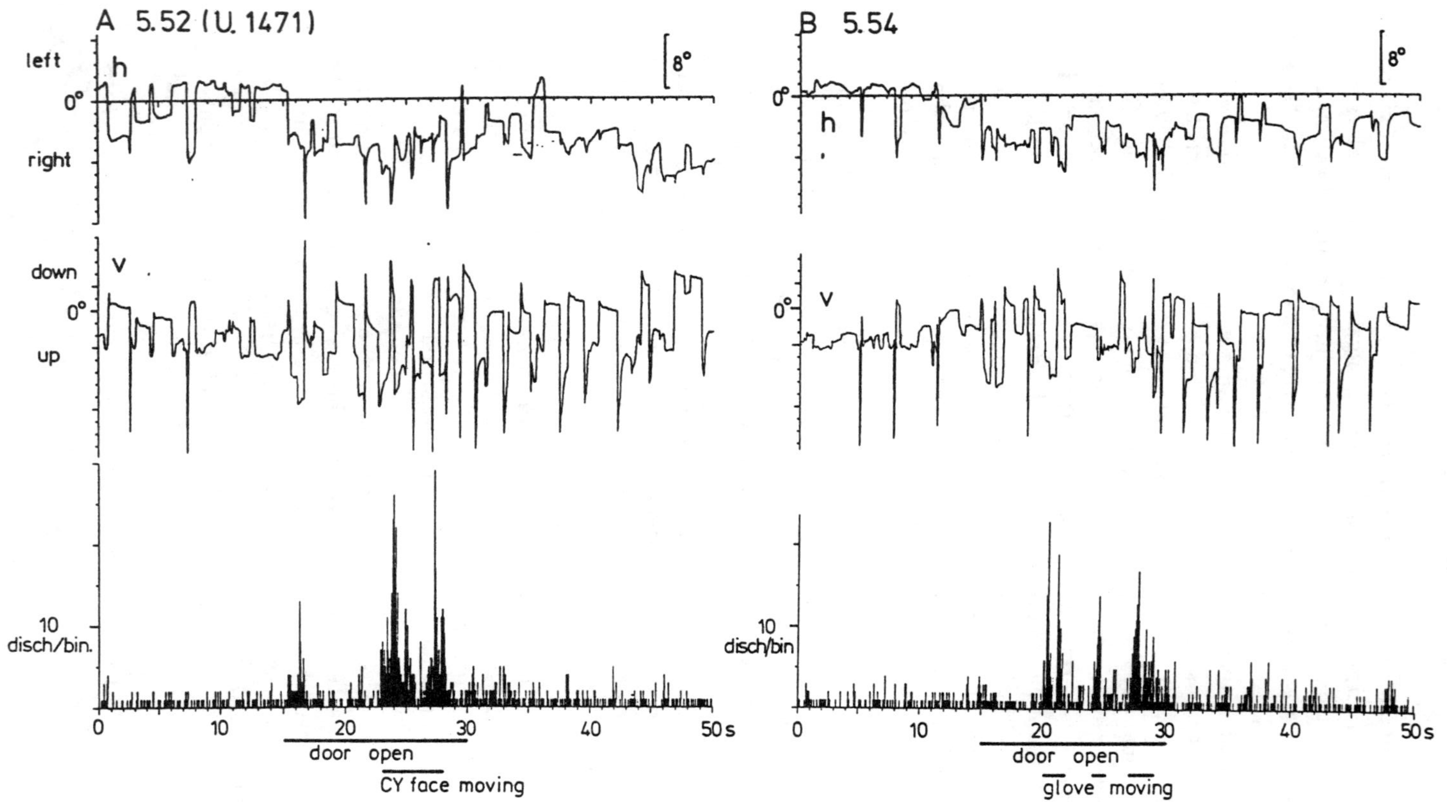

Fig. 7: Activation of a neuron in the dorsal prelunate area (DP) of a monkey. The monkey sits in a chair with his head fixed. **A**: When the door to his experimental room is openend he looks at the door (eye movement record on top, h, to the right). The unit (histogram, bottom) is shortly activated. When the face of the experimenter appears in the door, the unit is stronger activated, although the eye position does not change significantly. **B**: This time, the door opening hardly activates the unit, although the monkey still shifts his gaze towards the door. If a new stimulus, a glove with which the monkey is usually handled, appears in the door, the cell is again activated although the gaze does not shift significantly. (From Li, Tanaka, & Creutzfeldt, in preparation).

From this we must conclude that the selection process for fixating a point in the visual environment takes place in area 17, and the holding phase must be related to some extent to the activation pattern of foveal neurons. One could then consider maximal activation of foveal cortical neurons elicited by oriented and crossing objects as hold signals for eye fixation. Decrease of such activities may unlock the fixation, so that the gaze shifts to a new contour boarder. Candidates for such a function could be "simple" cortical neurons, which are specifically sensitive to oriented contours and whose activation typically decreases after a few 100 ms. While this hold function would have to be the task mainly of simple cells in the foveal region of area 17, simple cells located in more peripheral parts of the visual field could have a function for selecting the next fixation point, i.e. an other contour corner (Creutzfeldt & Nothdurft, 1978). In the *prelunate association field V4*, one group of neurons are specifically activated by stimuli which are rich in detail (Tanaka et al., 1986). Activation of such units may also contribute to the command signals for fixation. Admittedly, this jumping of the gaze from one contrast and contour corner to the next and from one finely detailed structure to another does not represent, as such, a cognitive map or structure of the explorative (attentive) gaze shifts, but it does, at least, give a hint to a mechanism on which such a cognitive structure may depend.

Another aspect, in which area 17 neurons may be directly involved in the control of eye movements is the imperative character of small moving objects for gaze shift: we can hardly resist to turn our eyes towards a fly running across a page we are reading or a cat running through the periphery of our visual field. Such stimuli excite predominantly the movement sensitive complex cells in area 17, and the cells projecting from area 17 into the superior colliculus are, in fact, all complex cells. It is reasonable to assume, that this cortico-collicular pathway is involved in gaze shifts towards objects moving in the peripheral field.

A further example in which area 17 and possibly area 18 (V2) may be directly involved is the fusion of the images from the two eyes. Binocular fusion is a formidable task of the visuo-motor system. It is obvious that the fusion signals must be related to activation of binocular neurons in area 17 (and maybe 18) which are excited from homonymous points on the two retinae. When binocular innervation of cortical neurons is eliminated in early childhood due to refraction anomalies or innervation problems of the eye muscles (squint), binocular fusion may become impossible because the input to cortical neurons from the "weaker" eye is suppressed. The following experiment illustrates that binocular fusion actually depends on the presence of identical contours in the visual field of the two eyes (Figure 8). If one presents each eye with a random dot pattern in which one central field of dots is systematically displaced by a few minutes of arc, this area will appear in front or behind the background as

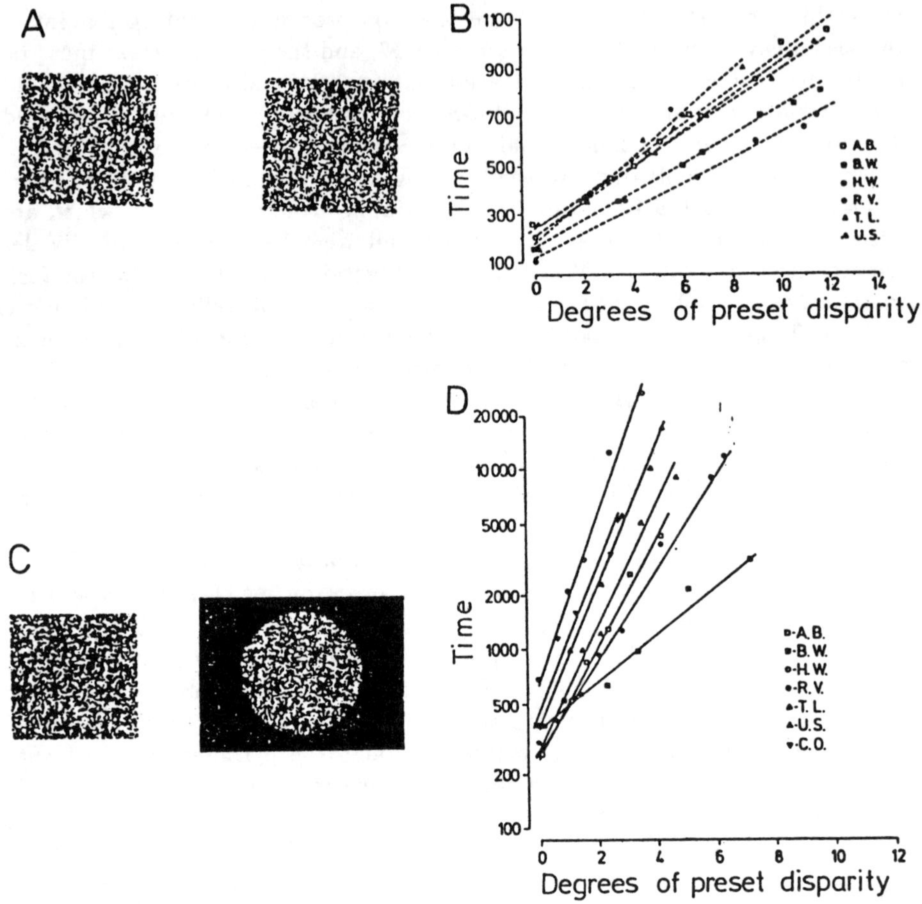

Fig. 8: Binocular fusion of random dot stereograms with identical (A) and different boarders (C). If the two dot displays are correctly fused, a small square pops out in the center. The time to fuse the two diagrams, until the stereo picture is recognized, depends on the disparity of the picture (B). When the diagrams have no common boarder, the time to fuse them is much longer (C). Note the different ordinates in B (linear) and D (logarithmic). Symbols and initials refer to different test subjects.

a stereo-image when the two images are correctly fused. We presented such dot patterns at different angles of disparity, so that the test subject had to converge his eyes (squint) in order to superimpose the two images. Correct superimposition was reached when the stereo image appeared. The time from the beginning of exposure of the two images to the moment in which they were correctly fused could be measured by exposing the two pictures for different lengths of time. As can be seen from Figure 8A, B, the time needed for fusion increases linearly with the initial disparity of the two images. However, the fusion time at any disparity angle depends also critically on whether the two random dot images have some prominent contours in common. Such prominent contours are usually the edges of the images, which are identical in Figure 8A. If one surrounds one image with a square and the other with a circular frame (Figure 8C), the fusion time increases, at all present disparities by a factor of ten and more. It increases exponentially and is not possible at all at large disparity angles (Figure 8D). By introducing identical contours into the two pictures, the fusion time can be reduced again. This experiment then suggests that fusion of the images from the two eyes depends on binocular excitation of neurons being excited by identical contours with the same orientation and in the same region in the visual field. This condition is fulfilled by the binocular simple and complex cells of area 17 and 18 (V1 and V2).

We realize that we have now assigned command tasks for visual behavior to the typically sensory neurons in the striate and prestriate cortex. This should not mean, however, that we have thus dismissed their sensory task, but by giving them also a function for motor command, we imply that their activation represents both, the presence of a sensory feature and command for appropriate visuo-motor responses, or action. The fact that visual perception is a continuous exploration of the visual environment by the gazing and thus, via the fovea, indicates, of course, that visual perception is an active process. The strategy for these explorative eye movements is layed down in the sensory properties of neurones in the primary visual cortex. It is in line with this that electrical stimulation of the points in one representation region of the visual field in the visual cortex induces a gaze shift towards that part of the visual field.

Let us now turn to the *frontal eye fields*. We had seen, already, that they are not necessary for saccadic exploration nor for fixation. On the other hand, activation of neurones in the frontal eye field are, of all motoneurons, most predictive for the appearance, size and direction of a saccade. Their activation clearly precedes all saccades during visual exploration. Can we consider them, then, as the final path for cortically induced eye movement commands? But how would that be compatible with the fact that we can dismiss them without eliminating visual exploration? Let us therefore look a bit closer into the activation pattern of frontal eye field neurons during visual oculomotor tasks (Goldberg & Bushnell, 1981; Bruce & Goldberg, 1984; Fischer, 1987). Then we discover different types of neurons and different responses in relation to the stimuli: pure visual responses, visuo-movement responses which last from the cueing stimulus to the execution of the eye movement, and those which discharge during the saccade. These types of activity then look similar to activities found elsewhere in the premotor cortex during delayed response tasks, as e.g.

in its hand-arm area during reaching tasks (Wise & Strick 1984; Creutzfeldt, 1983). One may interpret such activities as being related to the motivation and intention to do a certain movement. These activities come closest to the actual voluntary command aspect of movements. Such commands have to take into account sensory stimuli as well as the present state of the system. The frontal eye field may then be involved predominantly in eye movements depending on voluntary or instructed commands. It is in line with such an interpretation, that patients with frontal eye field lesions may fail to respond to the verbal demand to move their eyes to the contralateral side (Foerster, 1936; Guitton et al., 1985). The frontal eye fields are not, however, the final common path of all cortically induced eye movements, and are only one of the many parallel cortical input-output loops feeding into the collicular and supranuclear mesencephalic interface in which all these commands are coordinated into purposeful movements of the eyes.

Conclusion

We have seen that not only the cortical fields considered as motor fields but also those necessary for visual perception are all involved in eye movements and they all appear to cooperate. However, different aspects are emphasized in the different areas and thus different emphasis may be given to the goal selection for an eye movement by each area depending on the situation and the state of the whole system. This we may call a parallel representation of active vision. Such a model does not dismiss completely the hierarchic organization, but only assumes that the top level may change from one area to another according to the demand of a visual task. The emphasis may be on exploration, discrimination and decision, on attention or on volition, and the highest command would then switch accordingly from the sensory to the association areas or to the frontal eye field. The parallel representation of cortical eye movement control also does not mean that these areas are completely independent of each other and that either this or that area is called upon by an agent of highest command in the brain. These areas are not isolated units but connected via association fibres leading messages in both ways or through convergence of outputs at different levels and feedback from different levels. The main connection between all areas is, however, that they are getting their input directly or indirectly from the same visual environment and that any command execution, i.e. any eye movement, changes the input and thus also the condition for further commands in all of them. They are thus connected through an external, extracerebral loop (Creutzfeldt, 1983). We may consider it to be the main unifying condition of the various parallel cortical eye movement systems that they share the same visual environment and that any change of the subjects relation to this visual environment either through eye or body movements affects each of these subsystems according to its access to the visual input. According to the situation induced by the demands of one system (or the motivation), another system may be called upon to induce a correction or a new situation thus keeping the subject in an appropriate relation with his environment, consistant with the goal and purpose of a behavior, and adapted to the environment.

Author Note

This article is dedicated to Hans Kornhuber on the occasion of his 60th birthday.

References

Andersen, R.A., *Inferior parietal lobule function in spatial perception and visuomotor integration*, in "V.B. Mountcastle, F. Plum, & St. R. Geiger (Eds.), Handbook of physiology - The nervous system, Vol. V," American Physiological Society, Maryland/USA, 1987, pp. 483-518.

Balint, R., *Seelenlähmung des "Schauens", optische Ataxie, räumliche Störung der Aufmerksamkeit*, Monatsschrift für Psychiatrie und Neurologie **25** (1909), 25-81.

Bender, M.B., *Brain control of conjugate horizontal and vertical eye movements. A survey of the structural and functional correlates*, Brain **103** (1980), 23-69.

Bianchi, L., *The functions of the frontal lobes*, Brain **18** (1895), 497-530.

Bizzi, E., *Discharge of frontal eye field neurons during saccadic and following eye movements in unanesthetized monkeys*, Experimental Brain Research **6** (1968), 69-80.

Bruce, C.J., & Goldberg, M.E., *Physiology of the frontal eye fields*, Trends in Neuroscience **7** (1984), 436-441.

Bruce, C.J., & Goldberg, M.E., *Primate frontal eye fields. I. Single neurons discharging before saccades*, Journal of Neurophysiology **53** (1985), 603-635.

Bushnell, M.C., Goldberg, M.E., & Robinson, D.L., *Behavioral enhancement of visual responses in monkey cerebral cortex. I. Modulation in posterior parietal cortex related to selective attention*, Journal of Neurophysiology **46** (1981), 755-772.

Cogan, D.G., *Ophthalmic manifestations of bilateral non-occipital cerebral lesions*, The British Journal of Opthalmology **49** (1965), 281-297.

Creutzfeldt, O.D., "Cortex Cerebri. Leistung, strukturelle und funktionelle Organisation der Hirnrinde," Springer-Verlag, Berlin, 1983.

Creutzfeldt, O.D., *Comparative aspects of representation in the visual system*, in "C. Chagas, R.Gattass, & C. Gross (Eds.), Pattern recognition mechanisms. Experimental brain research, Suppl. 11," Springer-Verlag, Berlin, 1985, pp. 53-81.

Creutzfeldt, O.D., & Nothdurft, H.C., *Representation of complex visual stimuli in the brain*, Naturwissenschaften **65** (1978), 307-318.

Fischer, B., & Boch, R., *Peripheral attention versus central fixation: modulation of the visual activity of prelunate cortical cells of the rhesus monkey*, Brain Research **345** (1985), 111-123.

Fischer, B., *Express saccades in man and monkey*, in "H.J. Freund, U. Büttner, B. Cohen, & J. Noth (Eds.), Progress in brain research, Vol. 64," Elsevier Science Publishers, 1986, pp. 155-174.

Fischer, B., *The preparation of visually guided saccades*, Reviews of Physiology, Biochemistry, and Pharmacology **106** (1987), 1-35.

Fischer, B., & Boch, R., *Enhanced activation of neurons in prelunate cortex before visually guided saccades of trained rhesus monkeys*, Experimental Brain Research **44** (1981a), 129-137.

Fischer, B., & Boch, R., *Selection of visual targets activates prelunate cortical cells in trained rhesus monkeys*, Experimental Brain Research **41** (1981b), 431-433.

Foerster, O., *Motorische Felder und Bahnen*, in "O. Bumke & O. Foerster (Eds.), Handbuch der Neurologie, Bd. 6," Springer-Verlag, Berlin, 1936, pp. 1-357.

Goldberg, M.E., & Wurtz, R.H., *Activity of superior colliculus in behaving monkey. I. Visual receptive fields of single neurons*, Journal of Neurophysiology **35** (1972a), 542-559.

Goldberg, M.E., & Wurtz, R.H., *Activity of superior colliculus in behaving monkey. II. Effect of attention on neuronal responses*, Journal of Neurophysiology **35** (1972b), 560-574.

Goldberg, M.E., & Bushnell, M.C., *Behavioral enhancement of visual responses in monkey cerebral cortex. II. Modulation in frontal eye fields specifically related to saccades*, Journal of Neurophysiology **46** (1981), 773-787.

Goldberg, M.E., & Bruce, C.J., *Cerebral cortical activity associated with the orientation of visual attention in the rhesus monkey*, Vision Research **25** (1985), 471-481.

Goldberg, M.E., & Bruce C.J., *The role of arcuate frontal eye fields in the generation of saccadic eye movements*, in "H.J. Freund, U. Büttner, B. Cohen, & J. Noth (Eds.), Progress in brain research, Vol. 64," Elsevier Science Publishers, 1986, pp. 143-154.

Goldberg, M.E., Bushnell, M.C., & Bruce, C.J., *The effect of attentive fixation on eye movements evoked by electrical stimulation of the frontal eye fields*, Experimental Brain Research **61** (1986), 579-584.

Gould, H.J., Cusick, C.G., Pons, T.P., & Kaas, J.H., *The relationship of corpus callosum connections to electrical stimulation maps of motor, supplementary motor, and the frontal eye fields in owl monkeys*, Journal of Comparative Neurology **247** (1986), 297-325.

Guitton, D., Buchtel, H.A., & Douglas, R.M., *Frontal lobe lesions in man cause difficulties in suppressing reflexive glances and in generating goal-directed saccades*, Experimental Brain Research **58** (1985), 455-472.

Haenny, P.E., & Schiller, P.H., *State dependent activity in the monkey visual cortex. I. Single cell activity in V1 and V4 on visual tasks*, Experimental Brain Research **69** (1988), 225-244.

Heilman, K.M., Valenstein, E., & Goldberg, M.E., *Attention: behavior and neural mechanisms*, in "V.B. Mountcastle, F. Plum, & St.R. Geiger (Eds)., Handbook of physiology - The nervous system, Vol. V," American Physiological Society, Maryland/USA, 1987, pp. 461-481.

Henn, V., & Cohen, B., *Coding of information about rapid eye movements in the pontine reticular formation of alert monkeys*, Brain Research **108** (1976), 307-325.

Henn, V., Büttner-Ennever, J.A., & Hepp, K., *The primate oculomotor system. I. Motoneurons. A synthesis of anatomical, physiological and clinical data*, Human Neurobiology **1** (1982a), 77-85.

Henn, V., Hepp, K., & Büttner-Ennever, J.A., *The primate oculomotor system. II. A synthesis of anatomical, physiological and clinical data*, Human Neurobiology **1** (1982b), 87-95.

Hepp, K., & Henn, V., *Spatio-temporal recording of rapid eye movement signals in the monkey paramedian pontine reticular formation (PPRF)*, Experimental Brain Research **52** (1983), 105-120.

Heywood, C.A., & Cowey, A., *On the role of cortical area V4 in the discrimination of hue and pattern in macaque monkeys*, Neuroscience (1987), 174-218.

Hoffmann, K.P., *The control of the optokinetic reflex by the nucleus of the optic tract in the cat (subcortical vs cortical nystagmus)*, in "G. Lennerstrand, D.S. Zee, & E.L. Keller (Eds.), Functional basis of ocular motility disorders," Pergamon Press, Oxford, 1982.

Holmes, G., *Disturbances of visual space perception*, British Medical Journal **II** (1919), 230-233.

Holmes, G., & Horrax, G., *Disturbances of spatial orientation and visual attention with loss of stereoscopic vision*, Archiv Psychiatrie und Nervenkrankheiten **1** (1919), 385-407.

Hyvärinen, J. (Ed.), "The parietal cortex of monkey and man," Springer-Verlag, Berlin, 1982.

Jackson, H., "Selected writings. Vol. II. J. Taylor (Ed.)," Hodder and Stoughton, London, 1932.

Julesz, B., *Preconscious and conscious processes in vision*, in "C. Chagas, R. Gattass, & C. Gross (Eds.), Pattern recognition mechanisms. Experimental brain research, Suppl. 11," Springer-Verlag, Berlin, 1985, pp. 333-359.

Jung, R., *Neuropsychologie und Neurophysiologie des Kontur - und Formsehens in Zeichnung und Malerei*, in "H.H. Wieck (Ed.), Psychopathologie musischer Gestaltungen," Schattauer Verlag, Stuttgart, 1974, pp. 29-88.

Keating, E.G., Gooley, S.G., Pratt, S.E., & Kelsey, J.E., *Removing the superior colliculus silences eye movements normally evoked from stimulation of the parietal and occipital eye fields*, Brain Research **269** (1983), 145-148.

Keller, E.L., *Colliculoreticular organization in the oculomotor system*, in "Progress in brain research," Elsevier, Amsterdam, 1980.

Kommerell, G., *Supranukleäre Augenbewegungsstörungen*, in "H. Kaufmann (Ed.), Strabismus," Enke Verlag, 1986, pp. 402-440.

Latto, R., *The effects of bilateral frontal eye field, posterior parietal or superior collicular lesions on visual search in the rhesus monkey*, Brain Research **146** (1978), 35-50.

Latto, R., & Cowey, A., *Visual field defect after frontal eye-field lesions in monkeys*, Brain Research **30** (1971), 1-24.

Lynch, J.C., *The role of parieto-occipital association cortex in oculomotor control*, Experimental Brain Research **41** (1980), p. A32.

Lynch, J.C., *Frontal eye field lesions in monkeys disrupt visual pursuit*, Experimental Brain Research **68** (1987), 437-441.

Lynch, J.C., & McLaren, J.W., *Effects of lesions of parieto-occipital association cortex upon performance of oculomotor and attention tasks in monkeys*, Neuroscience Abstracts **5** (1979), p. 794.

Lynch, J.C., & Allison, J.C., *A quantitative study of visual pursuit deficits following lesions of the frontal eye fields in rhesus monkeys*, Society for Neuroscience Abstracts **11** (1985), p. 473.

Lynch, J.C., Mountcastle, V.B., Talbot, W.H., & Yin, T.C.T., *Parietal lobe mechanisms for directed visual attention*, Journal of Neurophysiology **40** (1977), 362-389.

Mitz, A.R., & Wise, St.P., *The somatotopic organization of the supplementary motor area: intracortical microstimulation mapping*, Journal of Neuroscience **7** (1987), 1010-1021.

Mohler, C.W., & Wurtz, R.H., *Organization of monkey superior colliculus: intermediate layer cells discharging before eye movement*, Journal of Neurophysiology **39** (1976), 722-744.

Moran, J., & Desimone, R., *Selective attention gates visual processing in the extrastriate cortex*, Science **229** (1985), 782-784.

Mountcastle, V.B., *The world around us. Neural command functions for selective attention*, Neurosciences Research Program · Bulletin **14**, Supplement (1976).

Mountcastle, V.B., *Functional properties of the light sensitive neurons of the posterior parietal cortex and their regulation by state controls: influence on excitability of interested fixation and the angle of gaze*, in "O. Pompeiano & C. Ajmone Marsan (Eds.), Brain mechanisms of perceptual awareness and purposeful behavior. IBRO Monograph Series, Vol. 8," Raven Press, New York, 1981, pp. 67-69.

Movshon, J.A., Adelson, E.H., Gizzi, M.S., & Newsome, W.T., *The analysis of moving visual patterns*, in "C. Chagas, R. Gattas, & C. Gross (Eds.), Pattern recognition mechanisms. Experimental brain research, Suppl. 11," Springer-Verlag, Berlin, 1985, pp. 117-152.

Pasik, T., Pasik, P., & Bender, M.B., *The superior colliculi and eye movements*, Archives of Neurology **15** (1966), 420-436.

Pöppel, E., Held, R. & Frost, D., *Residual visual functions after brain wounds involving the central visual pathway in man*, Nature **243** (1973), 295-296.

Posner, M.I., Walker, J.A., Friedrich, F.J., & Rafal, R.D., *Effects of parietal injury on covert orienting of attention*, Journal of Neuroscience **7** (1984), 1863-1874.

Precht, W., *Cerebellar influences on eye movements*, in "G. Lennerstrand & P. Bachey-Rita (Eds.), Basic mechanisms of ocular motility and their clinical implications," Pergamon Press, Oxford, NY, 1975, pp. 261-280.

Precht, W., *Anatomical and functional organization of optokinetic pathways*, in "G. Lennerstrand, D.S. Zee, & E.L. Keller (Eds.), Functional basis of ocular motility disorders," Pergamon Press, New York, 1982.

Robinson, D.A., & Fuchs, A.F., *Eye movements evoked by stimulation of frontal eye fields*, Journal of Neurophysiology **32** (1969), 637-648.

Robinson, D.A., Goldberg, M.E., & Stanton, G.B., *Parietal association cortex in the primate: Sensory mechanisms and behavioral modulations*, Journal of Neurophysiology **41** (1978), 910-932.

Robinson, D.A., *Control of eye movements*, in "J.M. Brookhart & V.B. Mountcastle (Eds.), Handbook of physiology. Vol. II: Motor control, Part 2," American Physiological Society, Bethesda/MA, 1981, pp. 1275-1320.

Schiller, P.H., *The superior colliculus and visual function*, in "J.M. Brookhart & V.B. Mountcastle (Eds.), Handbook of Physiology. Vol III: Sensory Processes, Part 1," American Physiological Society, Bethesda/MA, 1984, pp. 457-505.

Schiller, P.H., Stryker, M., Cynader, M., & Berman, N., *Response characteristics of single cells in the monkey colliculus following ablation or cooling of visual cortex*, Journal of Neurophysiology **37** (1974), 181-194.

Schiller, P.H., True, S.D., & Conway, J.L., *Paired stimulation of the frontal eye fields and the superior colliculus of the rhesus monkey*, Brain Research **179** (1979), 162-164.

Schiller, P.H., Sandell, J.H., & Maunsell, J.H.R., *The effect of frontal eye field and superior colliculus lesions on saccadic latencies in the rhesus monkey*, Journal of Neurophysiology **57** (1987), p. 1033.

Schlag, J., & Schlag-Rey, M., *Visuomotor functions of central thalamus in monkey. II. Unit activity related to visual events, targeting, and fixation*, Journal of Neurophysiology **51** (1984), 1175-1195.

Schlag, J., & Schlag-Rey, M., *Unit activity related to spontaneous saccades in frontal dorsomedial cortex of monkey*, Experimental Brain Research **58** (1985), 208-211.

Schlag, J., & Schlag-Rey, M., *Eye fixation units in the supplementary eye field of monkey*, Neuroscience Abstracts **25** (1985), 23-82.

Schlag, J., & Schlag-Rey, M., *Evidence for a supplementary eye field*, Journal of Neuroscience **57** (1987a), 179ff.

Schlag, J., & Schlag-Rey, M., *Does microstimulation evoke fixed-vector saccades by generating their vector or by specifying their goal?*, Experimental Brain Research **68** (1987b), 442-444.

Sparks, D.L., Holland, R., & Guthrie, B.L., *Size and distribution of movement fields in the monkey superior colliculus*, Brain Research **113** (1976), 21-34.

Sparks, D.L., Mays, L.E., & Pollak, J.G., *Saccade-related unit activity in the monkey superior colliculus*, in "R. Baker & B.A. Brooks (Eds.), Control of gaze by brainstem neurons," Elsevier, Amsterdam, 1977, pp. 437-444.

Stein, J., *The effect of parietal lobe cooling on manipulative behavior in the conscious monkey*, in "G. Gordon (Ed.), Active touch," Pergamon Press, Oxford, 1978, pp. 79-90.

Straschill, M., & Rieger, P., *Eye movements evoked by focal stimulation of cat's superior colliculus*, Brain Research **59** (1973), 221-227.

Tanaka, M., Weber, H., & Creutzfeldt, O.D., *Visual properties and spatial distribution of neurons in the visual association area on the prelunate gyrus of the awake monkey*, Experimental Brain Research **63** (1986), 11-37.

Vogt, C., & Vogt, O., *Allgemeinere Ergebnisse unserer Hirnforschung. IV. Die physiologische Bedeutung der architektonischen Rindenfelderung aufgrund unserer Rindenreizungen*, Journal of Psychology and Neurology **25** (1919), 401-461.

Wagman, I.H., *Eye movements induced by electric stimulation of cerebrum in monkeys and their relationship to bodily movements*, in "M.B. Bender (Ed.), The oculomotor system," Hoeber, New York, 1964, pp. 18-39.

Weiskrantz, L., Warrington, E.K., Sanders, M.D., & Marshall, J., *Visual capacity in the hemianopic field following a restricted occipital ablation*, Brain **97** (1974), 709-728.

Wise, S.P., & Strick, P.L., *Anatomical and physiological organization of the non-primary motor cortex*, Trends in Neuroscience **7** (1984), 442 ff.

Wurtz, R.H., & Albano, J.E., *Visual-motor function of the primate superior colliculus*, Annual Review of Neuroscience **3** (1980), 189-226.

Wurtz, R.H., Goldberg, M.E., & Robinson, D.L., *Behavioral modulation of visual responses in the monkey: stimulus selection for attention and movement*, in "J.M. Sprague & A.N. Epstein (Eds.), Progress in Psychobiology and Physiological Psychology, Vol. 9," Academic Press, New York, 1980, pp. 43-83.

Wurtz, R.H., Goldberg, M.E., & Robinson, D.L., *Brain mechanisms of visual attention*, in "R.F. Thompson (Ed.), Progress in neuroscience," Readings from Scientific American, 1982, pp. 82-90.

Wurtz, R.H., & Hikosaka, O., *Role of the basal ganglia in the initiation of saccadic eye movements*, in "H.J. Freund, U. Büttner, B. Cohen, & J. Noth (Eds.), Progress in brain research, Vol. 64," Elsevier Science Publishers, 1986, pp. 175-190.

Yarbus, A.L. (Ed.), "Eye movements and vision," Plenum Press, New York, 1967.

3
History of Eye Movement Research

ON THE HISTORY OF EYE MOVEMENT RECORDING

DIETER HELLER

Psychologisches Institut, Universität Fribourg

INTRODUCTION

Eye movement monitoring today is an area of scientific inquiry with multiple branches and sophisticated measurement techniques. As such, it appears to be a typical product of the second half of the 20th century, with some original forerunners in the founding years of experimental psychology, for instance, Helmholtz, Javal, and Dodge. For this reason, the historical discussion of this subject has concentrated on the developments since the turn of the century (e.g. Taylor, 1937; Woodworth, 1938; Woodworth & Schlosberg, 1954; Venetzky, 1977).

Ever since Ebbinghaus (1908) introduced his convenient distinction between the "long past" and the "short history," hinting that the former could be largely ignored, this restricted historical perspective has been accepted without question by many in the field. We have become accustomed to dating the beginnings of modern psychology in the second half of the 19th century, for instance, with the publication of Fechner's *Elements of Psychophysics* (1860) or Wundt's *Contributions to a Theory of Sensory Perception* (1862a) which introduced and attempted to substantiate the idea and programme of "Experimental Psychology."

It is now clear that this restricted historical treatment neglects important findings and lines of development that substantially contributed to the current understanding of our subject.

Indeed, a broad range of current issues in, amongst others, eye movement research had been under vigorous investigation during the first half of the 19th century, and a number of questions (particularly in the area of perception) can be traced back to the Middle Ages, and in some cases, to Greek antiquity (Grüsser, 1986). Some of these investigations have rightly fallen into oblivion and might be of interest only to the historian. However, this "long past" could still provide an interesting perspective for our present discussions. To uncover such aspects should be the prime concern of any historical treatment, i.e. what is called for is a "history for the present" (Traxel, 1986).

The methodological problems in the recording and analysis of eye movements are still a prominent issue in current research and have received little historical attention. Techniques and apparatuses need to be discussed in their own right because of their essential part in the development of our field. The availability or non-availability of certain apparatuses and methodological tools determines how one approaches a subject and in turn the development of a theory.

In view of the interaction between subject and method, any historical discussion concentrating only on the development of theoretical formulations in a given field to the neglect of a discussion about the apparatus available before development of a theory is bound to remain incomplete. An apparatus not only defines a subject in operational terms but also serves to focus attention on specific facets. However, that the apparatus thereby acts to direct attention away from other aspects is often overlooked.

The tachistoscope (invented by Volkmann in 1850) is one of the most striking examples in point. Methodologically, its purpose is the accurate measurement of exposure times. However, it led to an emphasis on to the unmoving eye and static objects. The common reference to the phi-phenomenon as "apparent motion" clearly points to the axiomatic importance of the static gaze and the unmoving object. Moreover, technical limitations of the apparatus, e.g. the so-called "window size," the minimum exposure duration or the maximum rate of successive frames, determined specific ways in which questions were formulated.

It should therefore be worthwhile to take a closer look at some of the major stations in the "long past" of eye movement research.

On the Medieval Pre-History of Eye Movement Research

Try to imagine a medieval treatment of eye movements and physiological optics and immediately an Anglo-Saxon or Franconian monk comes to mind, who, in his cell, reasons about the experience of the "outer" world and whether universals pre-exist before the thing itself or are derived therefrom. If this monk took up the question of vision, you would expect him to produce mystical speculations - for instance, about the eye as the light of heaven or as a mirror of the mind, psyche and medium of knowledge about other humans. Examples of such a medieval mysticism and physiognomics can be found in the works of Konrad von Megenberg or Albertus Magnus (Schleusener-Eichholz, 1985).

Such notions were preserved well into the 19th century and can still be found, in almost identical formulations, in psychological treatises of this time which regarded themselves as empirical and scientific. Scheidler, for example, states in 1833: "The organ of vision, the eye, is favoured above all other senses in that it most clearly expresses the state of the psyche and acts as a mirror both of the world and of inner life" (p. 402). Such statements might have contributed to our impression that the 19th-century revival of physiological research on this subject represents a fundamentally new development.

The existence, of a differentiated experimental science of physiological psychology in the earlier Middle Ages, is largely ignored because of our fixation on the Modern Age and Christian West. Until today, medieval Arabic science, which we must focus upon in this context, has been regarded mainly as the mediator of classical Greek knowledge, but has not been credited with its many own scientific achievements, or if acknowledged, they were persistently underrated. This can be seen, among others, in Crombies's statement: "Of the actual knowledge from the stores of Greek learning which was transmitted to Western Christendom by the Arabs together with some additional observations and comments of their own, some of the most important were the new Ptolemaic astronomy and its associated trigonometry ... What the Arabs did was to improve observing instruments ..." (1952, p. 31).

Elsewhere, though, Crombie writes: "The original Arabic contribution was more important in the study of optics and perspective for here, though the works of Euclid, Hero and Ptolemy had dealt with the subject. Alkindi (about 870) and Alhazen (c. 965-1039) mad a big advance on what had been known by the Greeks ... Alhazen discussed, among other things, spherical and parabolic mirrors, the camera obscura, lenses and vision."

Despite this positive appraisal, especially of Ibn al Haytham (Alhazen), Crombie fails to recognize the real importance of the Arabs for their development of the experimental sciences in general and the foundation of physiological optics in particular. They linked a mathematical and an experimental optics with an empirical anatomy. They developed a theory of visual perception and subjected it to experimental tests, for instance, by applying it to optical illusions. For example, detailed anatomical investigations with animals were carried out to determine the properties of the various light-refractive media of the eye, and the results were compared with hypotheses derived from a theoretical model (camera obscura) or observations of the human eye. A variety of translucent media were investigated and manifold instruments developed and employed to aid experimenting, for example, "tachistoscopic" exposure, colour discs and the use of afterimages.

The establishment of this science and its presentation on a comprehensive treatise is the achievement of Ibn al Haytham (Alhazen, who was born in Basra in 965 and died in Cairo in 1039). The *Kitab al Manazir*, the book on light, his main work published between 1025 and 1030, must be regarded as the first "Handbook of Physiological Optics." It contains a stunning wealth of observations and experimental findings which we regard as - supposed - discoveries or results of 19th-century science.

Unfortunately, this is not the occasion to discuss the importance of the *Kitab al Manazir* in more detail. But it must be stated that its extraordinary impact on the advance of the sciences can hardly be overrated. Presumably, neither the telescope nor the microscope, the two main instruments of scientific progress, would have been invented without this work. As regards to the investigation of visual perception, only Helmholtz's *Handbook of Physiologi-*

cal Optics (1866) could again approach the rank of the *Opticae - Thesaurus Alhazeni*, as Friedrich Risner entitled his Latin edition of 1572 (OPTICAE THESVRVS ALHAZENI ARABIS libri septem, nunc primum editi. EIVS-DEM liber DE CREPVSCVLIS Nubium ascensionibus ITEM VITELLONIS THVRINGOPOLONI LIBRI X).

The following drawings (Figure 1) are particularly interesting as they illustrate Ibn al Haytham's (Alhazen's) conception of the eye and anatomical properties of the visual system. The drawing of the eye is taken from the *Tanqih al-Manazir* by Kamal al-Din al Farisi, an early 14th-century (1316) commentary to Ibn al Haytham's *Kitab al Manazir*. According to the text, this is a copy of Alhazen's drawing. The drawing of the visual system is taken from a copy of the *Kitab al Manazir* owned by the Süleymaniye Library Istanbul. These illustrations are examples of the detailed knowledge available at that time not only of the anatomy of the eye but also of the whole visual system, including the visual pathways.

The page of the *Opticae Thesaurus Alhazeni* shown in Figure 2 contains the most interesting section with regard to visual resolution and eye movements. It says, in brief, than an object can be clearly perceived if the axes of the eyes intersect at the object's location. The parts of the object immediately surrounding the ocular axes can be seen clearly; however, towards the periphery, perception of detail decreases. For the ocular axes to intersect at an object, both eyes must be moved in a coordinated fashion. This is achieved "reflexively," as formulated by Ibn al Haytham in a different paragraph: One cannot intentionally prevent one eye from following the other; only mechanical constraints can do this. Such a prevention gives rise to double images.

Ibn al Haytham also addressed the issue of reading, still a central issue of today's eye movement research. He stated that recognition of familiar words does not require that all characters are seen in detail; rather, they can be recognized on the basis of their global appearance. Further, he distinguished between recognition and naming times in reading.

Ibn al Haytham's (Alhazen's) optics played an important role, (until the beginning of the Modern Age) in the development of Western science and was completely assimilated, among others, by Witelo (Risner, 1572) and by Roger Bacon in his opus majus. However, Ibn al Haytham's (Alhazen's) observations relating to eye movements were apparently forgotten, despite the fact that many eminent scientists to the Modern Age (e.g. Galileo, Harvey and Descartes) concerned themselves with vision. Accordingly, Kepler, for example, is credited with the discovery of the reversed retinal image.

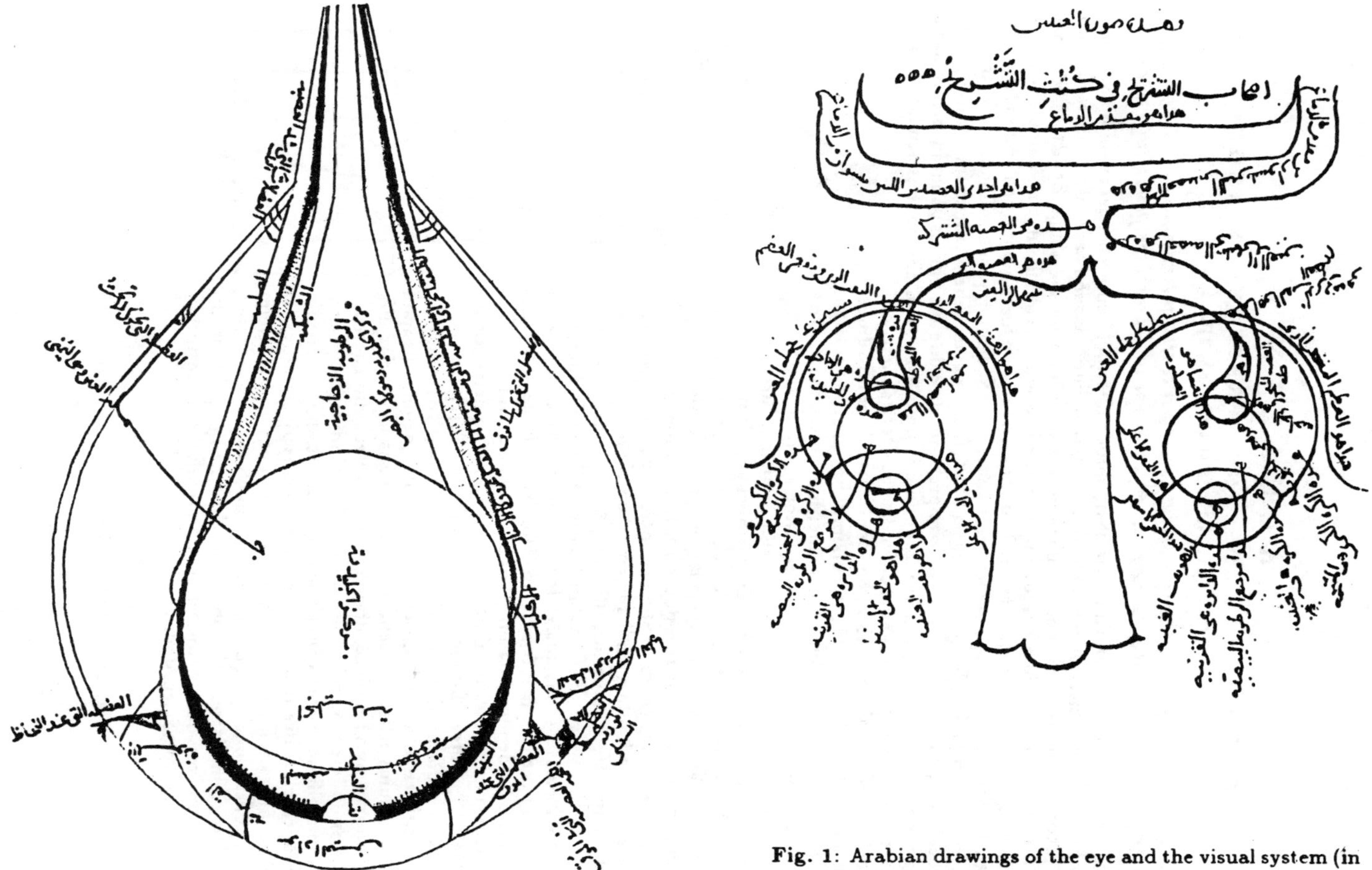

Fig. 1: Arabian drawings of the eye and the visual system (in Kamal al-Din al Farisi commentary).

76 ALHAZEN

DE IIS QVAE DEBENT PRAEPONI SERMONI in deceptionibus uisus. Cap. II.

2. Axes pyramidum opticarum utriusq; uisus per centrum foraminis uueæ transeuntes, in uno uisibilis puncto semper concurrunt: & sunt perpendiculares superficiei uisus. 32. 35 p 3.

DEclaratum est in primo tractatu [18 n] quòd uisus nihil comprehendat ex uisibilibus, nisi secundum uerticationes refractas linearum radialium: & quòd ordo uisibilium & partium eorum non comprehenditur, nisi ex ordinatione linearum radialium. Et dictum est etiam [27 n 1] quòd unum uisum, quod comprehenditur duobus oculis simul, non comprehenditur unum, nisi quando positio eius in respectu duorum oculorum fuerit positio consimilis: & quòd si positio fuerit diuersa: tunc comprehendetur unum duo. Sed unumquodq; uisibilium assuetorum, quæ semper comprehenduntur à duobus uisibus, semper comprehendetur unum. Vnde oportet nos declarare, quomodo unum uisum comprehendatur à duobus uisibus unum in maiore parte temporis & in pluribus positionibus: & quomodo positio unius uisi ab ambobus oculis in maiore parte temporis, & in pluribus erit consimilis. Et declarabimus etiã quomodo positio unius uisi ab ambobus uisibus erit positio diuersa, & quomodo accidat hoc. Et iam diximus hoc in primo tractatu [27 n] & declarauimus ipsum uniuersaliter, non determinatè. Dicamus ergo quòd cum inspiciẽs inspexerit aliquod uisum, tunc uterq; uisus erit in oppositione illius uisi: & cum inspiciens direxerit pupillam ad illud uisum: tunc uterq; uisus diriget pupillam ad illud uisum directione æquali. Et cum uisus fuerit motus super rem uisam: tunc uterq; uisus mouebitur super illud. Et cum uisus direxerit pupillam ad rem uisam: tunc axes duorum uisuum congregabuntur in illa re uisa, & coniungentur in aliquo puncto illius superficiei. Et si inspiciens mouerit uisum per illam rem uisam: tũc illi duo axes mouebuntur simul super superficiẽ illius uisi, & per omnes partes eius. Et uniuersaliter duo oculi sunt æquales in omnibus suis dispositionibus: & uirtus sensibilis, quæ est in eis, est eadem, & actio & passio eorum semper est æqualis & omnino cõsimilis. Et si alter uisus fuerit motus ad uidendum, statim reliquus mouebitur ad illud uisum illo eodem motu: & si alter uisus quieuerit, reliquus quiescit. Et impossibile est, ut alter uisus moueatur ad uidẽdum, & reliquus quiescat, nisi impediatur. Et declaratũ est in præteritis [19 n 1] quòd inter quodlibet uisum & cẽtrum uisus est pyramis imaginabilis apud uisionem, cuius uertex est centrum uisus, & basis superficies uisi, quod uisus comprehendit: & ista pyramis continet omnes uerticationes, ex quibus comprehendit illã rem uisam. Cum ergo duo axes amborum uisuum fuerint cõiuncti in aliquo puncto superficiei uisi: tunc superficies uisi erit basis communis ambabus pyramidibus radialibus, figuratis inter duo cẽtra amborum uisuum & illud uisum: & tunc positio puncti, in quo axes sunt cõiuncti apud ambos uisus, est positio cõsimilis: quia est oppositũ duobus medijs amborum uisuum, & duo axes, qui sunt inter illud & duos uisus, sunt perpendiculares super superficiem duorum uisuum.

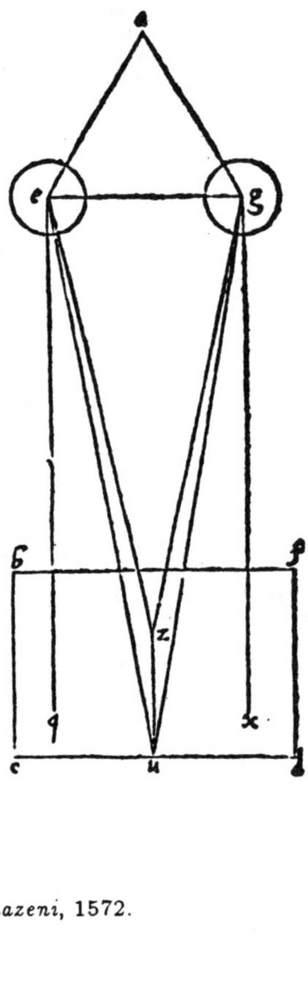

Fig. 2: Text from the *Opticae Thesaurus Alhazeni*, 1572.

The Revival of Eye Movement Research in the 19th Century

New interest in this issue did not reemerge before the beginning of the 19th century. By then, Ibn al Haytham had long been forgotten and his name did not even receive mention in the "real-encyclopedias" which originate from that time. Charles Bell (1823) and Johannes Müller (1826), the two founders of modern physiology, "discovered" this subject anew. Both devoted special treatises to eye movements marking the beginning of their systematic study. At the outset, these studies involved, above all, a more accurate determination of eye motion characteristics, particularly, of the centre of rotation, which Müller had localized in the rear wall of the eye.

"Wheel-like" ocular rotations, also described by Müller, were systematically investigated by Hueck (1838) who tried to show that head movements to one side result in (compensatory) rotations of the eyes in the opposite direction.

Ruete's (1845) development of the first technique for observating the state of the ocular rotation produced the greatest impetus in the founding phase of eye movement research. Ruete produced strong afterimages of, for example, vertical lines and observed their orientation as a function of head orientation.

Volkmann (1846) carried out the first attempt to determine more accurately the velocity of eye movements. He tested how often in the course of 1800 "Tertien" (i.e. 30 s) he could move his eyes to an fro between two pins which were placed at various distances from each other. Volkmann discovered that vertical movements can be executed faster than horizontal movements, that differential (unequal) distances of the pins from the eye result in slowed movements and that monocular movements can be carried out faster than binocular movements. He found, further, that the ocular musculi recti can be influenced voluntarily in contrast to the musculi obliqui. He demonstrated this in several afterimage experiments.

Also using the afterimage technique, Donders (1847) provided the first comprehensive description of ocular movements and confirmed, in part, Listing's (1845) laws of motion. Donder's findings were later replicated and further extended by Meissner (1855). However, the final experimental confirmation of the laws of motion was only achieved by Helmholtz (1863) who had earlier succeeded in describing the accommodation movements and associated changes of the eye, e.g. narrowing of the pupil, curvature of the lens, etc. (Helmholtz, 1855).

Building on Hueck's (1840) attempt to determine the decrement of visual acuity on the extrafoveal field, E.H. Weber (1846) proposed that the size of the retinal area allocated to a single fibre of the optical nerve varies as a function of the distance from the fovea ("... that the terminators of the elementary threads of the optic nerve are extremely dense only at the location of the central depression and are the more widely spaced the further away a retinal part from the centre (is)," 1846, p. 531). He attempted to determine the size of the fovea using a letter recognition technique. To exclude eye movements, he briefly illuminated words of a language unknown to the subject by means of the spark discharge of a Leidner-bottle (i.e. 320 to 350 ms exposure). He found that about three letters could be recognized in a single fixation. With regard to eye movements, he drew the following conclusion: "In vision I can demonstrate that the extent of that part of the retina with which we see clearly is only about 1/3 Parisian Line (1 Parisian Line = 2.2558 mm). Therefore, we have to shift our eye from one part to the next, so that little by little each part of a bigger object is represented at this small, most sensitive locus of the retina. However, we believe, we view simultaneously physical bodies which cannot be represented at once at this retinal part. We believe, we perform simultaneously what we carry out successively" (1846, p. 488).

In short, Weber's (1846) investigations and conclusions anticipated the lines along which subsequent research developed in eye movement and reading.

In retrospect, it is difficult to understand why Weber's proposals, which anticipated the work of Javal (1878), Lamare (1893) and Cattell (1885, 1886), failed to have an immediate impact. The fact that no one before Erdmann and Dodge (1898), some 50 years later, referred to Weber's findings cannot be blamed on Wagner's *Hand-Dictionary of Physiology* in which Weber's contribution was published. Since this was the standard text of his time, read by every worker in the field. If one does not want to hold Boring's "Zeitgeist" responsible, the only explanation remaining is that at that time the mechanical and physiological properties of eye movements still absorbed too much of the researchers' attention for them to realise the potential use of eye movements for the study of psychological processes.

Wundt's contribution to eye movement research, it appears, also fell into oblivion. In his monography *Contributions to the Theory of Sensory Perception* (1862a), he introduced the term of "experimental psychology" and his research program in Leipzig. Wundt concerned himself in detail (on more than 100 pages) with issues of eye movements and their implications for psychological questions. His treatment refers to two of his own articles publish[Bed in the same year in Graefe's "Archiv": *On movements of the eyes* (1862b), and *The description of an artificial system of the ocular muscles for investigating the laws of motion of the human eye in a healthy condition and a condition of disorder* (1862c).

Wundt tried to show in his monography that eye movements are not primarily determined by optical laws, but rather by mechanical principles; that is, an eye movement reaches the intended fixation location at the minimum expenditure of muscular action. To test this idea, Wundt developed an artificial system of the ocular muscles which is illustrated in Figure 3. This apparatus was designed to

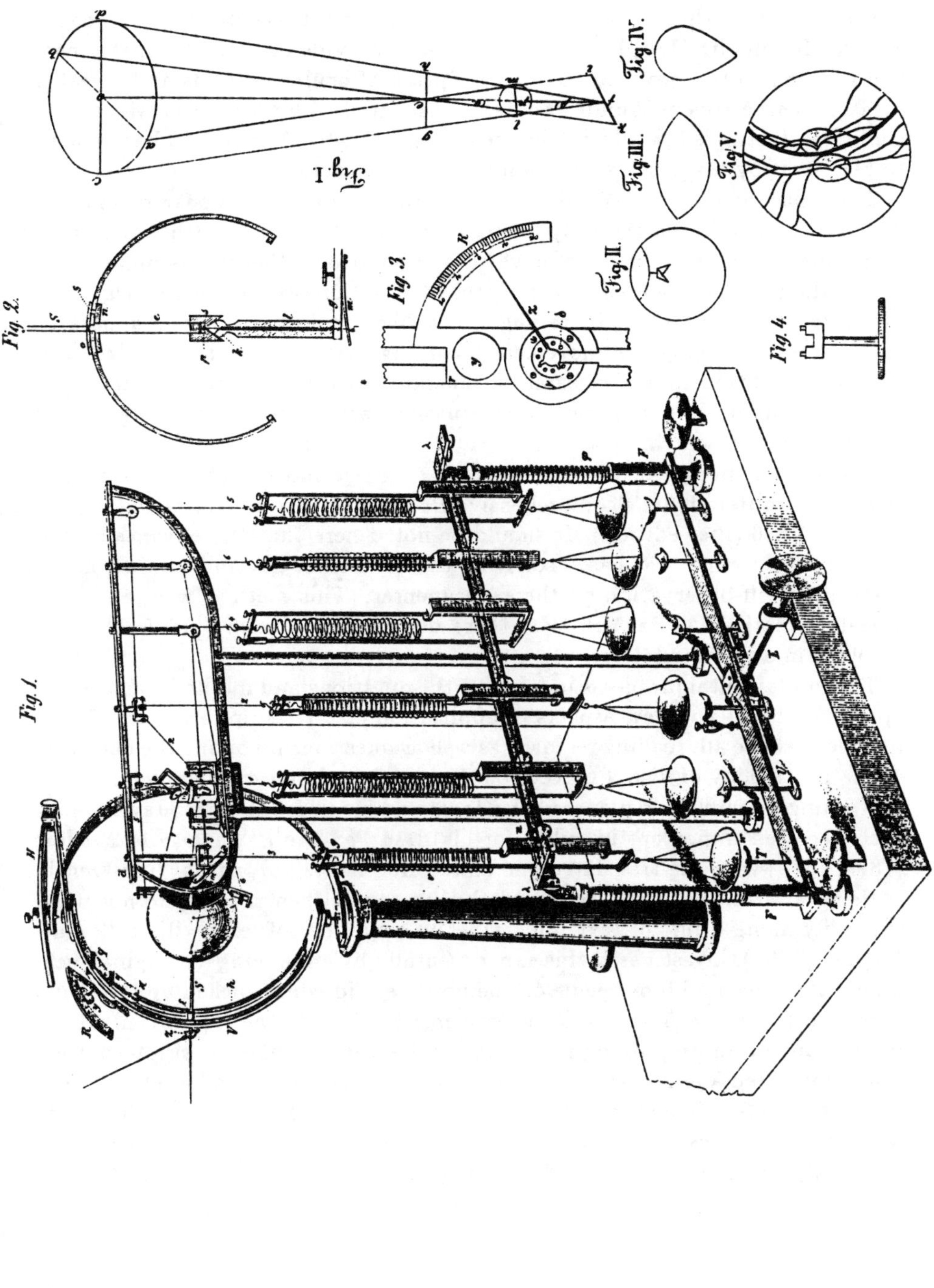

Fig. 3: Eye movement simulator developed by Wundt (1862).

simulate all possible eye movement situations as a function of acting muscular forces (i.e. weights). Wundt believed that this device would also prove useful for the diagnosis and modelling of eye movement disorders.

Unfortunately, this apparatus failed to gain practical acceptance, presumably because Helmholtz (1863), only one year later, provided a (largely) mathematical solution to the problem of the description of ocular motions and revealed measurement errors in Wundt's observations of up to 1.5 ° Moreover, Helmholtz confirmed Listing's law which had been questioned by Wundt who had wanted to replace it by his principle of minimal muscular action.

This must have made Wundt's eye movement simulator appear redundant. This is regrettable, particularly for methodological reasons. If this apparatus had gained acceptance, it might have been developed further with similar intensity as the tachistoscope, of which dozens of variations existed at the beginning of the 20th century. Thus, there might have been available today an apparatus to calibrate the many eye movement recording systems currently in use. Despite the long tradition of research in this area, such a calibration system is as yet non-existent. In my opinion, this situation casts doubt on the reliability of eye movement research.

The 40-year period of intense study on pure eye movements found its first conclusion in Helmholtz's comprehensive *Handbook of Physiological Optics* published in 1866 (first edition). It should be noted here that the advance knowledge up to this time was based solely on the method of afterimages, i.e. on the systematic self-observation by the experimenter. This method was capable of revealing motion laws as subtle as those described by Listing (1845, 1851) or involved in accommodation.

The fundamental problems in terms of the questions and methods of his time, appeared solved and new aspects of application could gain prominence. These included, above all, reading research as well as questions involving the questions of the psychology of visual perception discussed in detail by Helmholtz.

Reading research was pioneered by Javal and his pupil Lamare. Javal apparently received important impulses for his *Essay on the Physiology of Reading* (1878, 1879) when he translated and edited Helmholtz's *Handbook* into French.

Using afterimages, Javal observed that the eyes when reading do not move smoothly along a line of text, but rather in a number of jerks. His colleague, Lamare (1893), investigated this experimentally by employing an original technique: He placed a blunt needle on the upper eyelid which picked up the sound produced by ocular movements and transmitted them to the experimenter's ear by meBans of an amplifying membrane and a rubber tube. A short-duration sound indicated a jerk within a line and a longer-duration sound a return sweep between lines. This device can bè regarded as the starting point of the search for apparatuses designed to record eye movements.

In this way Lamare observed that readers divide lines into subsections of about 10 characters which are read during rhythmical intervals (i.e. fixations). The transition from one section to the next is accomplished by energetic jerks during which reading cannot occur. Further, the number of fixations did not vary as a function of eye-text distance (0.3 to 1 m).

Independently of Javal, Erdmann and Dodge (1898) commenced investigations of reading eye movements. Their starting point was the question raised by Cattell (1885, 1886), whether reading is based on a letter-by-letter process or the simultaneous recognition of words as whole entities. Given the small area used for detailed vision, reading could be expected to involve a great number of rightwards eye movements. Erdmann and Dodge tested this by using a mirror placed on one side of the text, in order that they could directly observe the eyes of the subject.

Erdmann and Dodge's findings were consitent with those of Lamare; that is, the number of characters per "reading interval," as they termed fixations, was approximately 12 and calculated values of interval durations varied between 250 and 400 ms. Experimentally determined durations of single saccades ranged from 15 to 30 ms. These values were in good agreement with Lamansky (1869) and Volkmann (1846) whose data were reanalysed according to a procedure developed by Dodge. Erdmann and Dodge concluded from the high velocity of ocular rotations that reading can take place only during the resting periods of the eyes.

Huey (1908) was the first to record eye movements in reading by using a technique developed by Delabarre (1898). Eye movements were recorded directly on the rotatable drum of a kymograph by means of a pointer system which was directly attached to the cornea and whose weight was reduced by Huey to a 1/2 g.

The first photographic recording technique was developed by Dodge and Cline (1901). A beam of light was used to illuminate the cornea, and the reflected light, focused by means of a lens system, was recorded on a moveable photographic plate. This technique was later developed into the photokymograph and played a significant role in early reading research, alongside Judd's (1905, 1907) recording technique by means of a film camera.

Using Dodge's technique, Dearborn (1906) found that for the reading of newspaper lines, the average number of fixations was 4.6 and the average fixation duration was 285 ms.

The last technique introduced, by Schott (1922), the electrical recording of the corneo-retinal potential, is still in use today. By means of a string galvanometer, Schott succeeded in describing a nystagmus. This technique was further studied by Meyers (1929) and Mowrer, Ruch, and Miller (1936). Mowrer et al. showed that the EOG is not, as originally believed, based on the summed action potentials of the ocular muscles but rather on the corneo-retinal potential.

The period of intensive reading research which began with the new techniques developed after the turn of the century has already been comprehensively reviewed, among others, by Taylor (1937), Woodworth (1938), Woodworth and Schlosberg (1954) and, recently, Venezky (1977). Therefore, there is no need to go into further detail.

Implications for Current Research

Some past achievements which could be profitably used today, such as Wundt's "ophthalmotrope," have been completely overlooked.

Also forgotten is the method of afterimages which was powerful enough to reveal such subtle laws of motion as those of Listing, but which failed to gain acceptance in modern psychology. This method could be profitably applied to a series of questions, e.g. calibration of eye movement registration, determination of fixation locations within words, etc. Presumably, this method has fallen victim to both the "cult of apparatuses" and the, in this regard, misleading or, respectively, misconceived discussion of the question concerning objectivity and selfobservation, which both accompanied psychology right from its outset.

It appears to be a consequence of this that renowed journals in perception today decline to publish studies based on the method of afterimages, stating as a reason that there are better methods of eye movement monitoring. (Personal report of P. Dunn-Rankin, University of Hawaii.)

To conclude, the current "renaissance" of discussing older eye movement research reveals that far fewer issues are outdated by the current state of knowledge.

Considering the course of research up to the beginning of our century, the broad wealth of knowledge that had been accumulated by that time is indeed astonishing. It is apparent that many more questions had been closely examined during the last century than is commonly believed. By comparison, relatively little has been added in the last 80 years, despite (or, in some cases, because of) the great technical progress.

References

Baarmann, J., *Abhandlung über das Licht von Ibn al Haitam*, Zeitschrift der deutsch - morgenlaendischen Gesellschaft **36** (1882), 195-237.

Bauer, H., *Die Psychologie Alhazens*, in "Beiträge zur Geschichte der Philosophie des Mittelalters (Bd. 10, Heft 5)," Aschendorffsche Verlagsbuchhandlung, Münster, 1911.

Bell, C., *On the motions of the eye, and illustration of the use of the muscles and nerves of the orbit*, Philosophical Transactions of the Royal Society (London) **113** (1823), 166-168.

Cattell, J. McK., *Über die Zeit der Erkennung und Benennung von Schriftzeichen, Bildern und Farben*, Philosophische Studien **2** (1885), 635-650.

Cattell, J. McK., *Über die Trägheit der Netzhaut und des Sehcentrums*, Philosophische Studien **3** (1886a), 94-127.

Cattell, J. McK., *Psychometrische Untersuchungen (2. Abteilung)*, Philosophische Studien **3** (1886b), 452-492.

Crombie, A.C., "Augustine to Galileo. The History of Science A.D. 400- 1650," Falcon Press, London, 1952.

Crombie, A.C., "Robert Grosseteste and the origins of experimental science 1100-1700," Clarendon Press, Oxford, 1953.

Delabarre, E.B., *A method of recording eye-movements*, American Journal of Psychology **9** (1898), 572-574.

Dodge, R., & Cline, T.S., *The angle velocity of eye-movements*, Psychological Review **8** (1901), 145-157.

Donders, F.C., *Beitrag zur Lehre von den Bewegungen des menschlichen Auges*, Holländische Beiträge zu den anatomischen und physiologischen Wissenschaften **1** (1847), 104-145, 384-386.

Ebbinghaus, H., "Abriß der Psychologie," Veit & Comp, Leipzig, 1908.

Erdmann, B., & Dodge, R., "Psychologische Untersuchung über das Lesen auf experimenteller Grundlage," Niemeyer, Halle, 1898.

Fechner, G. Th., "Elemente der Psychophysik," Breitkopf & Härtel, Leipzig, 1860.

Froebes, J., *Aus der Vorgeschichte der psychologischen Optik*, Zeitschrift für Psychologie **85** (1920), 1-36.

Gruesser, O.-J., *Interaction of efferent and afferent signals in visual perception. A history of ideas and experimental paradigms*, Acta Psychologica **63** (1986), 3-21.

Helmholtz, H., *Über die Accomodation des Auges*, Archiv für Ophthalmologie **1/II** (1855), 1-74.

Helmholtz, H., *Über die normalen Bewegungen des menschlichen Auges*, Archiv für Ophthalmologie **9/II** (1863), 153-214.

Helmholtz, H., "Handbuch der Physiologischen Optik (2. Aufl.)," Voss, Hamburg, 1896.

Hirschberg, J., *Geschichte der Augenheilkunde bei den Arabern*, in "Th. Saemisch (Hrsg.), Handbuch der Gesamten Augenheilkunde (Bd. 13, 2. Aufl.)," Engelmann, Leipzig, 1908.

Hueck, A., "Die Achsendrehung des Auges," Kluge, Dorpat, 1838.

Hueck, A., *Von den Grenzen des Sehvermögens*, in "J. Mueller (Hrsg.), Archiv für Anatomie, Physiologie und Wissenschaftliche Medicin," Veit, Berlin, 1840, p. 82.

Huey, E.B., "The psychology and pedagogy of reading," MIT Press, New York, 1968. (Originally published 1908).

Javal, E., *Essai sur la physiologie de la lecture*, Annales d'Oculistique. **79** (1878), 97-117, 240-274, 155-167; **80** (1879), 61-73, 157- 162, 72-81, 159-170, 242-253.

Javal, E., "Die Physiologie des Lesens und Schreibens," Engelmann, Leipzig, 1907.

Judd, C.H., *Movement and consciousness*, Psychological Review Monograph Supplements **29** (1905).

Judd, C.H., *Photographic records of convergence and divergence*, Psychological Review Monograph Supplements **34** (1907), 370-423.

Kepler, J., "J. Keplers Grundlagen der geometrischen Optik (Übersetzung von F. Plehn). Ostwalds Klassiker der exakten Wissenschaften (Bd. 198)," Akademische Verlagsgesellschaft, Leipzig, 1922.

Lamansky, S., *Bestimmung der Winkelgeschwindigkeit der Blickbewegung, resp. Augenbewegung*, Pflüger's Archiv f. die gesamte Physiologie **2** (1869), 418-422.

Lamare, M., *Des mouvements des yeux pendants la lecture*, Comptes rendus de la société française d'ophthalmologie (1893), 354-364.

Lindberg, D.C., *Alhazen's Theory of Vision and Its Reception in the West*, ISIS **58** (1967), 321-341.

Lindberg, D.C., "Theories of vision from al-Kindi to Kepler," University Press, Chicago, 1976.

Listing, J.B., "Beitrag zur physiologischen Optik," Vandenhoeck & Ruprecht, Göttingen, 1845.

Listing, J.B., *Dioptrik des Auges*, in "R. Wagner (Hrsg.), Handwörterbuch der Physiologie (Bd. 4)," Vieweg, Braunschweig, 1851, pp. 451-504.

Meissner, G., *Zur Lehre von den Bewegungen des Auges*, Archiv für Opthalmologie **2** (1855), 1-123.

Mowrer, O.H., Ruch, T.C., & Miller, N.E., *The corneo-retinal potential difference as the basis of the galvanometric method of recording eye- movements*, American Journal of Physiology **114** (1936), 423-428.

Mueller, J., "Zur vergleichenden Physiologie des Gesichtssinnes des Menschen und der Tiere nebst einem Versuch über die Bewegungen der Augen und über den menschlichen Blick," Cnobloch, Leipzig, 1826.

Risner, F., "Opticae thesaurus alhazeni. Basileae: Episcopios. Ruete, Th. (1845a). Lehrbuch der Ophthalmologie," Vieweg, Braunschweig, 1572.

Ruete, Th., "Das Ophthalmotrop," Vandenhoeck & Ruprecht, Göttingen, 1845b.

Schapurian, R., "Die deskriptive Bedeutung von Ibn-al-Haithams Optik 'Kitab - al - Manazir' für die Wahrnehmungslehre," Dissertation, Bonn, 1960.

Scheidler, C.H., "Handbuch der Psychologie zum Gebrauch bei akademischen Vorlesungen und zum Selbststudium (2. Aufl.)," Carl Wilhelm Leske, Darmstadt, 1833.

Schleusener-Eichholz. G., "Das Auge im Mittelalter (2 Bände)," Fink - Verlag, München, 1985.

Schnaase, L., *Alhazen. Ein Beitrag zur Geschichte der Physik*, Schriften der Naturforschenden Gesellschaft in Danzig, Neue Folge **7** (1890), 140-164.

Schott, E., *Über die Registrierung des Nystagmus und anderer Augenbewegungen vermittels des Saitengalvanometers*, Deutsches Archiv für klinische Medizin **140** (1922), 79-90.

Schramm, M., *Zur Entwicklung der physiologischen Optik in der arabischen Literatur*, Sudhoffs Archiv für Geschichte der Medizin und der Naturwissenschaften **43** (1959), 289-316.

Schramm, M., "Ibn al-Haythams Weg zur Physik," Franz Steiner, Wiesbaden, 1963.

Taylor, E.A., "Controlled reading," University of Chicago Press, Chicago, 1937.

Traxel, W., "Geschichte für die Gegenwart," Passavia Universitätsverlag, Passau, 1985.

Venetzky, R.L., *Research on Reading Processes. A Historical Perspective*, American Psychologist, May (1977), 339-345.

Volkmann, A.W., *Sehen*, in "R. Wagner (Hrsg.), Handwörterbuch der Physiologie (3. Bd., 1. Abteilung)," Vieweg, Braunschweig, 1846, pp. 265-351.

Volkmann, A.W., *Das Tachistoskop, ein Instrument welches bei Untersuchung des momentanen Sehens den Gebrauch des electrischen Funkens ersetzt*, Berichte der königlichen sächsischen Gesellschaft der Wissenschaften zu Leipzig (1850), 90-98.

Weber, E.H., *Der Tastsinn und das Gemeingefühl*, in "R. Wagner (Hrsg.), Handwörterbuch der Physiologie (3. Bd., 2. Abteilung)," Vieweg, Braunschweig, 1846, pp. 481-588.

Wiedemann, E., *Beiträge zur Geschichte der Naturwissenschaften bei den Arabern*, J.C. Poggendorf's Annalen der Physik und Chemie **165** (1876), 656-658.

Wiedemann, E., "Über die Naturwissenschaften bei den Arabern," Verlags- und Druckerei AG (vormals J.F. Richter), Hamburg, 1890a.

Wiedemann, E., *Zur Geschichte der Lehre vom Sehen*, Annalen der Physik und Chemie, Neue Folge 39 (1890b), 470-474.

Wiedemann, E., *Ibn al Haitam, ein arabischer Gelehrter*, in "Festschrift für J. Rosenthal zur Vollendung seines siebzigsten Lebensjahres. In zwei Teilen (Teil 1)," Thieme, Leipzig, 1906, pp. 147-178.

Wiedemann, E., *Zu Ibn al Haitams Optik*, Archiv für die Geschichte der Naturwissenschaften und der Technik 3 (1910), 1-53.

Woodworth, R.S., "Experimental Psychology," Holt, New York, 1938.

Woodworth, R.S., & Schlosberg, H., "Experimental Psychology," Holt, Rinehart & Winston, New York, 1954.

Wundt, W., "Beiträge zur Theorie der Sinneswahrnehmung," Winter'sche Verlagsbuchhandlung, Leipzig und Heidelberg, 1862a.

Wundt, W., *Über die Bewegung der Augen*, Archiv für Ophthalmologie 8/II (1862b), 1-87.

Wundt, W., *Beschreibung eines künstlichen Augenmuskelsystems zur Untersuchung der Bewegungsgesetze des menschlichen Auges im gesunden und kranken Zustande*, Archiv für Opthalmologie 8/II (1862c), 88-114.

4
Basic Findings in Smooth Pursuit and Saccadic Eye Movements

PREDICTION AND STRATEGY IN HUMAN SMOOTH PURSUIT EYE MOVEMENTS

REINHART JÜRGENS, ANSELM W. KORNHUBER, AND WOLFGANG BECKER

Sektion Neurophysiologie, Universität Ulm

Introduction

The present paper reports on a number of recent findings regarding pursuit eye movements which have been made in our laboratory and which, we feel, require a reconsideration of some of the current concepts of the human smooth pursuit system. We will divide the presentation into two parts. First we will summarize a variety of observations from this and other laboratories which stress the importance of prediction and discontinuous and non-linear processes in the generation of smooth pursuit eye movements. Subsequently, we shall report, in some detail. on a set of experiments aimed at a comparison of the role of prediction for smooth pursuit and optokinetic responses and shall discuss our results with regard to the conceptual mechanisms of prediction.

The role of visual feedback and prediction

When we pursue a smoothly moving object, we do so by smooth eye movements (as opposed to the discontinuous, saccadic eye movements), which stabilize the image of the target on our retina. It is generally *not* possible to initiate such smooth pursuit eye movements (SPEM) without the presence of a moving object, e.g. in the dark; the SPEM system is, therefore, often considered as a "velocity servo" which uses the target's retinal slip velocity to adjust eye velocity until it approximately matches the target velocity. Although a number of authors have demonstrated that inputs other than the slip velocity can influence the SPEM response (retinal target position, Pola & Wyatt, 1980; target acceleration, Lisberger et al., 1981; proprioceptive inputs, Gauthier & Hofferer, 1976; perceptually constructed target movements, Steinbach, 1976), it is still generally held that retinal target velocity (i.e. slip) is the major source that evokes SPEM.

For a time, it was thougt that the velocity servo of the SPEM system might work in the manner of a "sampled data" system (Young & Stark, 1963). In its simplest form, the sampled data notion, (which proved to be an adequate description for the saccadic system), would imply that SPEM consist of a series of constant velocity epochs, each corresponding to a discrete sample of the instantaneous slip velocity. This was contradicted by Robinson (1965) who demonstrated that the SPEM system starts to oscillate if a positive feedback is artificially introduced, a property that would be avoided by sampling. Accordingly, it is now generally assumed that the SPEM system operates continuously in time, i.e. that it is always ready to react, within a constant delay, to changes of the target. However, observations in our laboratory indicate that the reaction time to changes of target motion may *not* be constant; while the SPEM system clearly has the ability to start its action with a latency of only about 100 ms, it may need 500 ms or longer, if it is to modify an ongoing sinusoidal movement. Results that will be presented below provide evidence that the latency of the SPEM reactions to changes of target movement depends on the system's actual state. Furthermore, whereas a continuously operating system will always respond to a smooth input signal, (e.g. a sine wave), by a smooth output signal, actual SPEM responses do exhibit abrupt changes which occur so systematically, that the concept of "temporal continuity" must be questioned (cf. Figure 2).

It is widely acknowledged that prediction of the target movement is an important feature of the SPEM system. Many quantitative studies of SPEM have used a linear systems approach in order to analyze the frequency characteristics (gain and phase) of smooth pursuit responses. It was a consistent finding that sinusoidal target movements can be pursued with a much smaller phase lag than irregular target waveforms (e.g. Dallos & Jones, 1963; Stark et al., 1962). This suggests that the unavoidable delays in the sensory and motor systems can be circumvented by a predictive mechanism which comes into play whenever the target moves in a periodic or "regular" fashion. However, the exact mechanism of the postulated predictor is far from being understood.

Recent attempts to identify the characteristics of the predictor by means of control systems methods have produced paradoxical results when the SPEM response to non-periodic, random target motions was considered. As long as the contribution of saccades to tracking is not eliminated, as was the case in the earlier work cited above, the response exhibits a clear phase lag at all frequencies. However, when the smooth component was isolated by removing the saccades, Yasui and Young (1984) found the expected phase lag only at medium and high stimulus frequencies, whereas a phase lead of the response emerged at low frequencies. For example, at 0.046 **Hz** the response advanced the stimulus by 84 °, which would correspond to an anticipation of an "unpredictable" target by as much as 5.1 s. Obviously, such an anticipation does not make sense and these authors explained the phase lead at low frequencies as the result of some compromise of the pursuit system to keep the average phase of the system small. Other authors (Collewijn, 1984; Barnes, 1987) also described the phase lead phenomenon but found it hard to explain. Similar results were obtained in our laboratory. Unlike Yasui and Young, however, we consider the phase lead phenomenon as an "artifact" arising from the inappropriate application of linear methods to a non-linear system as the following example illustrates.

We presented a bandlimited white noise with 1 Hz bandwidth to three Subjects (Ss) and recorded the eye movements using a search coil. Figure 1 shows a typical segment from our recording protocol, including an epoch of weak and irregular target motion followed by an impulse-like deviation to the left (downward deflection, upper trace, t1-t3). The eye position trace shows that the leading edge of the target "impulse," t1-t2, was responded to mainly by saccades whereas the trailing edge of the target "impulse," t2-t3, evoked an epoch of almost perfect smooth pursuit. This kind of response pattern was observed repeatedly in all three Ss.

To account for this behavior we hypothesize that the smooth pursuit system takes into account the finite horizontal range of the display. Accordingly, when the system perceives a rapid centrifugal movement of the target, it expects that the target, in order to avoid a collision with the limits of the display, will soon have to reverse its direction and return towards the center. Conceivably, it is a general strategy of the SPEM system to "observe" the target while it moves in *one* direction in order to prepare a smooth return movement to be started at the reversal of the target movement. The observed target movement pattern serves as a guess for the return movement. Although such a strategy may have been devised primarily for the pursuit of periodic target movements, it appears to be also operative in the case of random events, as in the above example. In the case of a random target movement as in Figure 1, the initial centrifugal movement is unexpected and, therefore, "missed" by the pursuit response so that saccades are needed to catch up with the target. By contrast, the subsequent centripetal movement evokes a segment of predominantly smooth pursuit. It is our impression that it is virtually impossible to prevent the pursuit system from making guesses of this kind even if the target movement is not fully predictable.

Independent of such speculations, however, the SPEM pattern in Figure 1 can be shown to correspond to a phase lead in the frequency domain. Indeed, the smooth component of the eye position curve has the shape of a rounded rightward step. A technical system that transforms a pulse to the left into a step to the right is an integrator with a negative sign and therefore produces a 90 ° lead. More generally, the response to any random waveform containing high and low frequencies, (and not only the particular one selected for Figure 1), will undergo a phase advance in the low frequency range if the system's gain is lower for rapid and unexpected centrifugal than for centripetal movements. This phase advance, however, does not constitute a prediction in the sense that the SPEM system would know the future course of the low frequency component; rather it is the indirect result of a complex pursuit strategy.

Whereas a sinusoidal target movement has been held to be best suited for prediction in SPEM, Bahill and McDonald (1983) demonstrated that a near zero phase lag can also be obtained with other target waveforms. The authors

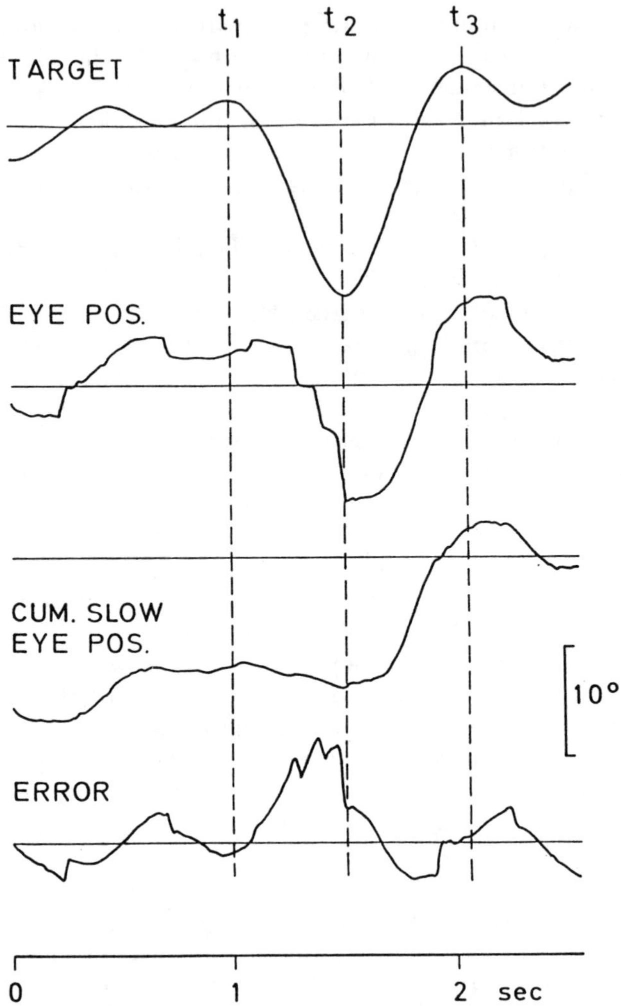

Fig. 1: Smooth pursuit tracking of an "unpredictable" target (sample epoch). Time course of target position, eye position, cumulative slow eye position (saccades removed), and position error (eye position minus target position). Upward excursions, movement to the right. Note poor SPEM during interval t1-t2 and good SPEM during t2-t3.

suggested that the pursuit system can be functionally divided into two components, a "direct" component driven by the visual error velocity on the retina and an "indirect" component, (the prediction mechanism), which generates an additional control signal for **SPEM**, once it has learned the target's movement pattern. They concluded that any periodical time pattern of the target can be learned equally well and that there is no preferred waveform for SPEM. In contrast to these observations, we have frequently observed that the SPEM velocity is *not* a good replica of the target velocity, in particular when high

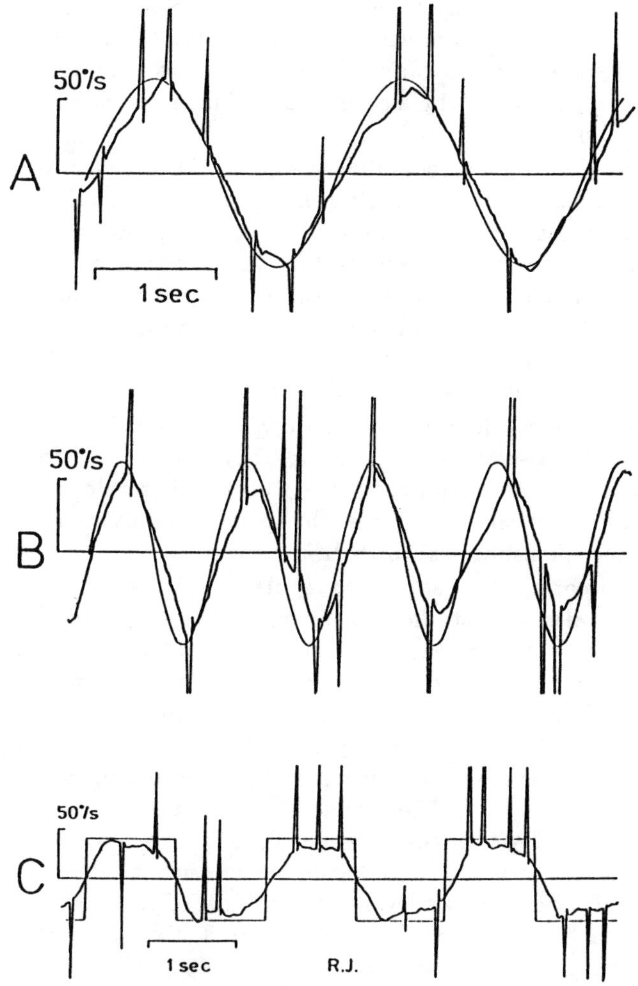

Fig. 2: Velocity profiles of periodic SPEM. **A** and **B**, target moves sinusoidally with 20 ° amplitude and 0.5 Hz (**A**) and 1.0 Hz (**B**). **C**, target velocity is a square wave function (i.e. target position profile is triangular). Target velocity indicated by thin lines. Note that SPEM velocity consists of velocity ramps (i.e. segments of almost constant acceleration), separated by sharp bends.

velocities are required. As an example, Figure 2 A and B show velocity profiles obtained with a target moving sinusoidally at an amplitude of 20 ° at 0.5 Hz (panel A) and 1.0 Hz (panel B). Note that the velocity pattern is almost triangular rather than sinusoidal.

It must be pointed out that when the peak velocity of the target movement shown in Figure 2 A is changed, the slope of the velocity ramps, which constitute the SPEM response, will vary correspondingly (Figure 2 B). Therefore, the occurrence of these ramps cannot be explained by a limitation in the rate of change of the velocity (i.e. by a saturation of the acceleration), but must be attributed to a "strategy."

Another example is presented in Figure 2 C. The target position had a triangular time course and therefore an alternating rectangular velocity profile but evoked a trapezoid pattern of eye velocity. It also appears that the eye anticipates the changes of the target by starting velocity ramps, (i.e. segments of constant accelerations), prior to each reversal of the target movement. These segments of constant acceleration are clearly not expectancy drifts (Kowler & Steinman, 1979) which are periods of low acceleration that can be seen to precede the steep velocity ramps in Figure 2 C.

Epochs of constant acceleration with abrupt transitions between epochs (corresponding to a polygone pattern in the velocity domain) are found in SPEM so regularly that we suggest that they constitute one basic element of the repertoire of the SPEM system. Of course, this is not its only mode of operation. In a large number of situations, the SPEM acceleration changes smoothly.

Instead of comparing the response to regular and irregular motions, the role of prediction has also been studied by having the target transiently disappear. The underlying assumption was that the amount of pursuit generated after the target's disappearance stems from a prediction mechanism. Whittaker and Eaholz (1982) demonstrated that humans are able to continue sinusoidal pursuit for, at least, 1 s even if the target disappears. Becker and Fuchs (1985) measured the smooth eye velocity during the transient disappearance of a target moving at constant velocity. They found that (1) after sudden disappearance of the target the SPEM can continue for as long as 4 s at up to 60% of its normal velocity and that (2) SPEM can even be initiated without vision at the beginning of an expected movement. In view of the concept that SPEM is generated by a "direct" and an "indirect" (predictive) component, this may suggest that the predictor contributed to the SPEM (in the particular case studied by Becker and Fuchs) by about 60%.

Differences between SPEM and OKN

It is commonly held that optokinetic (optokinetic nystagmus, OKN) and smooth pursuit responses are produced by similar, albeit not identical, mechanisms. The question as to whether OKN also has predictive properties has been considered only by Yasui and Young (1984). They noted a slightly smaller phase lag of sinusoidal OKN as compared to an OKN elicited by the pseudo-random motion of a visual pattern. However, as stated above, their results were difficult to explain as they used a method which is only appropriate for linear systems and therefore, possibly not for OKN. The behaviour of the OKN system after transient disappearance of the OKN stimulus has not yet been investigated. In the following, we report on a series of experiments that are aimed at a comparison of SPEM and OKN under conditions that are thought to reveal the contribution of predictive mechanisms. Specifically, we addressed the following questions:

(1) Is prediction also involved in OKN responses?
(2) How do SPEM and OKN interact with regard to prediction?

These questions also have a clinical significance. A number of quite different neurological diseases (e.g. lesions in the cerebellum, the basal ganglia, or the cortex) are known to impair SPEM. We wondered whether some diseases would impair more or less specifically only the prediction mechanism. Furthermore, we thought that the quantitative differences between pursuit and OKN which exist in certain patients (Barrat et al., 1985) might be enhanced under conditions that call for the assistance of predictive mechanisms. Ideally, of course, one would like to relate the prediction component of the SPEM response to a location in the brain by demonstrating that certain lesions specifically affect the prediction mechanism.

METHODS

In Experiment 1, 12 normal subjects (Ss, paid volunteers) sat in complete darkness in the center of a drum that could be rotated horizontally about the Ss (Figure 3). The drum was driven by a torque motor under control of a microcomputer. In the pursuit (PUR) paradigm, the Ss had to pursue a red light emitting diode (LED) mounted on the inner surface of the drum which moved sinusoidally back and forth with the drum while the lights were off so that the surface of the drum was invisible. In the OKN paradigm, a Julesz pattern painted on the inner drum surface was illuminated by a bright yellow LED array which could be rapidly (< 1 ms) switched on and off; the red target LED was not visible in this condition and the Ss were instructed to look straight ahead at the pattern without pursuing its details. Finally, in the OKN-plus-pursuit (OKP) paradigm, both the Julesz pattern and the target LED were visible and the Ss had to pursue the target LED as in the PUR paradigm. The drum rotated with the following frequencies, amplitudes, and peak velocities:

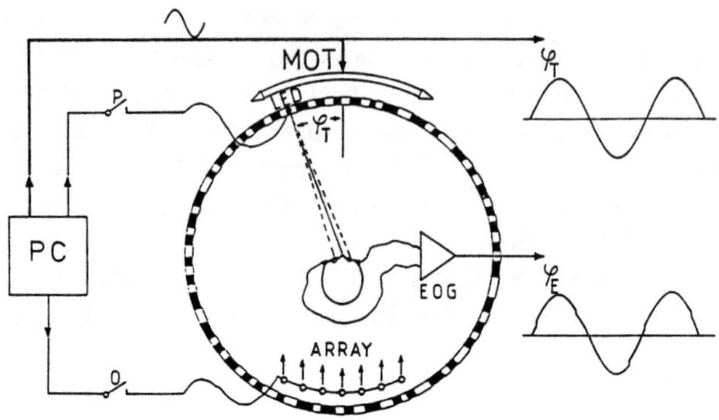

Fig. 3: Experimental design for comparison of SPEM and OKN (see text for details). φ_T, target position; φ_E, eye position.

(1) 0.31 Hz, 20.2 °, 39.4 °/s, or (2) 0.65 Hz, 18.9 °, 77.2 °/s, or (3) 1.12 Hz, 15.8 °, 111.2 °/s.

In each of the three paradigms the target or the Julesz pattern was first continuously visible for about 20 cycles of rotation. Thereafter, it disappeared transiently for 2 s or for 4 s while the drum continued to oscillate; each of the two blanking periods was repeated four times. The onset and duration of blanking was determined by a computer program and could not be predicted by the Ss. The Ss were instructed to "mentally continue" the target movement when it became invisible and to pursue the imagined target motion.

Data acquisition and analysis

Horizontal eye movements were recorded by bi-temporal EOG which was recalibrated every 3 min (as this experiment was also intended for use with patients, a search coil was not employed). The eye movement recordings were electronically filtered with an upper limit of 30 Hz and differentiated. The thus obtained eye position and velocity signals, together with the control signals for the drum and the on/off for the LEDs were (a) displayed on an oscilloscope, (b) written on a stripchart recorder (Mingograph), and (c) recorded on analogue tape for further analysis.

The recorded eye movements were analyzed on a laboratory computer (DEC PDP-12). In a first step, we eliminated the saccades (or quick phases) from the records, replacing them by a linear fit through the epochs of smooth velocity preceding and following the saccade. This was done interactively with the eye velocity curves displayed on the computer scope. The algorithm was based on a "velocity window" which moved along the smooth epochs in the velocity trace and which automatically detected saccades when there were deviations from the current smooth velocity. Epochs containing artifacts (e.g. eye blinks) were "desaccaded" by hand (via cursors which could be controlled by potentiometers). From the thus obtained curves of smooth eye velocity (SEV), we calculated three different averages for each S, paradigm, and frequency, which corresponded to the following conditions: (a) epochs that were continuously visible, (b) epochs containing a 2 s blanking period, and (c) the same for 4 s blanking periods. Averages of type (a) were fitted by a sine wave (fundamental wave) yielding the gain and phase of the SEV with visible target or Julesz pattern. Subsequently, the average (a) was used as a template against which we compared the SEV during periods in which the target (Julesz pattern) was invisible.

Results

Responses with the target continuously visible

The average SEV from the Ss tested in Experiment 1 is given in Table 1 in terms of gain and phase as a function of the stimulus frequency. PUR and OKN responses had similar amplitudes. As expected, the amplitude was clearly larger in the OKP paradigm (co-stimulation of pursuit and OKN responses). A phase lag was found in all paradigms and at all frequencies. It is true that in individual Ss a small phase lead would exceptionally appear during a few cycles of the stimulus, yet, all individual averages across 6 cycles or more always lagged the target. In the PUR paradigm, the phase lag was remarkably small. Given that the SPEM system has a reaction time in the order of 100 ms, one would expect, for example, a phase lag of 24 ° at 0.65 Hz. However, the actual lag of the pursuit system at this frequency amounted to only 7.2 °. The lag was much larger in the OKN paradigm, whereas the OKP paradigm, surprisingly, yielded lag values that were intermediate between those of PUR and OKN (instead of being smaller or as small as those of the PUR condition).

Tab. 1: Frequency responses (neg. sign = phase lag).

	PUR		OKN		OKP	
Freq	Gain	Phase	Gain	Phase	Gain	Phase
0.31	0.89	- 0.7	0.89	- 3.3	0.93	- 2.5
0.65	0.70	- 7.2	0.68	-14.9	0.81	-10.6
1.12	0.44	-20.6	0.44	-29.3	0.56	-26.0

Responses with blanking of the target

A general observation was that our Ss were able to continue, although at a much reduced velocity, their pursuit of a sinusoidally moving target even after the target disappeared. A representative example (U.C., average of 4 sweeps) is given in Figure 4. The sinusoidal trace represents a fit of the S's average eye velocity when the target is visible, whereas the second (noisy) trace gives the time course of the eye velocity during the disappearance of the target. In the light, U.C. followed the target with a peak velocity of about 58 °/s, i.e. he had a pursuit gain of 0.71. After the target disappeared (left vertical line in Figure 4), we can differentiate between three epochs in the response: (1) the "normal" pursuit continues for a short period (about 200 ms in this particular example), (2) the pursuit amplitude decays (during half a cycle), and (3) a regime of "residual oscillation" in the dark is entered (with an almost constant amplitude of roughly 8 °/s in the given example). Note that the residual oscillation has the same phase as the sinusoid (normal pursuit). We did not study dark epochs longer than 4s, but it was our impression that some Ss, as the one presented here, would have been able to pursue an imagined target in the dark for an even longer time. Other Ss showed a damped oscillation in the dark with time constants ranging from 5 to 10 s. The residual pursuit oscillation was generally larger at 0.31 Hz but poor and variable at 1.12 Hz; the latter will, therefore, not be further considered.

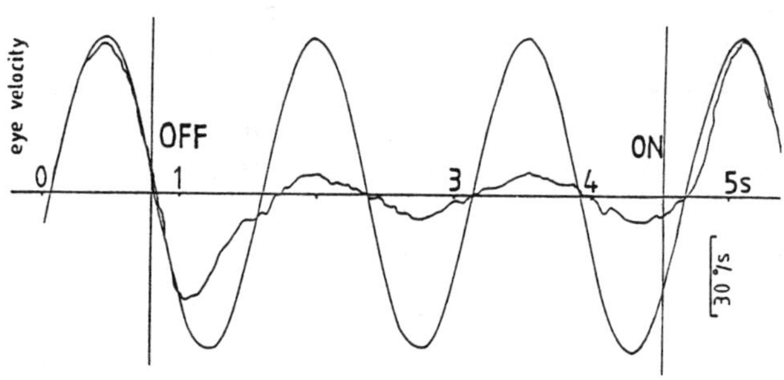

Fig. 4: Effect of target blanking on SPEM velocity. Target moved sinusoidally with 20 ° amplitude and 0.65 Hz and was blanked at the instant marked by the left vertical bar; the right vertical bar indicates reappearance of the target. One Subject, average of 4 sweeps. Sinusoid shows fundamental wave fitted to SPEM velocity from periods during which target was continuously visible.

Figure 5 compares the effect of target blanking upon SPEM and OKN at a frequency of 0.31 Hz. The response of all Ss was qualitatively similar, and Figure 5 gives the grand averages across all of them. In the left (pursuit) panel, the amplitude of the oscillation in the dark reaches about 25% of that obtained with a countinuously visible target (indicated by the sinusoidal fit). In the right (optokinetic) panel, the decay of the eye velocity is steeper and the oscillation in the dark reaches only about 5% of the amplitude evoked when the Julesz pattern is visible.

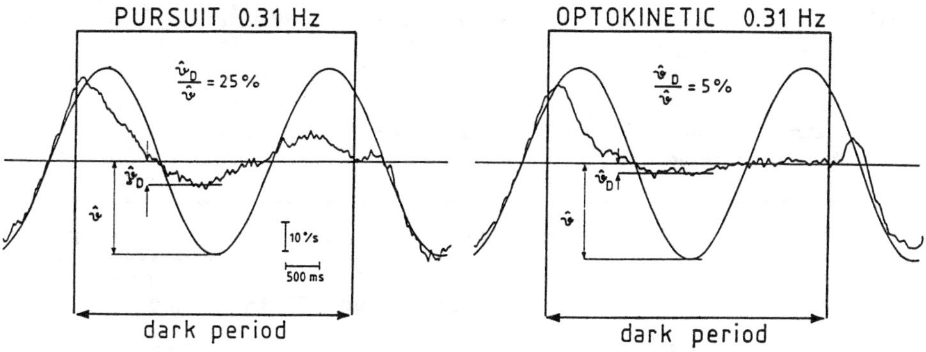

Fig. 5: Effect of target blanking on SPEM (left panel) and OKN velocity (right panel). Sinusoidal stimulation, 0.31 Hz. Grand averages across 12 Ss. Sinusoids show fit for average SPEM or OKN velocity, respectively, during periods of continuous target visibility. $\hat{v}$, average peak velocity with target continuously visible; $\hat{v}_D$, peak velocity of residual pursuit in the dark.

Another interesting difference between SPEM and OKN can be seen in Figure 5 in the behaviour of the eye velocity after the reappearance of the target. While the SPEM system "waits" until a pursuit movement to the left is due, the OKN system immediately starts to the right, and is then forced to change quickly to the left. Furthermore, the SPEM system, after having resumed its motion, is immediately in phase, whereas, the OKN system still has a delay in relation to the response in light.

Table 2 gives the amplitudes of residual oscillations in the dark obtained in the three paradigms and at the frequencies of 0.31 and 0.65 Hz. These results suggest that the mechanism (presumably the prediction) which generates the SPEM velocity in the dark is not (or to a very small extent) involved in the OKN response. Although the Ss were instructed not to follow a particular point on the Julesz pattern and although we rejected data which did not show the typical saw-tooth shaped OKN response, we cannot exclude that some Ss did, to some degree, pursue details of the pattern with their fovea. It is, therefore, possible that the small oscillation in the dark, seen in the OKN paradigm, stems from the pursuit system and not from the OKN system.

In the OKP paradigm, the amplitudes of residual oscillations ranged inbetween the two other paradigms. The finding that co-stimulation of both the foveal pursuit and OKN systems elicits a smaller residual oscillation as compared to the foveal pursuit system alone is surprising and not easy to understand. The Ss were well able to pursue the red LED, and there was no conflict with the Julesz pattern. We had, therefore, expected that the eye velocity in the dark would have, at least, the same characteristics as in the PUR paradigm. Instead, the residual oscillations were a "compromise" between those of the PUR and OKN conditions, much as the phase lag recorded in Table 1 was intermediate between that of PUR and OKN.

Tab. 2: Amplitude of residual-oscillation (in percent of response in light).

Freq	PUR	OKN	OKP
0.31	25	5	17
0.65	14	4	10

Tab. 3: OFF latencies (ms).

Freq	A	B	C	D
0.31	550	315	260	130
0.65	395	290	188	80

Experiment 2

Experiment 1 confirmed Becker and Fuchs' notion that the pursuit system does not only "hold" a part of the velocity reached by the instant of target disappearance, but that it is also able to accelerate without seeing a target motion when a target movement is expected. We qualify these two aspects of prediction as a "short term" and a "long term" behaviour. While the short term component simply continues an ongoing movement, the long term component determines the time of onset and the magnitude of eye acceleration or velocity, i.e. it predicts a pattern.

In Experiment 2, we manipulated the short term and the long term aspects of prediction separately by systematically varying the phase angle, and thereby, the instantaneous velocity at which the target disappeared. To this end, we expanded on the PUR condition and had the target disappear at instants corresponding to a -45, 0, 45, or 90 ° phase difference with respect to the zero crossing of the target velocity. In other words, the target was switched off either when its velocity had reached zero (0 °), or when it peaked (90 °), or half way in between (± 45 °). Otherwise, the conditions were identical to Experiment 1, PUR. Four Ss participated in Experiment 2. Their responses were averaged separately for each value of the switching phase.

We then tested whether (a) the amplitude of the residual oscillation in the dark and (b) the transition from the normal regime with visible target to that of residual oscillation in the dark was a function of the phase angle at which the target was blanked. The four velocity curves A, B, C, and D, depicted in

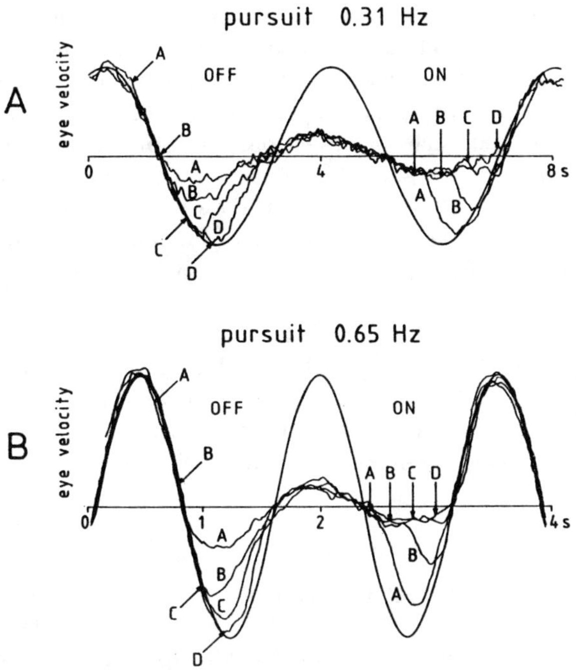

Fig. 6: Effect of the instant of target blanking upon SPEM response to sinusoidal stimulation, stimulus frequency 0.31 Hz (**A**) and 0.65 Hz (**B**). Curves A, B, C, and D show SPEM velocity corresponding to target blanking at instants marked by arrows A, B, C, D (left part), respectively, and to target reappearance as marked by arrows A, B, C, D, on the right. Grand averages across 4 Ss. Sinusoids show fit as in Figure 4.

both Figures 6 A and B represent grand averages obtained with 0.31 Hz and 0.65 Hz stimuli from the 4s dark intervals for the four phase angles of -45, 0, 45, and 90 °. The averages demonstrate that the amplitude of the residual oscillation does not depend on the instant of target blanking. Interestingly, however, a clear dependence of the short term behaviour on the phase angle is evident. Consider curve A in Figure 6 A, which shows the SEV resulting when the target disappears at the instant marked by the arrow A. The curve does not deviate from the time course corresponding to the pursuit of a visible target (sinusoid) until the velocity crosses zero. The effect of target disappearance in this instance has a latency of 550 ms. Curve D, which is the other extreme, results when the target disappears at the instant of peak velocity (arrow D). It deviates after a latency of only 130 ms from normal. The latencies of curve B and C range in between the two extremes.

One might object that the long latency of the target-off-effect in the case of curve A may be trivial since it is difficult to decide whether the SEV deceleration seen in curve A after the target's disappearance is related to the off-stimulus or whether it represents the continuation of active pursuit. There are two arguments against such an objection: (1) Simulation studies in our laboratory demonstrated that the sudden onset of a velocity decay should be sharp enough to be noticeable even during the descending part of a sinusoid. (2) If the deceleration of curve A in Figure 6 B did reflect the velocity decay due to the off stimulus, why, then, does curve A in Figure 6 B decelerate at double the rate of that in Figure 6 A?

Interestingly, the latencies in Figure 6 B, in which the stimulus frequency is twice that of Figure 6 A, are roughly half as long as those seen in Figure 6 A. We infer that the pursuit movement is continued for a fixed fraction of the stimulus cycle and that this fraction is a function of the instant at which the target disappears and independent of the stimulus frequency.

EXPERIMENT 3

We have attempted to carry out Experiment 1 also in neurological patients. It turned out, however, that it was too difficult for some of the patients to imagine a continuation of the target movement in the dark and to track the imagined target with their eyes. Instead, they tended to look around irregularly, making exceptionally large saccades. Moreover, it was sometimes difficult to explain the task to some of the patients with deficits in communication.

We, therefore, devised a slightly different version of the experiment which proved to be easier for the patients. We used the PUR, OKN, and OKP stimuli. After an initial run of 16 cycles with the target continuously visible (condition A), two further runs were presented (B, C) of 16 cycles each, in which the target was switched off and on periodically during each cycle. In (B), the target disappeared always at a phase angle of 45 ° preceding peak stimulus velocity and reappeared at a phase of 45 ° thereafter. The epoch covering the peak velocity was, thus, always invisible while the epochs covering peak stimulus excursions were visible. In (C), the reverse was true. Amplitudes and frequencies were the same as in the other two experiments.

The periodical disappearance and reappearance of the target had the advantage of automatically attracting the Ss' attention. The Ss were simply instructed to "look at the target (or Julesz pattern), even if it disappears for a while." The periodicity of the target disappearance and reappearance was predictable and could be learned easily. Experiment 3 was carried out in 7 normals and, so far, in 17 patients. Our data were analyzed in a manner similar to Experiments 1 and 2, but using a fully automatic procedure running on a VAX II/GPX workstation (Digital Equipment). It was ascertained that the automatic program yielded values identical to those obtained by the interactive program on the PDP-12.

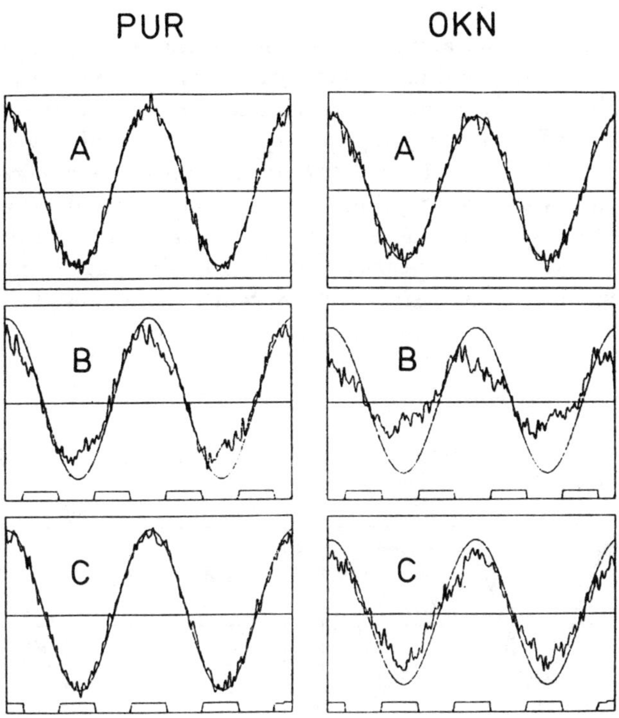

Fig. 7: Velocity profiles of SPEM (PUR paradigm) and OKN during periodic disappearance of the stimulus. One normal Subject. Sinusoidal stimulus, amplitude 20 °, frequency 0.31 Hz. Upper margins of panels correspond to 39.4 °/s (i.e. stimulus peak velocity). Trace above lower margins in each panel indicates stimulus visibility (no trace: stimulus invisible). **A**, stimulus continuously visible; **B**, stimulus blanked about its peak velocity; **C**, stimulus blanked about its peak excursion.

Normal Subjects

A typical result for normals is given in Figure 7. The left panels show averaged SPEM velocities, and the right ones give the corresponding curves for OKN. The figure illustrates the following consistent observations: (1) SPEM was not or only very slightly affected if the target disappeared during its peak excursion (bottom left panel), (2) SPEM and in particular, its peak velocity, was clearly reduced if the target disappeared while it reached its peak velocity (center left), and (3) the disappearance had a stronger effect on OKN than on SPEM. This was qualitatively true for all the normal Ss investigated. The grand averages for all Ss are shown in Table 4.

Patients

The group of neurological patients studied so far, is heterogeneous, and the experiments are being continued; therefore we will present only some preliminary results here. One group of patients had cortical lesions. These patients appear to have difficulties bridging the gaps in target visibility which occur in condition B and C, whereas their SPEM in A, (which is equivalent to the pendular test routinely used during clinical examination), was about normal. Quite interestingly, their OKN responses were less severely impaired than SPEM reponses by the periodic disappearance of the stimulus pattern in conditions B and C. An example is given in Figure 8, which shows results obtained in a

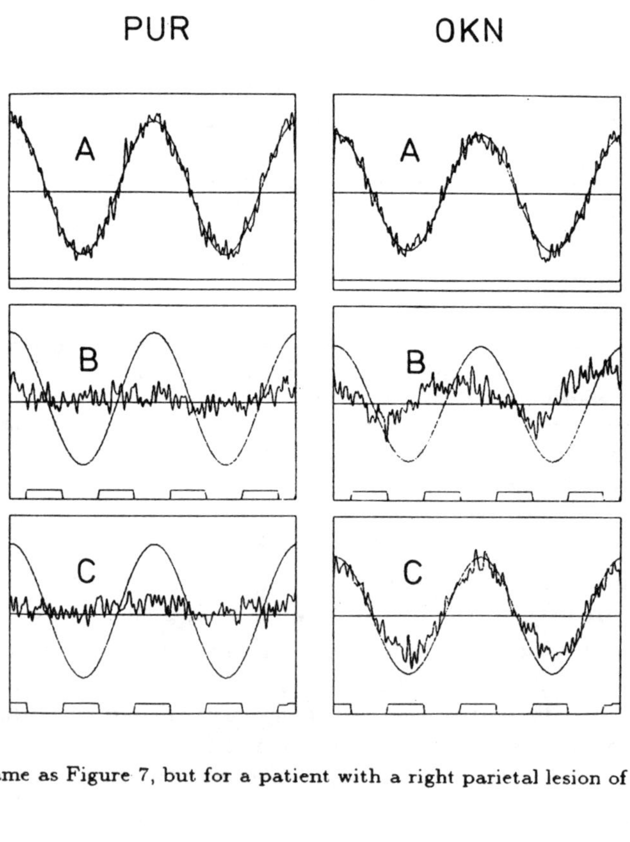

Fig. 8: Same as Figure 7, but for a patient with a right parietal lesion of the cortex.

patient with a lesion in the right occipital lobe. In condition A, pursuit and OKN were normal. In condition B and C, by contrast, we had only an OKN response, whereas the pursuit was almost abolished. We recall that in normal Ss the reverse occurs, in that, the OKN is more severely affected than the SPEM. From these preliminary results, we suggest that measuring the pursuit of an intermittantly blanked target is a more sensitive test than the pendular test with a permanently visible target. At present, however, it can not yet be concluded whether such experiments will help to localize the hypothetical prediction mechanism.

Tab. 4: Amplitudes of SPEMs in Experiment 3.

	PUR		OKN		OKP	
	0.31	0.65	0.31	0.65	0.31	0.65
A	0.84	0.76	0.80	0.70	0.89	0.83
B	0.65	0.55	0.44	0.35	0.69	0.57
C	0.74	0.58	0.68	0.47	0.80	0.68

Discussion

Differences between SPEM and OKN

In agreement with Yasui and Young, we found that the phase lag of OKN responses relative to the target was considerably larger than for foveal pursuit (when the stimulus is continuously visible). This is in line with our observation that a significant residual oscillation during periods in which the stimulus was invisible does occur in the pursuit (PUR) but almost never in the OKN paradigm. We, therefore, confirm (with an approach that does not depend on the systems' linearity) the conclusion drawn by Yasui and Young that prediction is of minor importance for the OKN system.

Prediction, in the sense used here, should not be confused with the "velocity storage" mechanism in the OKN system (Cohen et al. 1981) which has a long time constant and which is "charged" only by a prolonged unidirectional drum rotation and not by the pendular stimulation used in our experiments.

We have no explanation, why, during combined stimulation of the pursuit and OKN systems (OKP), the phase lag of the response becomes larger than for pursuit alone (PUR). If we assume that both SPEM and OKN contribute, synergistically, to the loop gain of a visual velocity tracking system, one would expect that the combined stimulation results in a better gain figure than the PUR condition, which was true, but also in a smaller lag, instead of a larger one.

Linear summation of direct and indirect sources?

Whereas the results reported by Becker and Fuchs are compatible with the view, (although they do not prove it), that the residual SPEM seen after target disappearance reflects the predictor's contribution to SPEM under normal vision, the characteristics of the residual oscillations in our PUR paradigm makes such a view unlikely. If these oscillations did, indeed, reflect the contribution of a predictor which, under conditions of normal target visibility, would be added to the output of a "direct" system processing the retinal error signal (Whittaker & Eaholtz, 1982), they should have a clearly smaller phase lag (or even a lead) than the normal responses resulting from the composite signal (i.e. predictor plus direct system).

Therefore, we deem the concept of a linear combination of a direct and an indirect signal unlikely. The fact that a SPEM can continue to proceed along a specific pattern for up to about 500 ms (Experiment 2) without being disturbed by the absence of a retinal signal, suggests that this SPEM is purely predictive rather than being the sum of a "direct" and a predictive component. Consequently, the sudden reduction of the SPEM amplitude that inevitably follows upon the disappearance of the target, does not reflect the removal of a direct component from a composite control signal but a parametric effect (reduction of gain) upon the predictive signal. Therefore, we conceive of a mechanism which is able to operate in a predictive mode, but requires frequent visual reinforcement. The idea of visual reinforcement is related to the notion that the actually existing error must be able to influence and correct the internally generated SPEM signal. Conceivably, this "updating" can be carried out discontinuously by adjusting the duration and amplitude of short epochs of constant acceleration. Our finding of SPEM responses composed of such epochs (cf. Figure 2) led us to consider the possibility that the predictive mechanism aims at the velocity peaks of the target signal. This means that it would predict their time of occurrence and their magnitude, and that it would generate segments of constant eye acceleration in order to meet the predicted peaks without bothering about the exact target motion *during* the execution of segments joining successive peaks.

An illustrative example for the notion that SPEM may be generated internally, in a purely predictive manner, (without contribution of a component reacting point-by-point to the current velocity error), is shown in Figure 9. Subject R.J. pursues a target which oscillates with 2 Hz and 5 ° of amplitude. Due to the high frequency of target oscillation the response is weak and has

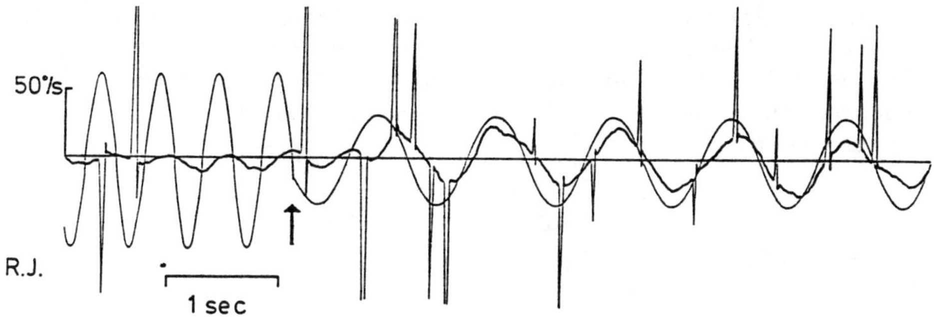

Fig. 9: Tracking of a sinusoidally moving target (amplitude 5 °) during a sudden change of the target frequency from 2 Hz to 1 Hz (arrow). Thin curve, target velocity; heavy curve, eye velocity. Note (1) that after the change of the target frequency, SPEM continues with the "old" frequency for about 700 ms, (2) that the change of the SPEM behaviour after that period is abrupt and occurs at the instant of peak target velocity, and (3) that after reaching the new target velocity, SPEM exhibits an almost triangular waveform.

a phase lag of roughly 90 °. After a sudden change of the target frequency (marked by the vertical arrow) from 2 Hz to 1 Hz, the S continues to generate a SPEM with unchanged amplitude and frequency for more than one period of oscillation (about 700 ms). The observation that the SPEM pattern remains constant for such a long time without an adequate visual stimulus does not only demonstrate that the SPEM is generated internally during the 700 ms latent period, but it also suggests that the internal generation was already operative during the normal "visual" pursuit, i.e. before the frequency was changed.

A further observation in Figure 9 supports the idea that pursuit may not be generated continuously. The transition from the pursuit of 2 Hz to the pursuit of 1 Hz occurs suddenly and at an instant where the velocity peaked. In terms of the hypothesis put forward in the first part of this paper, the SPEM system "analyzed" the new target for about half a cycle of the new stimulus frequency while it continued to oscillate with 2 Hz. At the instant of peak target velocity, it then generated a velocity ramp aimed at the new target velocity profile. Thereafter, a new regime of regular pursuit was installed, again, with a suspiciously triangular velocity pattern as already demonstrated above.

It is true that the example in Figure 9 is extreme because of the high target frequency. Our impression is that the suggested strategy of the SPEM system to generate its response by means of segments of constant accelerations is related to situations in which the visual pursuit of the target is difficult (high frequencies and velocities or abrupt changes). However, we do by no means deny that SPEM can also result from a servo controlling retinal slip velocity and position. The latter mode certainly takes over during slow and probably during unpredictable epochs of the target motion. The difficult question of how these two different modes of SPEM control could be coordinated must be left open at present.

ACKNOWLEDGEMENT

Supported by DFG Grant Be 783/2-2.

REFERENCES

Bahill, A.T., & McDonald, J.D., *Model emulates human smooth pursuit system producing zero-latency target tracking*, Biological Cybernetics **48** (1983), 213-222.

Barnes, G.R., Donnelly, S.F., & Eason, R.D., *Predictive velocity estimation in the pursuit reflex response to pseudo-random and step displacement stimuli in man*, Journal of Physiology (London) **389** (1987), 111-136.

Barratt, H., Gresty, M.A., & Page, N.G.R., *Neurological evidence for dissociation of pursuit and optokinetic systems*, Acta Otolaryngologica (Stockholm) **100** (1985), 89-97.

Becker, W., & Fuchs, A.F., *Prediction in the oculomotorsystem: Smooth pursuit during transient disappearance of a visual target*, Experimental Brain Research **57** (1985), 562-575.

Cohen, B., Henn, V., Raphan, T., & Dennett, R., *Velocity storage, nystagmus, and visual-vestibular interactions in humans*, in "B. Cohen (Ed.), Vestibular and oculomotor physiology," The New York Academy of Sciences, New York, 1981, pp. 421-431.

Collewijn, H., & Tamminga, E.P., *Human smooth and saccadic eye movements during voluntary pursuit of different target motions on different backgrounds*, Journal of Physiology (London) **351** (1984), 217-250.

Dallos, P.J, & Jones, R.W., *Learning behaviour of eye fixation control system*, IEEE Transactions on Automatic Control **8** (1963), 218-227.

Gauthier, G.M., & Hofferer, J.M., *Eye tracking of self-moved targets in the absence of vision*, Experimental Brain Research **26** (1976), 121-139.

Kowler, E., & Steinman, R.M., *The effect of expectations on slow oculomotor control. I. Periodic target steps*, Vision Research **19** (1979), 619-632.

Lisberger, S.G., Evinger, C., Johanson, G.W., & Fuchs, A.F., *Relationship between eye acceleration and retinal image velocity during foveal smooth pursuit in man and monkey*, Journal of Neurophysiology **46** (1981), 229-249.

Pola, J., & Wyatt, H.J., *Target position and velocity: the stimuli for smooth pursuit eye movements*, Vision Reserach **20** (1980), 523-534.

Robinson, D.A., *The mechanics of human smooth pursuit eye movements*, Journal of Physiology **180** (1965), 569-591.

Steinbach, M.J., *Pursuing the perceptual rather than the retinal stimulus*, Vision Research **16** (1976), 1371-1376.

Whittaker, S.G., & Eaholtz,G., *Learning patterns of eye motion for foveal pursuit*, Investigative Ophthalmology and Visual Science **23** (1982), 393-397.

Yasui, S., & Young, L.R., *On the predictive control of foveal eye tracking and slow phases of optokinetic and vestibular nystagmus*, Journal of Physiology (London) **347** (1984), 17-33.

Young, L.R., & Stark, L., *Variable feedback experiment testing a sampled data model for eye-tracking movements*, IEEE Transactions on Human Factors in Electronics **4** (1963), 38-51.

INVESTIGATION OF THE MUTUAL INTERACTION OF HUMAN SMOOTH PURSUIT AND SACCADIC EYE MOVEMENTS WITH PHASE PLANE ANALYSIS

LO J. BOUR

Department of Clinical Neurophysiology
Academic Medical Centre, University of Amsterdam

INTRODUCTION

In response to continuous target motion, eye movements in humans consist of a continuous (smooth) and a discontinuous (saccadic) component. The characteristics of both components are assigned to two separate systems. The smooth pursuit and saccadic systems, which are functionally thought of to be independent and complementary (Rashbass, 1961). Properties of the saccadic system, on the one hand, have been derived from experiments with discontinuously moving targets in time and in space. The determination of the properties of the smooth pursuit system, on the other hand, is far more complicated since in response to continuously moving targets, smooth eye movements are interrupted by saccades. Therefore, one has to separate smooth eye movements from the saccadic responses (Yasui & Young, 1984; Collewijn & Tamminga, 1984; Buizza & Schmidt, 1986). When successive stimulation of different parts of the retina takes place by smooth movements of a visual target, tracking can be accomplished by both systems. The function of the saccadic system is to foveate the target while the smooth pursuit system stabilizes it on the retina. The pursuit system seems to be mainly driven by the motion of a retinal image (Rashbass, 1961). However, several authors have shown that positional error can also elicit pursuit eye movements (Robinson, 1965; Pola & Wyatt, 1980; Pola & Wyatt, 1985; Carl & Gellman, 1987). The idea is that saccades are made when smooth pursuit is not sufficient. Under normal conditions, positional error drives the saccadic system and therefore, it is interesting to know which visual information and at what time, leads to the initiation of saccades when target position is continuously changing. The minimum latency of primary saccades to single target jumps (when the stimulus is previously unknown to the subject) is about 150 ms. However, when previously unknown continuously moving targets are presented, intersaccadic intervals can be found which are much less than 100 ms. Frequently, a repetitive pattern of several saccades can be observed. In this case, saccades seem to have no obligatory refractory period and evidence is given for parallel processing (Leigh & Zee, 1983). Experiments have demonstrated (Becker & Jürgens, 1979) that the size of saccades is processed about 70 ms before saccade onset. On the other hand, the results of Rashbass (1961) and Robinson (1965) also have shown that saccades can be completely inhibited in response to certain step-ramp target movements. Given these different saccadic latencies under different stimulus conditions and the sometimes absent saccadic responses, the question arises which cues lead to the initiation of saccades during continuous target motion. Moreover, since both the saccadic and smooth pursuit systems make use of the same external visual information (such as retinal error and error velocity) and influence the target position on the retina, a mutual interaction and information exchange would be advantageous. The aim of this study is to achieve more insight in the initiation of saccades when both the saccadic and the pursuit system are simultaneously active. Two dimensional phase plane plots were used to analyze the eye movement responses, with retinal error and error velocity displayed on the horizontal and vertical axis respectively. In order to achieve more information about the possible non-linear characteristics of the saccadic and pursuit system and their interactions under conditions of continuous target motion, a phase plane analysis was employed. For both the saccadic and pursuit systems separate linear models have been derived (Robinson, 1981; Robinson et al., 1986). However, if there should exist a mutual interaction as such, that parameters of each individual system may be updated by the state of the other system, essential non-linearities would be introduced. For instance, the internal gain or the amount of internal positive feedback of one system may depend on the performance of the other system. In this case, system parameters would not be constant and should change in a fairly short time (i.e. no long term adaptive changes). Phase plane analysis may reveal the existence and the characteristics of possible essential non-linearities. Special attention was paid to the saccadic behavior during pursuit. Therefore, retinal error and error velocity just before saccade onset and just after saccade offset were plotted in the phase plane. Due to the continuous character of stimulation, the analysis was restricted to these onset and offset moments, since no *a priori* estimation could be made as to which time before the saccade onset the target motion would lead to a saccade. If one attempts to characterize input-output relationships in terms of the velocity and position of retinal images, stimulation must be such that the subject can only rely on external retinal information. This means that one must randomize the stimulus presentation in order to avoid prediction or anticipatory effects. Although it is virtually impossible to exclude all prediction or anticipation (Kowler & Steinman, 1979; Kowler & Steinman, 1981; Young, 1977) much care was taken to decrease these effects as much as possible. Two sets of stimuli were applied. The first set consisted of pseudo-randomly smoothly moving targets which were a superposition of sinusoids. They did not exceed +10 or −10 degrees from primary horizontal position and they only moved in the horizontal plane. The second set of stimuli consisted of growing and decaying exponentials. The growing exponential motion started at primary position.

The decaying exponential stimulus was a step-ramp motion that started at primary position, suddenly jumped to the periphery and then again exponentially decayed to primary position. The objective for the application of these stimuli was to achieve various trajectories through the phase plane. While the first set describes complex motions in this plane, the exponential stimuli describe straight lines starting or ending at the origin. It can be concluded from the phase plane plots of both sets of stimuli that the initiation of a saccade firstly is influenced by the direction of error velocity and secondly by the ratio of error velocity and retinal error. In the case of pseudo-random stimuli, when the target is moving away from the fovea, the ratio of error velocity and retinal error just before the onset of a saccade must be smaller than about 12 s^{-1} in order to have a saccade onset. This means that the larger the error velocity, the larger the minimal retinal error will be at the moment of saccade onset, irrespective of the fact that the target passed the fovea before this onset. When positional error was larger than 10 degrees for the growing exponentials, this ratio depended on target eccentricity, i.e. the time constant of the exponential. When the target is moving towards the fovea, saccades are inhibited and only occur if error velocity is smaller than 25 $^{\circ}/s$ for both sets of stimuli. For the growing exponentials with a time constant of 125-175 ms, smooth pursuit responses were frequently found that even after 800 ms were not interrupted by catch-up saccades. In this case, "ringing" of the smooth pursuit response could be observed with a frequency of about 3 Hz. For the decaying exponentials with a time constant between -100 and -30 ms a bimodal distribution of saccadic latencies has been observed. The first group consists of "fast" and inaccurate saccades with latencies between 150 ms and 200 ms. The second group are "inhibited" saccades ("slow" and accurate) with prolonged latencies larger than 300 ms and occur only when error velocity is less than about 25 $^{\circ}/s$. The smooth pursuit latency for these decaying exponentials always lay between 150 ms and 200 ms and most of the primary saccades to these stimuli belonged to the second group of inhibited saccades. This last finding means that a time interval of, at least, 100 ms was found between initial smooth pursuit response and primary saccade onset, although during this time a substantial retinal error is present. These smooth pursuit responses also demonstrate that small targets moving very fast in the periphery may elicit the same smooth pursuit response as slowly moving targets of the same size in the fovea.

METHODS

Subjects

Four subjects with normal vision participated in the experiments. Both sets of stimuli were applied to subject LB, aged 33 and subject JVG, aged 40. The first set of stimuli was applied to subject HG, aged 25 and the second set to subject JDV, aged 24. Subjects were experienced with oculomotor tasks, but were unfamiliar with the outcome of the experiments.

Apparatus

After the subjects were dark adapted, they were asked to pursue, as accurately as possible, a single white circular spot of light that was back- projected on a translucent screen. The spot diameter was 0.4 ° and its luminance was 20 cd/m^2. To avoid multiple target selection no background was used. Vision was binocular and eye recordings were made from the left eye. It was supposed that both eyes made conjugate movements. At the beginning of each experimental session, a calibration experiment was carried out (Bour et. al., 1984).

Eye movement recording

The eye movement of the subject's left eye was measured with the double magnetic induction method (DMI) described by Bour et al. (1984). The subject's head was positioned in a homogeneous alternating primary magnetic field with a constant amplitude. Horizontal, as well as vertical eye position, were derived from a secondary magnetic field picked up by a detection coil placed in front of the eye. A metallic ring attached to the subjects eye generated this secondary field and its strength is related to the position of the ring. Beyond the range of -10 to 10 degrees, raw eye signals were corrected for non-linearity. The average resolution was 5'. The subject's head was stabilized by a deep bite board and a head rest in order to reduce drift and head movements. Data that contained drifts larger than 0.25 degree during one trial were rejected. Horizontal and vertical eye position signals were low-pass filtered (-3 dB at 150 Hz), digitized with a sample frequency of 500 Hz and stored in a computer.

Stimuli

The projected spots were moved by means of a scanning mirror device driven by a computer. Two sets of stimuli were generated by the computer. The first set consisted of quasi-random signals in the horizontal plane and were never beyond 10 degrees from primary position. These noise signals were a superposition of more than 20 single sine waves with a randomly distributed phase. The bandwidth of the noise signals lay between 1 and 1.5 Hz with a centre frequency between 0.7 and 1.15 Hz. A sample was computed every 10 ms. The D/A converted signals were low-pass filtered (-3 dB at 30 Hz). The total stimulus duration was 20.5 seconds. Head and tail (10% of total stimulus duration) were multiplied with increasing and decreasing gain in order to avoid sudden onsets and offsets of the stimulus. The second set of stimuli consisted of growing and decaying exponentials with time constants that ranged from 30 ms to 200 ms for the growing exponentials and -200 ms to -30 ms for the decaying exponentials. The eccentricity of these signals never exceeded 40 degrees from primary position. Every 1 ms a sample was computed. The duration of one exponential stimulus depended on the time constant. The growing exponentials started at primary position and initially a small offset, (smaller than 20 arcs of a second), was given because at t=0 this exponential function has a finite value. The decaying exponential was a step-ramp motion that started at primary position and then suddenly jumped to the periphery where it started to move back to primary position with an exponential decay. In order to avoid a visible streak, which could have an effect on the response during the stimulus jump to the periphery, the target was blanked. In one experimental trial, 10 exponentials were used which were randomized in direction (upward, downward, to the left and to the right) and time constant. Due to the variable duration of each exponential, the interval of stimulus presentation also changed pseudo-randomly.

Phase plane analysis

As was mentioned in the Introduction, phase plane analysis was applied. Restriction was made to a 2-dimensional phase plane analysis with retinal error, e, and error velocity, de/dt, as relative coordinates. In this phase plane, results are presented as retinal events or retinal trajectories. Retinal error is defined as the difference between target and eye position and will be negative as the target is at the left of the fovea. As a consequence, trajectories in this plane intend to move in a clockwise sense (see Figure 1). In the first quadrant the target is to the right of the fovea and is moving away from it, in the fourth quadrant the target is to the right of the fovea and is moving towards it. In the third quadrant the target is to the left of the fovea and is moving away from it and in the second quadrant the target is to the left of the fovea and moving towards it. If trajectories are located in the first and the third quadrant the match of target and eye position deteriorates and in the second and fourth quadrant this match improves. The ordinate represents the fovea. In the origin there is a perfect match of position and velocity. Retinal error and error velocity at the moment of the onset and offset of saccades are events and plotted as points in this e, de/dt plane. Therefore, all these onset events of saccades during pursuit of the different trials will be presented as clusters. Onset events of saccades to the right and to the left are called ONR and ONL respectively. Error velocity was digitally calculated (Usui & Amidror, 1982) with a second order low-pass differentiation using the algorithm :

$$\frac{de(n)}{dt} = \frac{e(n+2) + e(n+1) - e(n-1) - e(n-2)}{6t} \qquad t = 2ms$$

An extra digital symmetrical low-pass filtering (-3 dB at 15 Hz) was performed (Rabiner et al., 1970) to reduce mains hum and high frequency noise. In this manner an accuracy of $1°/s$ in error velocity was achieved. Due to this filtering, the saccadic velocity profiles were artificially broadened out. Therefore, error velocity during the onset of the saccade was computed as the average

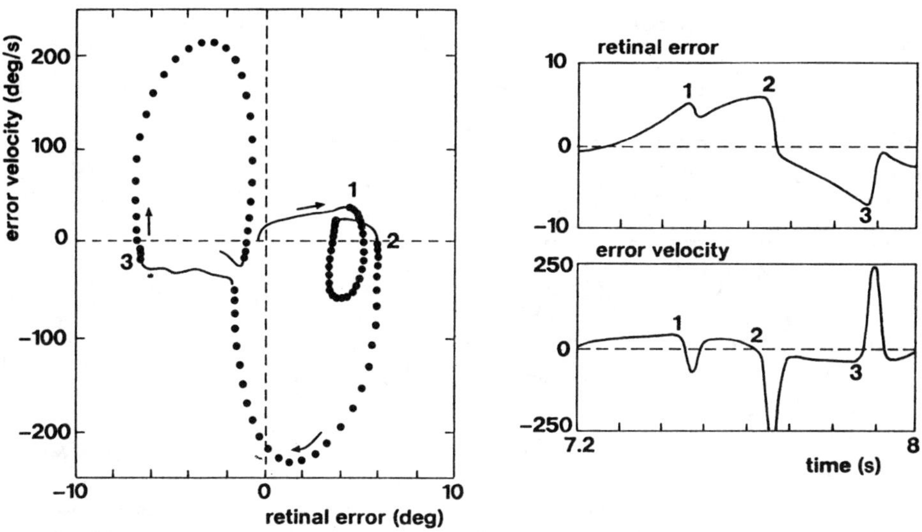

Fig. 1: The upper and lower panel at the right show a trajectory of simultaneously calculated retinal error and error velocity respectively. The left panel shows the corresponding phase plane plot. The numbers 1,2,3 indicate onsets of saccades. The arrows in the left panel refer to the movement direction of the trajectory.

error velocity between 40 and 20 ms before saccadic onset. Error velocity at the moment of saccadic offset was computed as the average error velocity between 20 and 40 ms after the saccade's offset. The frequency content of the stimulus and the frequency response of the eye are such that these velocities are approximately the same as the actual velocities at the onset and offset of the saccade. Artifacts in the determination of error velocity due to intersaccadic intervals shorter than 60 ms were removed from the results.

Results

Figure 2 shows an example of a response to a quasi-random target motion. Target position, eye position as well as retinal error are shown. At the moment of each saccade onset retinal error and error velocity were determined (see Methods). These values were plotted as events in the phase plane. The onset events of all trials of quasi-random stimuli form clusters, which for three subjects are shown in the left panels of Figure 3. The right panels of Figure 3 form the offset clusters, which represent the retinal error and error velocity just after the offset of the saccade. Squares in the left panels of Figure 3 indicate saccades to the right (ONR-cluster), the stars represent saccades to the left (ONL-cluster). Since the ONR-clusters are almost completely located to the

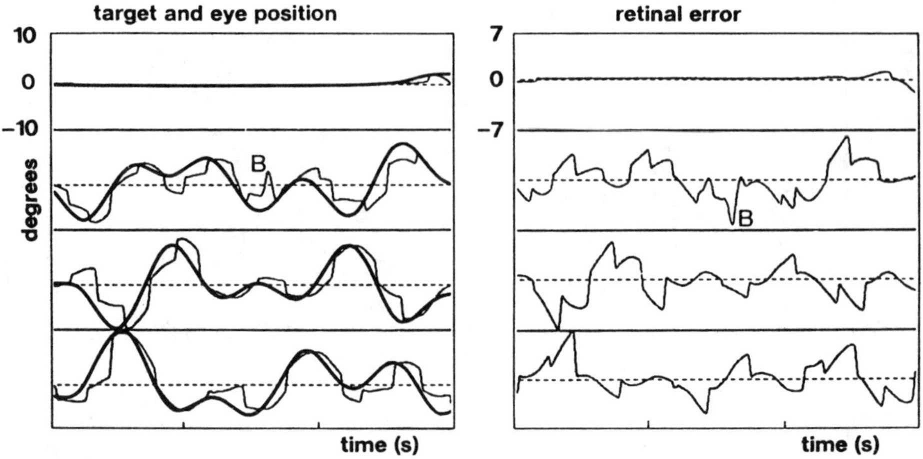

Fig. 2: The left panel shows a part of a quasi-random target motion (continuous trajectory) and the corresponding horizontal eye movement of the left eye. Positive values are movements to the right. Within each panel the top trajectory is continued in the trajectories below. The horizontal time scale indicates one second distances. The right panel represents retinal error. Note the different vertical scales between left and right panel. The disruption in eye tracking during the blink (B) is not an artifact but represents the actual eye movement.

right of the ordinate (fovea is left of the target) and the ONL-clusters are almost completely located to the left of the ordinate (fovea is right of the target), this indicates that for quasi-random stimuli saccadic eye movements are mostly goal-directed and can be classified as 'corrective.' The fact that ONR-clusters are rather located above than under the abscissa and ONL-clusters are located rather under than above the abscissa means that most saccades are initiated when the target is moving away from the fovea. When the target is moving towards the fovea, saccades are inhibited and error velocity must be less than about 25 $^\circ/s$ in order to have a saccade onset. In the first and third quadrant of the left panels of Figure 3 the ONR-clusters and ONL-clusters have relatively sharp boundaries to the side of the ordinate. The areas between these boundaries and the ordinate are empty of onset events. However, in these areas, there is still pursuit behavior. This can be deduced from the overlap between the onset and offset clusters shown in the insets of the left panels. In these insets, the dashed areas indicate regions with offset events but empty of onset events. After a saccade offset, smooth pursuit will continue. The observed boundaries indicate, that above a certain ratio of error velocity and retinal error an initiation of a saccadic eye movement is very improbable. For example, if we have a retinal target moving away from the fovea, the chance for a saccade will be practically zero when the ratio between error velocity and retinal error is larger

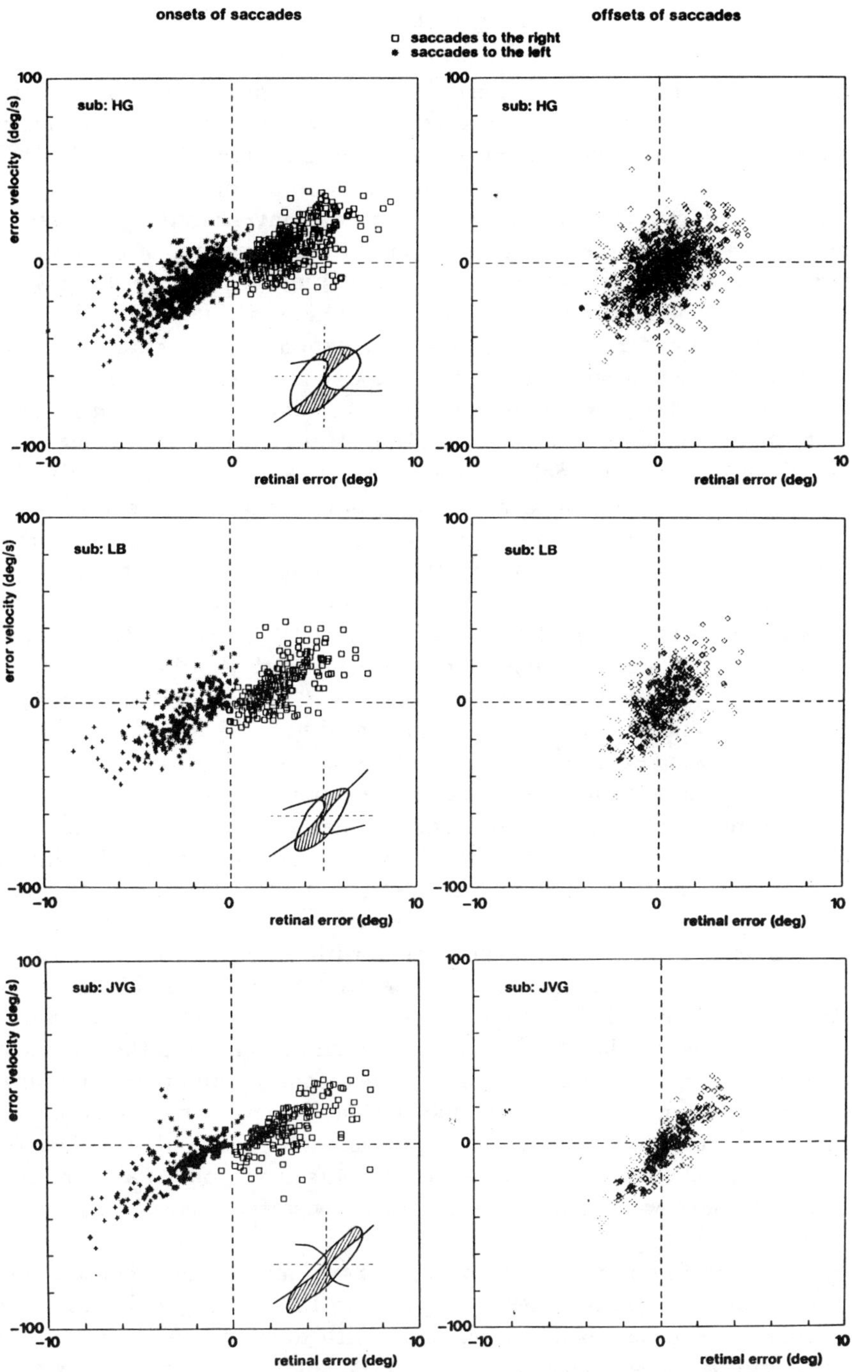

Fig. 3: The retinal error/error velocity phase plane plots at the moment of saccade onset (left panels) and saccade offset (right panels) in response to the quasi-random stimuli for three subjects are shown. Squares and stars refer to saccades to the right (ONR-cluster) and left (ONL-cluster) respectively. The inset in the left panels outlines the boundaries of the onset and offset clusters. The dashed area in these insets depicts the area where offsets of saccades but no onsets are found.

than 12 s^{-1}. In this case, retinal error will increase proportionally with error velocity. The value of 12 s^{-1} can be derived from the tangent of a straight line through the origin, which approximates the sharp boundaries of the ONR- and ONL-clusters. The first set of stimuli led to random trajectories through the phase plane in a clockwise sense. In order to investigate the behavior in this phase plane in another way, the second set of exponential stimuli was employed. These exponential stimuli (see Methods) initially lead to straight lines in the phase plane starting or ending at the origin, since the first derivative of retinal error, i.e. target velocity, is also an exponential function. Then, the ratio between target position and target velocity is equal to the time constant of the growing or decaying exponential. If the eye did not respond with smooth pursuit, this stimulus should lead to a straight line in the phase plane with a tangent inversely proportional with the time constant of the exponential.

The results for the growing exponentials can be summarized as follows. Figure 4 shows some responses of two subjects to growing and decaying exponentials for two time constants. When the time constant was small, a smooth pursuit response could hardly be observed, while the end points of the saccadic responses always missed the target (lagged behind). When the time constant was about 125 ms, smooth pursuit was adequate, such that even after 800 ms no catch-up saccades were observed. In this case, "ringing" of the smooth pursuit response could be seen with a frequency of about 3 Hz. When the time constant of growing exponentials was larger than 175 ms, within 200 - 300 ms after stimulus onset, corrective saccades were again observed.

Some examples of responses to decaying exponentials are shown in Figure 5. This figure demonstrates that smooth pursuit starts at about 150 ms, initially driven by the positional error and later on by the direction of the target velocity, i.e. in a direction away from target position. The latencies of the primary saccades to decaying exponentials with a time constant more than -100 ms, show a bimodal distribution. The results for three subjects are plotted together in Figure 6. The bimodal distribution consisted of a first group of "fast" saccades with a latency in between 150 and 200 ms and they were completely inaccurate and always too large. The second group of saccades always had prolonged latencies (larger than 300 ms) and were much more accurate. Between 200 ms and 300 ms, no saccadic responses were observed, although there was a substantial retinal error and a smooth pursuit response was seen. Thus, accurate saccades were inhibited when target velocity was too large (about 25 $^{\circ}/s$).

Figure 7 shows again a phase plane plot for two subjects of the onsets events of the primary saccade but now in response to the growing and decaying exponentials. Responses to all exponentials with different time constants and different directions are plotted in the same plane. The similarity with the phase plane plots of the first set of stimuli in Figure 3 is striking and the onsets

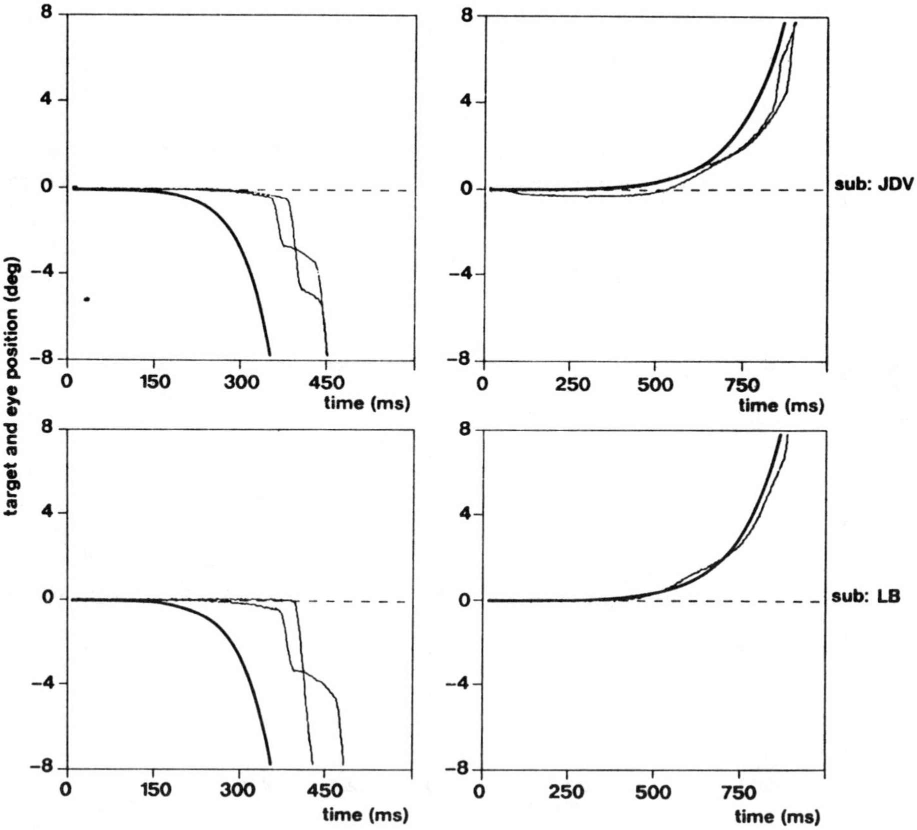

Fig. 4: This figure shows the exponentially growing target motion (thick continuous trajectory) and the eye movement response for two subjects (upper and lower panels). The left and right panels refer to a growing exponential with a time constant of 50 ms (to the left) and a time constant of 125 ms (to the right) respectively. Note the ringing of the smooth pursuit response in the right panel.

events of Figure 7 seem to be located along the boundaries of the ONL- and ONR-clusters of Figure 3. The reason why these onsets are only located along the boundaries may be caused by the fact that for Figure 7 target motion always was in one direction and by the fact that for the exponential stimuli only the onsets to the primary saccade are plotted. In the first and third quadrant mainly the onset of saccades to growing exponentials are located. Again there seems to be a constant relationship between error velocity and retinal error. However, this might be due to the kind of stimulus applied and not to the eye

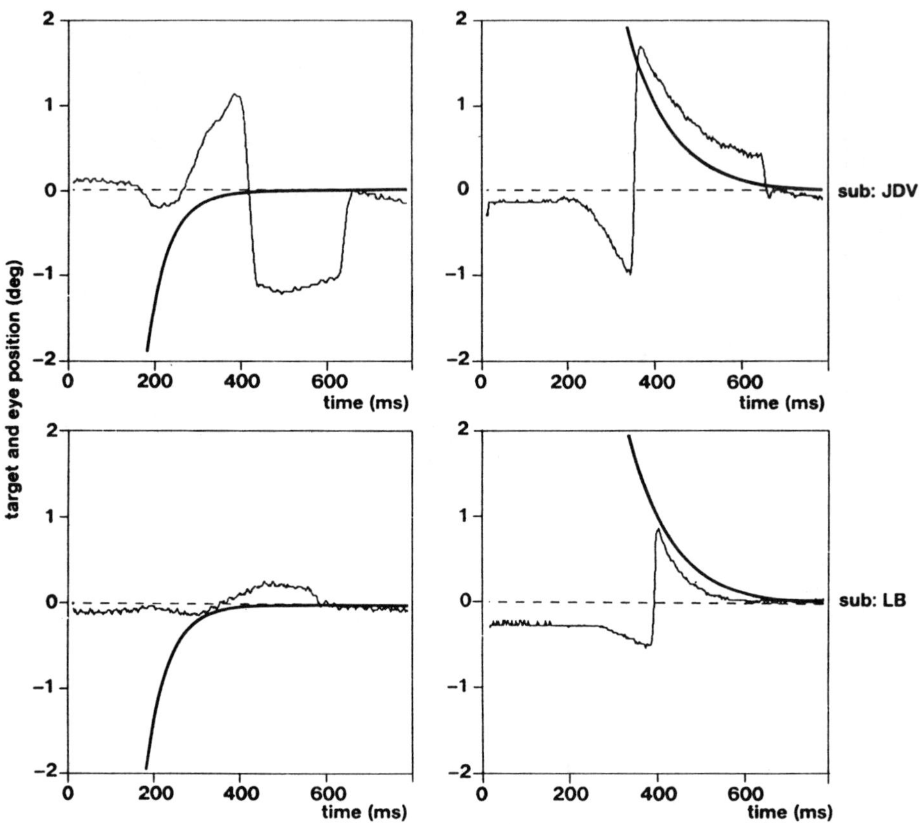

Fig. 5: This figure shows the exponentially decaying target motion (thick continuous trajectory) and the eye movement response for two subjects (upper and lower panels). The left and right panels refer to a decaying exponential with a time constant of -50 ms (negative vertical scale corresponds to downward position) and -100 ms (positive vertical scale corresponds to right position) respectively. Note the initial smooth pursuit response to positional error in the left panels and the prolonged saccadic latencies in all the responses.

movement response (see also Discussion). Smooth pursuit responses to growing exponentials with a small time constant were much less than required, so that the retinal error and retinal velocity at saccade onset were mainly determined by the stimulus. This is especially the case for onset events located at higher eccentricities. These onsets originate all from responses to stimuli with a time constant of 60 ms or less. Onset events related to the decaying exponentials are mainly located in the second and fourth quadrant. For stimuli with a small time constant, the onset events are located near the origin and only have a

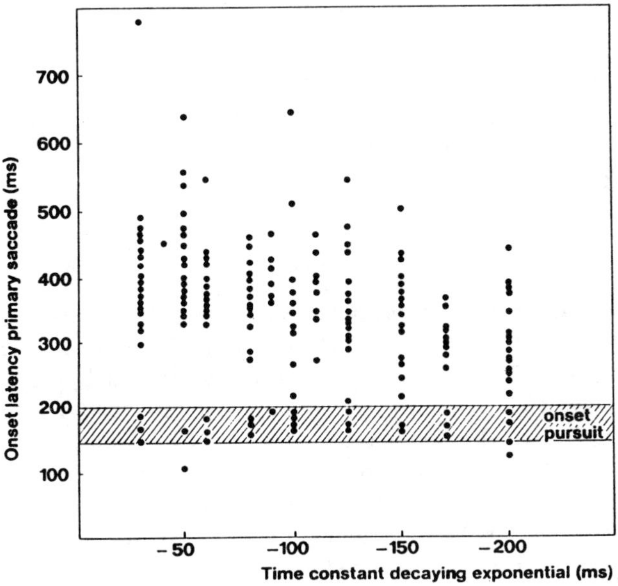

Fig. 6: The figure represents the onset latencies of the primary saccades in response to decaying exponentials with different time constants for three subjects. Note the bimodal distribution for time constants more than -100 ms.

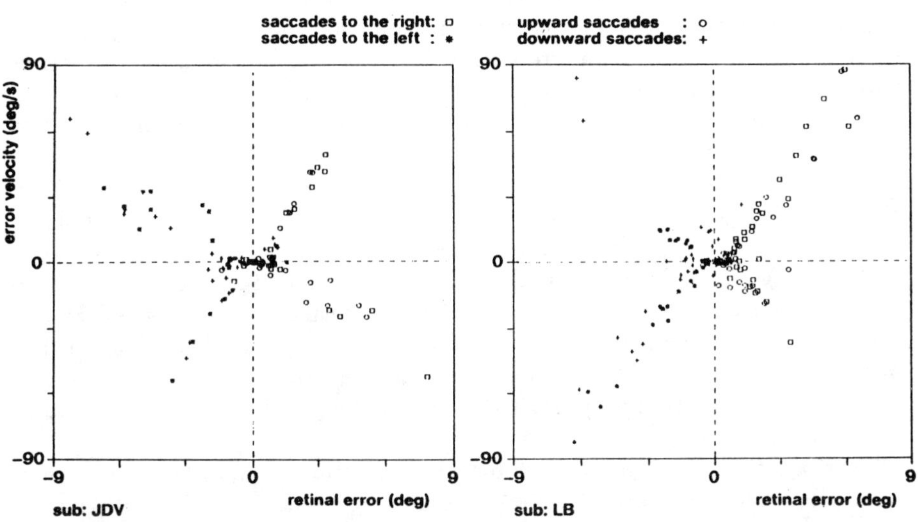

Fig. 7: Phase plane representations of onset events of the primary saccades in response to growing and decaying exponentials with different time constants and different directions plotted in the same plane. Left and right panel refer to different subjects. Open squares, stars, open circles and crosses indicate rightward, leftward, upward and downward saccades respectively.

difference in retinal error. For the larger time constants (larger than 100 ms), there can be a difference in error velocity, but this is not larger than about 25 $^\circ/s$. Onset events with a very large difference in error velocity refer to the "fast" saccadic responses with short latency.

Discussion

When targets are moving away from the fovea, it has been demonstrated that the initiation of saccades not only is determined by retinal error but also by the magnitude and direction of error velocity, provided target motions are previously unknown to the subject. There is a symmetry with respect to the fovea. With respect to the responses to random target motion, a threshold is observed for the ratio between error velocity and retinal error at the moment of the saccade's onset. This threshold is not necessarily related to a minimum latency as is the case for discontinuously moving targets. For example, if at a certain moment, the ratio of error velocity and retinal error reaches a supra-threshold value, a saccade may be generated. Then, the saccadic amplitude can fall short. Therefore, within a relatively short time, the ratio again becomes supra-threshold and another saccade will be generated. The difference between experiments with discontinuously moving targets is that before and after the saccade, the continuously moving target can fall within the same receptive field. Therefore, an initiation of a successive saccade could be facilitated by the successive stimulation of the same receptive field. This may explain why the time between two successive saccades can be as short as 60 ms. If, after a saccade, the target falls in another receptive field, a new build up of saccadic initiation is necessary. In this view, the inverse of the threshold-ratio of error velocity and retinal error (which has the dimension of time), might reflect something as a minimum integration-time of receptive fields. Given the logarithmic mapping between the retina and visual maps in the brain, it seems likely that the size of these receptive fields increases with eccentricity. This might explain that this threshold for saccade initiation is expressed by retinal velocity scaled to target's eccentricity. The fact that for growing exponentials with very small time constants this threshold is not independent of eccentricity may be explained by a deviation of the actual mapping from the ideal logarithmic mapping at large eccentricities.

Another difference with the second set of stimuli is that the onset events to primary saccades are plotted only, while this is not true for the first set of quasi-random stimuli. However, the most important reason might be that the phase plane analysis was restricted to a 2-dimensional plane with only retinal error and error velocity as coordinates. Several authors (Lisberger et al., 1981; Carl & Gellman, 1987) have demonstrated that acceleration plays an important role in the initiation of smooth pursuit. It is not unlikely that if retinal target acceleration as an additional dimension is taken into account, phase plane plots could become more stimulus-independent. For both sets of stimuli, retinal target acceleration is not constant and for the first set the sign continuously changes. However, for the sake of clarity, 3-dimensional phase plane plots were avoided.

When targets are moving towards the fovea, saccadic responses are clearly inhibited. This is true for both sets of stimuli. The similarity between these findings and the step-ramp experiments of Rashbass (1961) and Robinson (1980) is clear. The phase plane plots of the exponential and quasi-random stimuli nicely demonstrate that the inhibition of saccades for targets moving towards the fovea is a more common rule and does not depend on a special kind of stimulus set-up. There seems to be even a threshold for error velocity, i.e. inhibition always takes place when the error velocity is higher than about 25 $^\circ/s$. This result is in accordance with some of the results of Heywood and Churcher (1981), who found a significant increase of saccadic latency for higher ramp speeds (backward step-ramp). However, the "fast" saccadic responses to decaying exponential stimuli do not show this inhibition. One could speculate that these responses are generated by a structure which localizes a target with a course visual map and therefore, is quite insensitive to the velocity of the target. The other structure with a more refined visual map must be velocity-sensitive, otherwise it cannot localize the target. The process of localization in this last structure requires some time and this may explain the occurrence of a bimodal distribution of saccadic latencies with small time constant exponential stimuli. It can be derived from Figure 6, that the time constant of this process of localization must be in the order of 100 ms, since for time constants smaller than this value, the bimodal distribution starts to appear. There seems to be some resemblance between these findings and the bimodal distribution found with the experimental paradigm of express saccades (Fischer, 1986). In fact, the step followed by an exponential decrease could create a short period of stimulus absence in the central visual field. Such a stimulus absence is not unlikely since small targets (0.4 degrees) were used, which, after the step, started at an eccentricity of 35 degrees. A difference with the gap-paradigm is that, after the step, the stimuli were moving. This may explain why no saccadic latencies as short as those of express saccades were found. Some remarks must be made with respect to the smooth pursuit response. The smooth pursuit latency of 150 ms, found for the decaying exponential stimuli, is not in accordance with the latest results of Carl and Gellman (1987). This might be due to the fact that the stimuli started in the periphery and that the smooth pursuit latency is longer for stimuli moving outside the parafoveal region. The smooth pursuit responses to decaying exponential stimuli confirm the results of other authors (Heywood & Churcher, 1971; Kommerell & Täumer, 1972; Pola & Wyatt, 1980; Carl & Gellman, 1987) in the sense that smooth pursuit may respond to target position. An interesting result is that smooth pursuit responses to very small moving targets in the periphery are found, provided they are moving very fast. Therefore, there seems to be an invariance in smooth pursuit response for foveally and peripherally moving targets if the target velocity is scaled to its peripheral position. Also interesting are the smooth pursuit responses to growing exponentials with time constants between 125 and 200 ms. The first 'catch-up' saccades were seen after 800 ms. During this first period of time, "ringing" was clearly seen with a frequency of about 3 Hz which indicates that this kind of stimulus might simulate an open-loop situation because derivatives of an exponential function are always exponentials with the same time constant. If the eye movement response has the same exponential shape (with the same time constant) as the stimulus, there exists only a small constant positional error between target motion and eye movement response. However, the frequency of 3 Hz does not correspond with the results of Robinson et al. (1986) who found a mean value of 3.8 Hz. The difference with their experiments is that the smooth pursuit response was not interrupted by 'catch-up' saccades.

Acknowledgement

The author is indebted to the Department of Medical Physics and Biophysics of the University of Nijmegen. This work was supported partly by the Dutch Organization for the Advancement of Pure Research (ZWO).

References

Becker, W., & Jürgens, R., *An analysis of the saccadic system by means of double step stimuli*, Vision Research **19** (1979), 967-983.

Bour, L.J., Van Gisbergen, J.A.M., Bruijns, J., & Ottes, F.P., *The double magnetic induction method for measuring eye movement - results in monkey and man*, IEEE Transactions on Biometrical Engineering, BME-31 **5** (1984), 419-427.

Buizza, A., & Schmidt, R., *Velocity characteristics of smooth pursuit eye movements to different patterns of target motion*, Experimental Brain Research **63** (1986), 395-401.

Carl, J.R., & Gellman, R.S., *Human smooth pursuit: stimulus-dependent responses*, Journal of Neurophysiology **57** (1987), 1446-1463.

Collewijn, H., & Tamminga, E.P., *Human smooth pursuit and saccadic eye movements during voluntary pursuit of different target motions on different backgrounds*, Journal of Physiology **351** (1984), 217-250.

Fischer, B., *Express saccades in man and monkey*, in "H.J. Freund, U. Büttner, B. Cohen, & J. Noth (Eds.), The oculomotor and skeletalmotor systems: differences and similarities," Elsevier/North-Holland, Amsterdam, 1986, pp. 155-160.

Heywood, S., & Churcher, J., *Eye movements and the afterimage - I. Tracking the afterimage*, Vision Research **11** (1971), 1163-1168.

Heywood, S., & Churcher, J., *Saccades to step-ramp stimuli*, Vision Research **21** (1981), 479-490.

Kommerell, G., & Täumer, R., *Investigations of the eye tracking system through stabilized retinal images*, Bibliotheca Ophthalmologica **82** (1972), 288-297.

Kowler, E., & Steinman, R.M., *The effect of expectations on slow oculomotor control - II. Single target displacements*, Vision Research **19** (1979), 633-646.

Kowler, E., & Steinman, R.M., *The effect of expectations on slow oculomotor control - III. Guessing unpredictable target displacements*, Vision Research **21** (1981), 191-203.

Lisberger, S.G., Evinger, C., Johnson, G.W., & Fuchs, A., *Relationship between eye acceleration and retinal image velocity during foveal smooth pursuit in man and monkey*, Journal of Neurophysiology **46** (1981), 229-249.

Leigh, R.J., & Zee, D.S., "The Neurology of eye movements," F.A. Davis Company, Philadelphia, 1983.

Pola, J., & Wyatt, H.J., *Target position and velocity: The stimuli for smooth pursuit eye movements*, Vision Research **20** (1980), 523-534.

Pola, J.,& Wyatt, H.J., *Active and passive smooth eye movements: effects of stimulus size and location*, Vision Research **25** (1985), 1063-1076.

Rabiner, L.R., Gold, B., & Mc Gonegal, C.A., *An approach to the approximation problems for nonrecursive digital filters*, IEEE Transactions on Audio and Electroacoustics **AV-18** (1970), 83-106.

Rashbass, C., *The relationship between saccadic and smooth tracking eye movements*, Journal of Physiology **159** (1961), 326-338.

Robinson, D.A., *The mechanics of human smooth pursuit eye movements*, Journal of Physiology **180** (1965), 569-591.

Robinson, D.A., *Control of eye movements*, in "J.M. Brookheart, V.B. Mountcastle, & V.B. Brooks (Eds.), Handbook of Physiology (sect. I, Vol. II, part 2)," American Physiological Society, Betheseda, 1981, pp. 1275-1320.

Robinson, D.A., Gordon, J.L., & Gordon, S.E., *A model of the smooth pursuit eye movement system*, Biological Cybernetics **55** (1986), 43-57.

Usui, S., & Amidror, I., *Digital low-pass differentiation for biological signal processing*, IEEE Transaction on Biomedical Engineering, BME- 29 **10** (1982), 686-693.

Yasui, Y., & Young, L.R., *On the predictive control of foveal eye tracking and slow phases of optokinetic and vestibular nystagmus*, Journal of Physiology **347** (1984), 17-33.

Young, L.R., *Pursuit eye movement - what is being pursued?*, in "R. Baker & A. Berthoz (Eds.), Control of gaze by brain stem neurons," Elsevier/North-Holland, Amsterdam, 1977, pp. 301-308.

AN ABRUPT SHORT-LATENCY INCREASE IN SACCADE SPEED DURING SQUARE-WAVE TRACKING

JAN A.M. VAN GISBERGEN, AREND C. SMIT, AND ROB J.W. BERG

Department of Medical Physics and Biophysics
University of Nijmegen

Although slight differences in saccade dynamics have been noticed in different experimental paradigms (Becker & Fuchs, 1969; Zambarbieri et al., 1982), one of the most striking properties of the saccadic systems has always been the stereotyped character of its movements. Accordingly, since paradigm-related differences in saccade dynamics seemed rather uninteresting and almost trivial, it is not too surprising that few attempts have been made to account for these effects. The internal-feedback model of the saccadic system (Robinson, 1975; Van Gisbergen et al., 1981), for example, proposes implicitly that saccades based on information of quite different origin (visual, auditory, tactile, vestibular, memory, predictive, cognitive) are all generated by the same pulse generator in the final common pathway of the motor system. By implication, all these saccades have an invariant amplitude/peak velocity/duration (main-sequence) relationship in the model.

Recent developments have revived the interest in the different saccade characteristics revealed in various experimental paradigms:

First, there is now evidence that various visuomotor areas in the brain play, in part, distinct roles in the generation of different saccade types. For example, the frontal eye fields seem to be essential for the control of so-called anti-saccades (movements away from a visual stimulus; Guitton et al., 1985) and predictive saccades (Bruce & Borden, 1986), but apparently play no role in the generation of spontaneous saccades (Bruce & Goldberg, 1985). Single-unit studies in the substantia nigra of the awake monkey (Hikosaka & Wurtz, 1983) have yielded further support for the notion that the control of different saccade types is based on a differential involvement of various visuomotor control areas in the brain. Very recently, Schiller et al. (1987) have found that the superior colliculus, unlike the frontal eye field, is essentially involved in the generation of very short-latency visually elicited saccades (express saccades; for a review see Fischer, 1987). Studies in neurological patients seem in line with this emerging picture. For example, it is known that in Parkinson's disease, a condition involving dysfunction of the substantia nigra, the capability to generate predictive saccades to a repetitive visual stimulus is significantly reduced (Bronstein & Kennard, 1985).

Second, recent studies have shown that the differences between the dynamic characteristics of memory-guided saccades (Hikosaka & Wurtz, 1985; Smit et al., 1987) and anti-saccades (Smit et al., 1987) on the one hand and visually elicited saccades on the other hand are quite substantial.

The latter finding, together with earlier reports indicating that visually-elicited saccades are faster than saccades made in the absence of a visual stimulus (Becker & Fuchs, 1969; Zambarbieri et al., 1982), leads one to expect that predictive saccades, made when tracking a regular square-wave stimulus (Stark et al., 1962; Dallos & Jones, 1963), may likewise have a reduced peak velocity. So far, reports on the dynamics of predictive saccades have not led to a clear picture. While Findlay (1981) found identical peak velocities in predictive and visually-elicited saccades, a recent report by Bronstein and Kennard (1987) indicates that predictive saccades are indeed slower.

If predictive and visually-guided saccades have different dynamic characteristics, two interesting questions can be raised. Can the time when the transition occurs be determined and, if so, can the transition latency be used as a criterion for separating predictive and visually-guided saccades? In this paper we report experiments on human subjects engaged in square-wave tracking which allow the complete saccade dynamics/latency relation to be determined. An attempt is made to interpret the results against the background of the Becker and Jürgens (1979) model of the saccadic system. The experimental data will be further put into perspective by comparison with the results of other groups which have quantified the latency dependence of other saccadic characteristics.

Methods

Experimental paradigms

Six subjects (5 males, 1 female; ages 20-44), four of whom were naive, participated in this study. Stimuli were rear-projected on a translucent screen, placed at 57 cm in front of the subject. Background illumination was kept as low as possible ($< 0.06\, cd/m^2$) so as to make the fine texture of the screen invisible. Fixation and target positions were indicated by a 0.4 ° white spot ($5\, cd/m^2$). After calibration of eye position (see below), three different stimulus paradigms were used in order to elicit horizontal predictive as well as visually-guided saccades to the right.

(1) *Main-sequence paradigm.* The data obtained in this experiment served to quantify the amplitude/peak-velocity relationship (main sequence; Bahill et al., 1975) of visually-guided saccades (see below). After central fixation, the target appeared at 3, 5, 10, 15, 20, 25, 30 or 35 ° to the right. Each target eccentricity was used five times with randomized initial fixation durations. The sequence of target positions was also randomized. The subject was instructed to refixate the target as quickly and as precisely as possible. To check whether subject behaviour was stationary, the same experiment was repeated near the

end of the session, which lasted up to 1 hour.

(2) *Regular square-wave stimulus paradigm.* After five fixation trials in the primary position (for calibration purposes), the target light jumped regularly up and down forty times between the primary position and 25 ° to the right at a rate of 0.67 Hz. To ensure the occurrence of predictive saccades, the subject was instructed to move the eyes as much as possible in synchrony with the stimulus and to blink only when fixating peripherally or during a centripetal saccade. For this reason only movements related to rightward movements were digitized by the computer for analysis. The regular square-wave stimulus was repeated up to 10 times in one session. A few subjects participated in up to three sessions.

(3) *Random-gap step stimulus paradigm.* After a fixation period with a variable duration (random 500, 750, 1000, 1250 or 2000 ms), a randomized dark gap lasting 0, 100, 200 or 800 ms was introduced before the target reappeared, always at 25 ° to the right. The stimulus was presented for 40 trials. This sequence was repeated up to 10 times in one session. The subject was instructed to make a saccade to the peripheral target as soon as it appeared. Three subjects participated in this paradigm. Throughout the session, subjects were kept alert and encouraged in order to avoid the slowing down of saccades as a consequence of drowsiness (Ron et al., 1972).

Recording of eye movements

Saccadic eye movements of the left eye were recorded using the double-magnetic induction method (Bour et al., 1984). Raw horizontal and vertical eye position signals were low-pass filtered (-3 dB at 150 Hz), digitized at a rate of 500 samples/s in each channel with a precision of 12 bits and stored on disk in a PDP 11/34 computer. Data were corrected off-line for the static nonlinearity inherent in the method based upon an extensive set of calibration data collected at the beginning of each session (see also Bour et al., 1984). Since the pick-up coil in front of the left eye was placed slightly off-center (towards the nose) the range for movements to the right, reported in this paper, extended up to 35 °. Resolution in this direction was 0.25, or better, in the range of 0 to 25 °.

Normalization of saccadic peak velocity

Using the linearized data, vectorial eye velocity was computed from the position signals by differentiation based on the central-difference algorithm (T= 2 ms; Bahill et al., 1982). Subsequently, a symmetrical digital low-pass filter was used to smooth the eye-velocity profile (-3 dB at 76 Hz; Rabiner et al., 1970). Saccade on- and offset were determined by computer from the vectorial eye-velocity signal using a 30 °/*s* level-crossing criterion.

The smoothed saccadic velocity profiles were used to determine the peak velocity (V_p) of the movement. It is well known that the so-called main-sequence parameters peak velocity and saccade amplitude (A_s) have a strong nonlinear relationship (Bahill et al., 1975). This so-called main-sequence relationship was characterized quantitatively by fitting the equation:

$$V_p = V_a[1 - exp(-A_s/A_o)] \qquad (1)$$

to the first-saccade data obtained in the main-sequence paradigm. In this equation, V_p represents vectorial peak velocity, V_a is the asymptotic peak velocity for very large saccades, A_s represents saccade amplitude and A_o is an angular constant (Van Gisbergen et al., 1985). Fitting this equation separately to data of both the first and the second main-sequence experiment in each session yielded two V_a values. If these values differed by less than 15%, equation (1) was fitted to the pooled data and the resulting fit was used for normalization (see below). If the difference exceeded 15%, the V_p data in the first and the second part of the session were normalized using the fit results of the corresponding main-sequence data.

The normalized peak velocity (V_{pn}) for a saccade with amplitude (A_s) was obtained by (see Figure 1):

$$V_{pn} = V_s/V_p \qquad (2)$$

where V_s is the peak velocity of the saccade under consideration and V_p is the best-fit main-sequence value for peak velocity at that amplitude. This normalization, applied to the first saccade of each trial, enabled us to compare the peak velocity values of saccades with unequal amplitudes directly. We used it mainly to side-step the danger of finding a lower peak velocity at short latency simply because predictive saccades may have lower gains (Findlay, 1981; Fischer & Ramsperger, 1986; Bronstein & Kennard, 1987).

Determination of peak-velocity transition latency

The transition in normalized peak velocity from slightly slower early saccades to the faster saccades later on (see Results) was determined by fitting a function V(t) which started rising from an initial value (V_{IN}) after a latency of τ ms (relative to peripheral stimulus onset) with a fast exponential time course (fixed time constant: 1 ms) to a final asymptotic peak velocity (V_{FIN}). The V_{IN} value was set equal to the mean V_{pn} value of all negative-latency saccades. Using a least-squares error criterion, the best-fit value for the transition latency (τ) could be found quickly and objectively.

Results

The main-sequence measurements indicated that subjects were able to maintain a stable level of performance: the asymptotic peak velocity in equation (1) computed from the two data sets was identical within 15% except in one

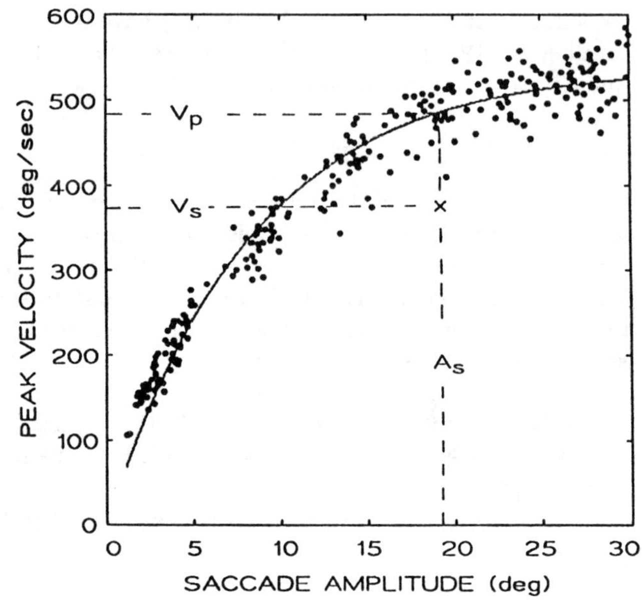

Fig. 1: Peak velocity/amplitude plot of main-sequence data (subject WBS) with best-fit curve [equation (1)] indicated by solid line through the data points. The hypothetical slow saccade, indicated by the cross, would have a normalized peak-velocity value (V_{pn}) of 0.78.

session (subject PVM, first session). With the exception of this case, main-sequence data obtained in one session were pooled and used for normalization of all first-saccade data in that session (see Methods).

Regular square wave stimulus

Plots of normalized peak velocity of first saccades against saccade onset latency are shown in Figure 2 for all six subjects. Saccadic latencies to the square-wave stimulus typically ranged from about -250 to 300 ms relative to peripheral stimulus onset. Although considerable differences in the amount of scatter were present among subjects, it is clear from Figure 2 that the mean normalized peak velocity of negative saccades (which are predictive by definition) was some 10% to 20% lower than in saccades with latencies beyond 150 ms, which are certainly of visual origin. This difference is in agreement with Bronstein and Kennard (1987). Our major new finding is that in all six subjects the transition from slower to faster saccades occurred at a very short latency (τ) and was sharply demarcated in most cases. The best-fit values of τ , found by fitting function V(t) to the data (see Methods) ranged from roughly 40-70 ms across subjects and had a mean of 50 ms (see Table 1). Since these values were unexpectedly short (see Discussion), all steps in the data-acquisition procedure, as well as the computation of latency and the

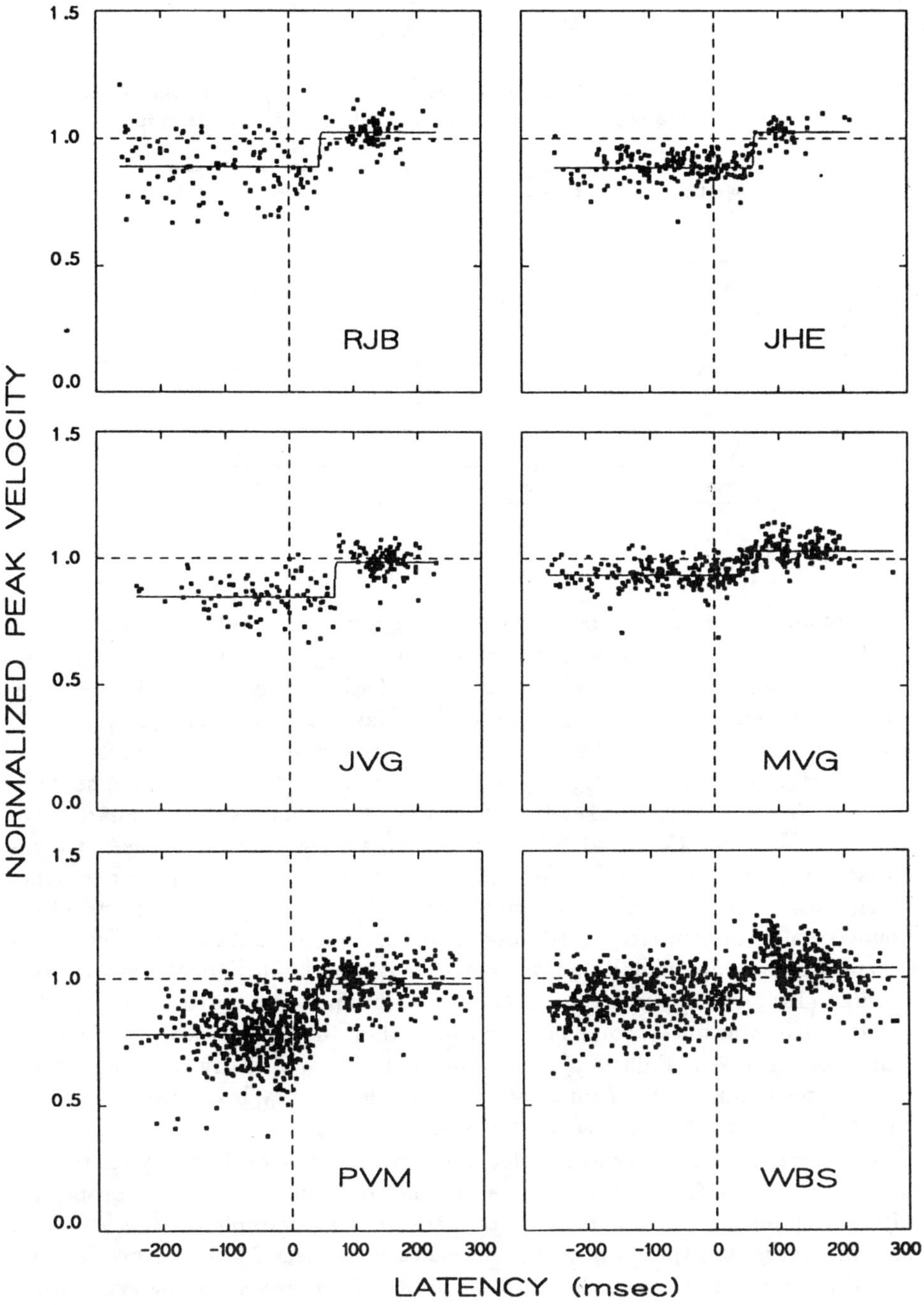

Fig. 2: Normalized peak velocity/latency plots for all six subjects in the square-wave paradigm. Horizontal dashed line indicates the best-fit peak velocity of visually-guided saccades in the main-sequence paradigm; the vertical dashed line indicates the peripheral stimulus onset. The best fit of the function V(t), see text, is indicated by a solid line through the data points. In all subjects, predictive saccades (negative latencies) are slower than visually-guided saccades (latency > 150 ms). The transition in peak velocity occurs remarkably early.

Tab. 1: Peak velocity transition latencies (τ ; ms) in two paradigms, determined by fitting function V(t) (see text) to the pooled data from each subject. ND: not determined.

subject	square wave	random-gap step
RJB	48	64
JHE	61	39
JVG	70	59
MVG	41	ND
PVM	39	ND
WBS	39	ND
mean	50	54

curve-fitting procedures were checked thoroughly to rule out artifacts.

Although we have reason to think that the sharp transition in normalized peak velocity represents an effect of peripheral stimulus onset (see below), this does not necessarily imply that the earliest fast saccades were *fully visually guided* (see Discussion). Therefore, we have looked at other measures of saccadic performance which might serve as indicators of visually-guided saccade latency. These measures, taken from first-saccadic responses to the square-wave stimulus (subjects JVG and RJB) are shown in Figure 3. For ease of comparison, the peak velocity/latency relation is again shown in the upper panel (Figure 3A). The latency histogram in both subjects (Figure 3B) shows a pronounced late peak superimposed upon a background level of earlier saccades. If this peak represents visually-guided saccades it would follow, in agreement with Findlay (1981), that predictive saccades may be initiated up to about 100-120 ms after stimulus onset, some 30-50 ms later than the normalized peak velocity transition visible in Figure 3A. We could not clearly identify a distinct early peak corresponding with express saccades in the latency histograms shown in Figure 3B, nor in the data of the other subjects.

Another measure of saccadic performance which may potentially yield further insight into the effect of the visual stimulus, concerns the metrical properties of the responses. As can be seen from the typical example on the left-hand side in Figure 3C, the gain of first saccades in subject JVG had no clear latency dependence in our experimental conditions. However, in one exceptional subject (RJB), about 30% of the early saccades had an abnormally low gain (< 0.8) whereas saccades with longer latencies had normal gains ranging mostly between 0.8 and 1.0 (Figure 3C, right-hand side).

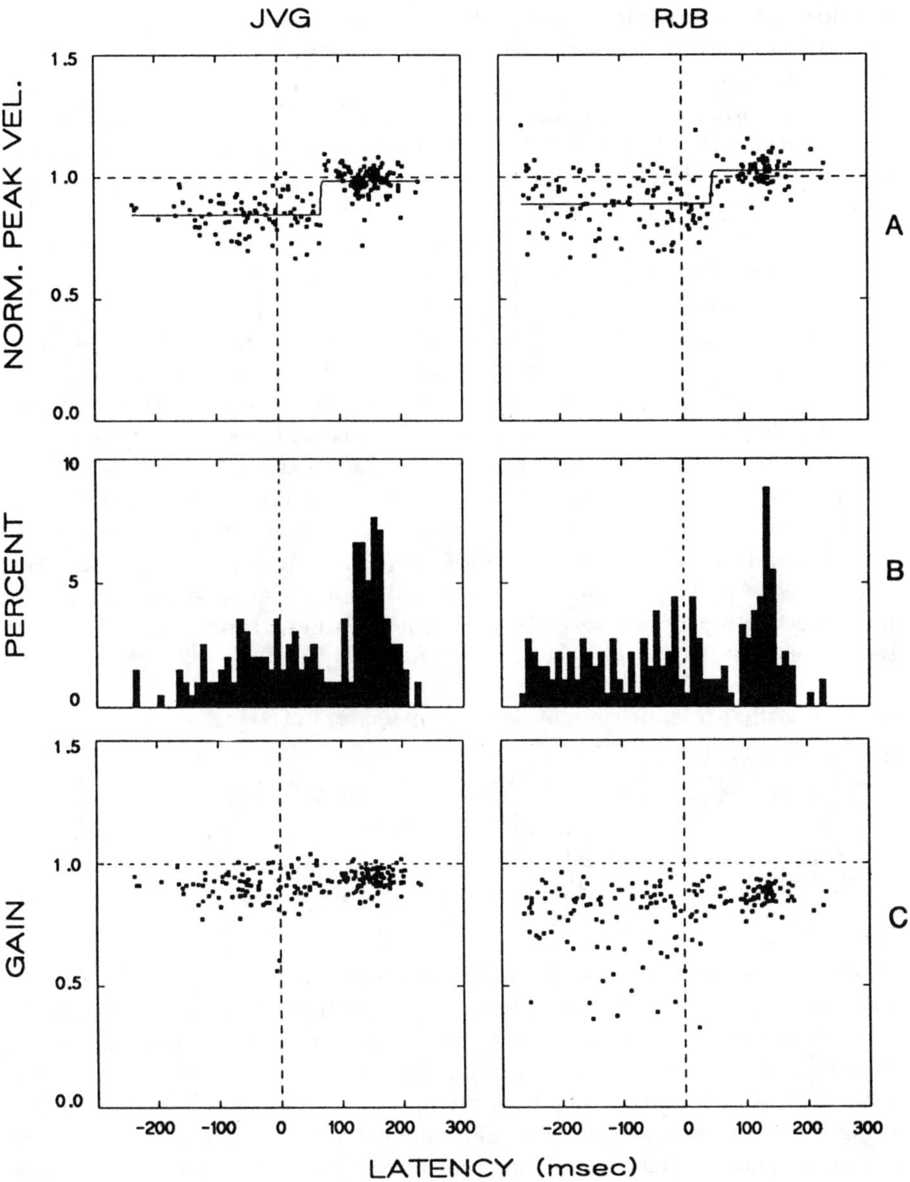

Fig. 3: Data of subject JVG (left-hand column) and RJB (right-hand column) in the square-wave paradigm. Vertical dashed lines indicate stimulus onset. A. Normalized peak velocity/latency relation, as in Figure 2. B. Latency histograms from data in A. Bin width: 10 ms. C. First-saccade gain as a function of latency. Horizontal dashed lines indicate normometric saccades (gain: 1.0).

Random-gap step stimulus results

We hoped that the use of the random-gap stimulus would permit us to identify express saccades which would provide a welcome opportunity to compare the τ values with what may be considered a lower bound on visually guided saccade latency (Fischer, 1987). Unfortunately, no sufficiently clear-cut express saccade peak could be identified in the latency histograms computed from the random-gap step results to allow this comparison.

In the longer gap-duration trials, subjects frequently made short-latency or even negative-latency (i.e. purely predictive) responses. This enabled us to look for a possible peak velocity/latency relationship also in these data. Again, in all three subjects tested, we observed a transition at very short latencies comparable to what was found in the regular square-wave paradigm (Figure 4 and Table 1). Since the data in Figure 4 were pooled across gap conditions, the possibility that the abrupt increase in normalized peak velocity is due to an arousal effect caused by the offset of the fixation stimulus can be excluded.

The first-saccade gain data of two subjects revealed no relation with latency at all. In the third subject tested in these experiments (RJB), we again noticed a proportion of low-gain saccades, which in these experiments occurred at latencies of up to 150 ms. This anecdotal finding is another indication that the earliest group of fast saccades may not have been (fully) visually guided (see Discussion).

Discussion

General remarks

We found that predictive saccades are up to 20% slower than visually-elicited saccades which is in agreement with Bronstein and Kennard (1987). The fact that Findlay (1981) was unable to find a similar difference in dynamics has been ascribed to the small saccadic amplitudes used in his study (see Bronstein & Kennard, 1987).

Minimum latency of visually-elicited saccades

Based on an analysis of metrical saccade properties, observed in experiments in which the target jumped either to the right or to the left, Kalesnykas and Hallett (1987) have been able to make a distinction in the short-latency range between predictive saccades (characterized by a considerable percentage of wrong-direction responses) and visually-guided saccades which bring the eye near to the target. They found that consistently correct saccades were made only at latencies beyond 120 ms. Several other groups had reported earlier that predictive saccades have, on average, smaller gains than later, visually-driven saccades (Saslow, 1967; Findlay, 1981; Fischer & Ramsperger, 1986). Kalesnykas and Hallett point out, however, that saccade size per se is not a reliable criterion for distinguishing between predictive and visually-guided sac-

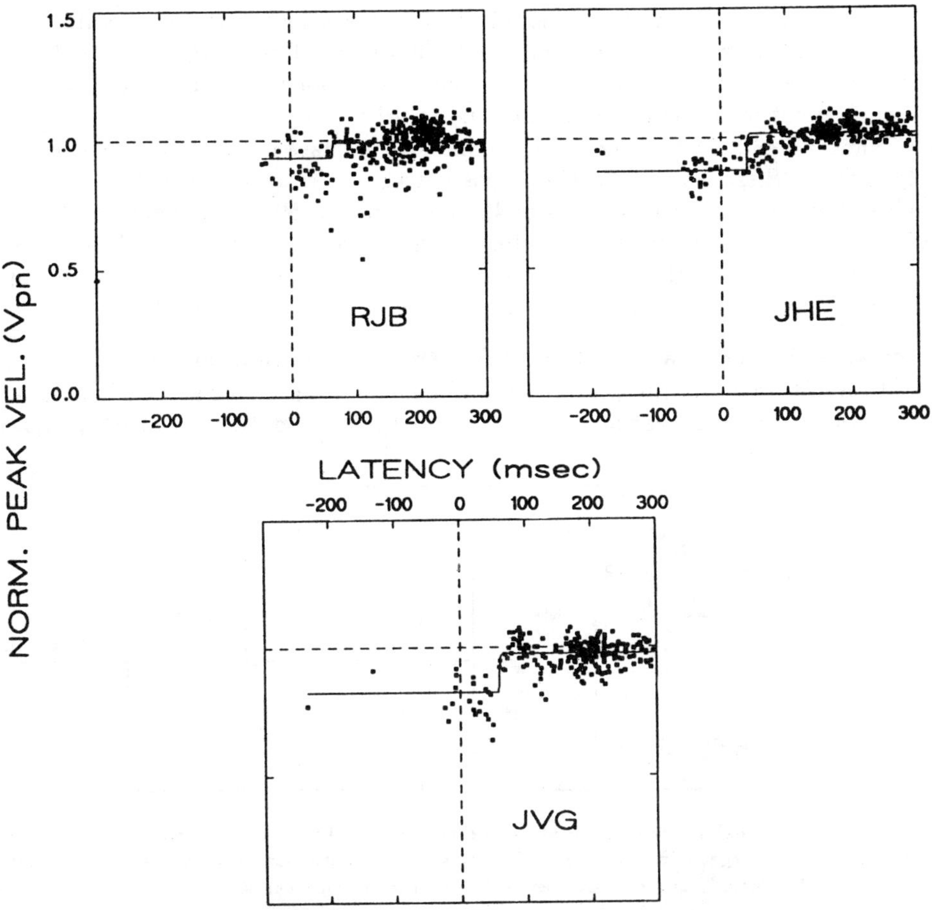

Fig. 4: Normalized peak velocity/latency plots of first saccade data obtained in random-gap step experiments from three subjects Data were pooled across gap conditions. Same conventions as in Figure 2.

cades: some very early responses in their experiments still had correct metrical properties.

Our failure to find a consistent reduction in saccade gain in short-latency or even negative latency saccades in most of our subjects (see e.g. Figure 3C, left-hand side) may be related to our experimental conditions. In our experiments the visual stimulus always had spatial predictibility so that both the prediction signal and the visual signal probably opted for the same saccade.

Also, studies relying on an analysis of latency histograms arrived at a minimum latency for visually-guided saccades which is considerably longer than the peak velocity transition latency reported in this paper. The first increase in saccade initiation probability thought to be caused by the visual stimulus can be detected near 100 ms (Findlay, 1981; Fischer & Ramsperger, 1984, 1986). In those cases in which this criterion could be applied to our own data, the results point in the same direction (Figure 3B).

Thus, taken together, the metrical and latency data in the literature suggest that the earliest time when (fully) visually-guided saccades first appear considerably exceeds the time span of 40-70 ms (mean: 50 ms) in which we found the first effect of the visual stimulus on the dynamical properties of saccades. If that is the case, the question arises how the visual stimulus can speed up saccades at an earlier time than when it can initiate and guide them.

Possible interpretation of the very short transition latencies

In an attempt to interpret these findings, we propose a model which is an extremely simplified version adapted from Becker and Jürgens (1979)(Figure 5).

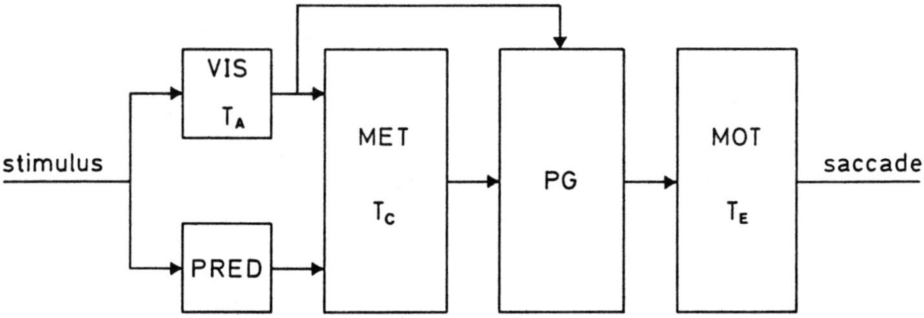

Fig. 5: Conceptual scheme, inspired by the Becker and Jürgens (1979) model, to explain how the visual target stimulus might already speed up anticipatory saccades before it can generate fully visually-guided movements. See text for further explanation.

In the scheme, the stimulus enters two pathways, denoted by VIS (visual system) and PRED (prediction system). The output signals of these two systems contain position information which is processed by a stage responsible for the computation of saccade metrics (MET) which corresponds with the central decision and computation stage in the Becker and Jürgens (1979) model. This computation takes a time of at least T_C ms. When the metrics computation, based on the VIS or the PRED signal (or both), has been completed, the saccade is executed by the saccadic pulse generator (PG) whose activity determines the metrical as well as the dynamical properties of the saccade (Robinson, 1975).

In addition to computation time T_C, the afferent delay (T_A) in the visual system and the efferent delay (T_E) in the motor system (MOT) also contribute to saccade latency (Becker & Jürgens, 1979). We propose that the visual system can influence the state of the pulse generator directly, without affecting the metrics of the movement, and thereby *speed up* saccades initiated by the prediction system (see upper pathway in Figure 5).

Thus, in this scheme, the shortest latency in which visually-guided saccades can be generated equals $T_A + T_C + T_E$ ms. Now consider the case, shortly after a stimulus step, when the metrics box, fed by the prediction signal, has already completed its computation. The earliest time when such a fully predictive saccade can be speeded up by the visual stimulus equals $T_A + T_E$ ms. If this interpretation is correct, saccades occurring at the peak velocity transition latency τ were still fully guided by the prediction system. Another implication is that τ (mean: 50 ms) equals the sum of afferent and efferent delays in the system. Assuming that the sum of all delays ($T_A + T_C + T_E$) is approximately 120 ms (Kalesnykas & Hallett, 1987), 70 ms for computation time T_C would be available in the earliest visually-guided saccades.

One way to evaluate our interpretation of τ is to ask whether 50 ms is reasonable for the sum of afferent and efferent delays, in view of other data from the literature. The problem in determining the value of afferent and efferent delays is that the result depends on how and where it is measured. It seems reasonable to suggest that values obtained from the primate collicular visuomotor system are the most relevant for an understanding of the timing of very early human saccades (Schiller et al., 1987). For this system estimates the afferent delay range of upward from 40 ms (Wurtz & Goldberg, 1972). The efferent delay has been estimated to be at least 20 ms (Robinson, 1972; Sparks, 1978; Mays & Sparks, 1980). Taken together, these data would indicate that the sum of T_A and T_E is at least 60 ms, which is in agreement with the range of τ values reported in this paper.

Based upon an analysis of responses to double-step stimuli, Becker and Jürgens (1979) arrived at a somewhat higher estimate (81 ms) for the sum of afferent and efferent delays. This result is a mean value (that is, in individual cases the delay ranged from 30 to 130 ms). Thus, in summary, our interpretation of τ as representing the sum of afferent and efferent delays is not in obvious disagreement with other data in the literature which were obtained in entirely different experiments and based on other criteria.

Finally, it is interesting to speculate on a possible neural basis for the proposed visual signal effect on the saccadic pulse generator. Recent experiments by Munoz and Guitton (1987) seem particularly relevant in this regard. They reported that the instantaneous firing frequency profile of collicular burst neurons in cats resembled the mean gaze velocity profile. This was true both for fast visually-guided movements and for slower predictive movements. It was observed repeatedly that the presentation of a visual target stimulus could speed up an ongoing low-frequency predictive burst signal after very short latencies. It is possible that a visual input to these neurons allowed them to respond more briskly to the prediction command signal.

Conclusion

We propose that the square-wave tracking paradigm may be used to obtain information on the sum of afferent and efferent delays in the visuomotor system controlling the generation of saccades. This paradigm is very straightforward and allows the necessary data to be collected very quickly: a total of about 200 saccades, requiring only some 15 minutes of recording time, is sufficient to determine the transition latency in one subject. The same criterion can be applied to data obtained with the random-gap step paradigm without the need for weeding out predictive saccades and without requiring an analysis of the shape of the latency histogram.

Acknowledgment

We would like to thank John van Opstal for his helpful suggestions and time in discussing the design of the curve-fitting procedures.

References

Bahill, A.T., Clark, M.R., & Stark, L., *The main sequence, a tool for studying human eye movements*, Mathematical Biosciences **24** (1975), 191-204.

Bahill, A.T., Kallman, J.S., & Lieberman, J.E., *Frequency limitations of the two points central difference differentiation algorithm*, Biological Cybernetics **45** (1982), 1-4.

Becker, W., & Fuchs, A.F., *Further properties of the human saccadic system: eye movements and correction saccades with and without visual fixation points*, Vision Research **9** (1969), 1247-1258.

Becker, W., & Jürgens, R., *An analysis of the saccadic system by means of double step stimuli*, Vision Research **19** (1979), 967-983.

Bour, L.J., Van Gisbergen, J.A.M., Bruijns, J., & Ottes, F.P., *The double magnetic induction method for measuring eye movements: results in monkey and man*, IEEE Transactions on Biomedical Engineering **BME-31** (1984), 419-427.

Bronstein, A.M., & Kennard, C., *Predictive ocular motor control in Parkinson's disease*, Brain **108** (1985), 925-940.

Bronstein, A.M., & Kennard, C., *Predictive saccades are different from visually triggered saccades*, Vision Research **27** (1987), 517-520.

Bruce, C.J., & Borden, J.A., *The primate frontal eye fields are necessary for predictive saccade tracking*, Society for Neuroscience, Abstracts **12 part 2** (1986), p. 1086.

Bruce, C.J., & Goldberg, M.E., *Primate frontal eye fields. I. Single neurons discharging before saccades*, Journal of Neurophysiology **53** (1985), 603-635.

Dallos, P.H., & Jones, R.W., *Learning behavior of the eye fixation control system*, IEEE Transactions on Automatic Control **AC-8** (1963), 218-227.

Findlay, J.M., *Spatial and temporal factors in the predictive generation of saccadic eye movements*, Vision Research **21** (1981), 347-354.

Fischer, B., *The preparation of visually guided saccades*, Review of Physiology, Biochemistry, and Pharmacology **106** (1987), 1-35.

Fischer, B., & Ramsperger, E., *Human express saccades: extremely short reaction times of goal directed eye movements*, Experimental Brain Research **57** (1984), 191-195.

Fischer, B., & Ramsperger, E., *Human express saccades: effects of randomization and daily practice*, Experimental Brain Research **64** (1986), 569-578.

Guitton, D., Buchtel, H.A., & Douglas, R.M., *Frontal lobe lesions in man cause difficulties in suppressing reflexive glances and in generating goal-directed saccades*, Experimental Brain Research **58** (1985), 455-472.

Hikosaka, O., & Wurtz, R.H., *Visual and oculomotor functions of monkey substantia nigra pars reticulata. I. Relation of visual and auditory responses to saccades*, Journal of Neurophysiology **49** (1983), 1230-1253.

Hikosaka, O., & Wurtz, R.H., *Modification of saccadic eye movements by GABA-related substances. I. Effects of muscimol and bicuculline in monkey superior colliculus*, Journal of Neurophysiology **53** (1985), 266-291.

Kalesnykas, R.P., & Hallett, P.E., *The differentiation of visually guided and anticipatory saccades in gap and overlap paradigms*, Experimental Brain Research **68** (1987), 115-121.

Mays, L.E., & Sparks, D.L., *Dissociation of visual and saccade-related responses in superior colliculus neurons*, Journal of Neurophysiology **43** (1980), 207-232.

Munoz, D.P., & Guitton, D., *Tecto-reticulo-spinal neurons have discharges coding the velocity profiles of eye and head orienting movements*, Society for Neuroscience, Abstracts **13 part 1** (1987), p. 393.

Rabiner, L.R., Gold, B., & McGonegal, C.A., *An approach to the approximation problem for nonrecursive digital filters*, IEEE Transactions on Audio and Electroacoustics **AU-18** (1970), 83-106.

Robinson, D.A., *Eye movements evoked by collicular stimulation in the alert monkey*, Vision Research **12** (1972), 1795-1808.

Robinson, D.A., *Oculomotor control signals*, in "G. Lennerstrand & P. Bach-y-Rita (Eds.), Basic mechanisms of ocular motility and their clinical implications," Pergamon Press, Oxford, 1975, pp. 337-374.

Ron, S., Robinson, D.A., & Skavenski, A.A., *Saccades and the quick phases of nystagmus*, Vision Research **12** (1972), 2015-2022.

Saslow, M.G., *Effects of components of displacement-step stimuli upon latency for saccadic eye movement*, Journal of the Optical Society of America **57** (1967), 1024-1029.

Schiller, P.H., Sandell, J.H., & Maunsell, J.H.R., *The effect of frontal eye field and superior colliculus lesions on saccadic latencies in the rhesus monkey*, Journal of Neurophysiology **57** (1987), 1033-1049.

Smit, A.C., Van Gisbergen, J.A.M., & Cools, A.R., *A parametric analysis of human saccades in different experimental paradigms*, Vision Research **27** (1987), 1745-1762.

Sparks, D.L., *Functional properties of neurons in the monkey superior colliculus: coupling of neuronal activity and saccade onset*, Brain Research **156** (1978), 1-16.

Stark, L., Vossius, G., & Young, R.L., *Predictive control of eye tracking movements*, IRE Transactions on Human Factors in Electronics **HFE-3** (1962), 52-57.

Van Gisbergen, J.A.M., Robinson, D.A., & Gielen, S., *A quantitative analysis of generation of saccadic eye movements by burst neurons*, Journal of Neurophysiology **45** (1981), 417-442.

Van Gisbergen, J.A.M, Van Opstal, A.J., & Schoenmakers, J.J.M., *Experimental test of two models for the generation of oblique saccades*, Experimental Brain Research **57** (1985), 321-336.

Wurtz, R.H., & Goldberg. M.E., *Activity of superior colliculus in behaving monkey. III. Cells discharging before eye movements*, Journal of Neurophysiology **35** (1972), 575-586.

Zambarbieri, D., Schmidt, R., Magenes, G., & Prablanc, C., *Saccadic responses evoked by presentation of visual and auditory targets*, Experimental Brain Research **47** (1982), 417-427.

SACCADIC EYE MOVEMENTS TO TARGETS DEFINED BY STRUCTURE DIFFERENCES

HEINER DEUBEL [1], JOHN FINDLAY [2],
ARTHUR M. JACOBS [3], AND DAVID BROGAN [2,4]

[1] Lehrstuhl für Nachrichtentechnik, Technische Universität München
[2] Department of Psychology, University of Durham
[3] Laboratoire de Psychologie Expérimentale, Université René Descartes, Paris
[4] Department of Experimental Psychology, University of Oxford

1. Introduction

The saccadic eye movement is an extremely simple response. For very many purposes, this response may be adequately specified by just three measures: the instant of initiation and the amplitude of rotation of the eye in horizontal and vertical components. Although other aspects are of considerable interest (torsional components of movement : Ferman, Collewijn, & van den Berg, 1987; variability in trajectory : Findlay & Harris, 1984; Smit, van Gisbergen, & Cools, 1987), they may safely be ignored for the present purpose since they contribute at most, a small perturbation of the effects we shall be describing which are large and systematic. Our aim is to elucidate the way the information from a visual target is processed in order to provide a meaningful signal for saccadic eye movement control.

It will be demonstrated that the signal specifying the required spatial parameters of the saccade shows several unexpected and highly interesting properties. Firstly, the signal depends on visual information which is processed "globally" from a wide area of the visual field. Secondly, the signal depends on simple physical stimulus properties such as target luminance. Thirdly, the signal will be shown to be affected by texture boundaries which means that higher-level visual information processing is also involved. We thus believe it possible that the signal relates to an important early stage in the evaluation of visual information (something similar to the primal sketch described by Marr, 1982) in which visual information is processed in a way which will be perceptually useful.

The essential, characteristic feature common to the experiments presented in the following is that saccadic eye movements have to be directed to targets embedded in a prominent background structure. The systematic investigation of the interaction between background and target in eye movement programming forms a novel aspect in research on sensorimotor processing. It will be suggested that the kind of experimental approach adopted, more than just yielding insights into motor programming, also allows a new, objective way of investigating early visual processing. Therefore, the next two sections will present, firstly, an outline of the evolution of current ideas on saccade programming, and, secondly, basic concepts on early visual processing.

Saccadic programming

Most early work on the control of saccades paid little attention to the spatial aspects of information processing. Two investigative lines can be traced from the classic paper of Westheimer (1954). Firstly, effort was directed to the specification of the control signals to the oculomotor neurons. Robinson's work over a long period (Robinson, 1964, 1982) has shown, in an elegant way, how the neural control systems are adaptively matched to the mechanical properties of the eye musculature. The way in which these signals are elaborated in the neural circuits of the brain stem is also well known (Fuchs, Kaneko, & Scudder, 1985). The second problem concerned the timing of saccades. Appreciating that some control process was in operation to prevent saccades occurring in too rapid succession, the suggestion of a "sampled data" system arose. In its most extreme form (Young & Stark, 1962), it suggested that the angle between desired angle of gaze (target position) and actual eye position is sampled every 200 ms and when this angle is sufficiently large (outside a postulated dead zone), a saccade results at about the time of the next sample (i.e. with a latency of 200 ms).

The "sampled data" model makes definite predictions concerning the outcome of when a target is tracked which is moving in a series of steps. Certain results from such studies are incompatible with the sampled data model. For example, Wheeless, Boynton, and Cohen (1966) showed that when tracking targets that jumped twice with an interval between the jumps of 100 ms, 77% of the saccades ignored the first target step and moved straight to the position after the end of the second step. Such a result suggests that information about target behaviour can influence a saccade if it occurs within 100 ms of its onset. A model with more flexibility was introduced by Becker and Jürgens (1979) which has strongly influenced subsequent thinking about the saccadic system.

The results on which this model is based come from experiments on tracking double steps with the eye. The cases of particular interest are those in which the second step of the target occurs while the saccade elicited by the first step is still in preparation. The second step may then be regarded as a perturbing influence on the process of saccade preparation. Becker and Jürgens (1979) pointed out that much of the variability that characterizes the responses can be accounted for by taking note of the exact point at which this perturbing influence occurs in the preparation process. This may be demonstrated as follows. If the time between the second (perturbing) target step and the first saccade is denoted by D, then a plot may be made in which the amplitude of the saccade is shown for each value of D. Such a plot, termed "amplitude transition function" shows how the perturbation systematically influences the saccade. The amplitude takes a range of values: for small values of D, the perturbing step has no effect and the saccades go to the first target position; for sufficiently large values of D, the saccades ignore the first step and go to the second target position. For intermediate values, saccades are found with intermediate amplitudes and a systematic transition between the two limits is evident.

The model postulates two stages in the preparation of a saccade. The first (decision process) decides when a saccade will occur and also which direction it will take (the saccades in Becker and Jürgens's study were all horizontal). The second process (amplitude computation) is activated by a trigger from the decision mechanism and is responsible for the programming of the amplitude of the saccade as described in the next paragraph. In addition to providing a good account of experimental results, the model bears promising correspondence with known physiological processing in the brainstem oculomotor areas (Fuchs, Kaneko, & Scudder, 1985).

The process of amplitude computation is modelled as an automatic piece of sensory input processing (see also Deubel, 1986). Becker and Jürgens (1979) viewed this process as one involving temporal integration. Rather than using instantaneous values of target position, the operation used an integrated value within a particular temporal window. When the window included the second target step, the window would include contributions from both target positions and thus arrive at an intermediate value for the saccade amplitude. The temporal integration can thus account for saccades directed to intermediate positions and also for the transition shown in the amplitude transition function.

Although Becker and Jürgens emphasized the temporal aspect of the integration, the model, in fact, involves a spatio-temporal integration since the parameter which is being integrated is the spatial target position. A slightly different paradigm shows clearly that spatial integration is an integral aspect of the programming of saccade amplitude. This comes from studies of saccades to targets which consist of two separate elements in neighbouring positions (double targets). In this situation, the first saccade made is directed to an intermediate position between the targets. This result, termed the "centre of gravity" effect or "global" effect, was first noted by Coren and Hoenig (1972).

The "global effect" forms a central aspect of the work presented in this paper. It is important to note from the previous investigations that the weight of an individual stimulus as reflected in the exact saccade landing position in between the targets depends systematically on various relative visual properties of the targets. So, if one target is made larger (Findlay, 1982), more intense (Deubel & Wolf, 1982; Deubel, Wolf, & Hauske, 1984), presented with higher contrast (Deubel & Hauske, 1988), or with a higher dot density (Menz & Groner, 1987), the first saccade lands closer to this target. Also, it has been demonstrated that the target weight depends critically on the spatial frequency content of the stimuli (Deubel, 1984) in a manner closely related to the modulation transfer function of the peripheral visual system (Koenderink & van Doorn, 1978). This observation leads to the idea that the saccadic response to spatial stimuli might elucidate properties of the sensory visual pathways. In fact, Deubel et al. (1984) proposed that the saccadic "amplitude transition function" found in double step experiments (Becker & Jürgens, 1979) is simply the result of spatio-temporal filtering in the sensory visual pathways.

The results presented above all show the influence exerted by sensory factors in the spatial averaging involved in saccade control. On the other hand, saccadic eye movements are clearly motor responses which can obviously be controlled at a volitional level. This might suggest that the direction of saccades to an intermediate position reflects some strategy designed to optimise visual information intake. However, the findings described above show that saccades land nearer to the target which should be most visible. This point is difficult to reconcile with such a strategic view. Further, a number of studies have examined the extent to which voluntary strategies can overcome the global tendency (Findlay, 1981, 1985; Ottes, van Gisbergen, & Eggermont, 1985; Coeffé & O'Regan, 1987; Jacobs, 1987). These demonstrate a very interesting pattern in which the global effect is present for short latency saccades but may be overridden by voluntary effort if there is a delay in the initiation of a saccade. In addition, extensive training produces some modification to the global effect (Findlay & Crawford, 1983). Nevertheless, the description given by Ottes et al. (1985) that the global effect is the default option for the saccadic system seems most in accordance with the findings.

Early visual processing

There has been much debate in recent years about the types of research strategy that are most useful in approaching early visual perception. The most traditional strategy has been to build on neurophysiological findings, taking into account the increasingly well documented properties of neurons in the visual pathways. An approach which was originally grounded in neurophysiological findings but which developed its own autonomy, has been the postulation of spatial frequency channels. An important advance in visual science has been the development of the channel concept and particularly, the suggestion that a set of spatial frequency channels is involved in spatial vision in a way analogous to the involvement of colour mechanisms in colour vision.

Marr (1976, 1982) argued convincingly that this channel approach on its own was inadequate. He pointed out the necessity of identifying the computational goals of vision, and then to develop suitable algorithms for the implementation of these goals. These algorithms would make use of the "hardware" revealed by neurophysiological work. In practice, his detailed work on the primal sketch (Marr & Hildreth, 1980) is characterized by a brilliant synthesis of the neurophysiological and the computational approaches into a theory in which the computational goal is to construct a "raw primal sketch," the function of which is to form a representation of an image in terms of its edges.

Another major contribution to the study of early visual perception has come from the work of Julesz. To an even greater extent than Marr, the approach of Julesz is deliberately independent of neurophysiological findings (e.g. Julesz & Schumer, 1981). Apart from the wellknown work in stereopsis, another thrust of Julesz's work has been concerned with the segmentation of the visual scene on the basis of differences in visual characteristics and particularly, differences in microtexture. These studies have led to a large body of work on human texture discrimination (for reviews see Julesz & Bergen, 1983; Julesz, 1986). A basic assumption is that human vision operates into two distinct modes which are denoted as *preattentive* and *attentive* vision. According to the definition given by Julesz, preattentive visual processing allows the instantaneous discrimination of different texture areas. Julesz uses the term texton to denote the micropatterns constituting textured areas. Preattentive vision then reflects a system working in parallel over a large part of the visual field, acting almost instantaneously, and indicating *where* texton gradients occur. Attentive vision, on the other hand, involves a serial stepwise search using a small focus of attention. Attentive vision is required to determine *what* the textons are. It is suggested that the essential functional role of preattentive vision is, through instantaneous texture discrimination, to direct focal attention to locations in the visual field where texture gradients occur, allowing subsequent analysis by the attentive system. This leads to the idea that preattentive processing should deliver essential signals for the guidance of the eye when viewing complex visual structures. The question thus arises whether preattentive texture discrimination can immediately affect the signals relevant for saccadic eye movement control.

Visual processing for target oriented eye movements

In this paper, we present results from two separate and largely independent experimental programmes which both address the problem of how visual information is processed in order to extract the appropriate signals for eye movement control. The first experiment (Durham experiment) is aimed at linking the "global effect" to work in the tradition of visual channels. The second set of experiments investigates the role of preattentive texture discrimination in saccade control. Although the two experimental approaches differ in detail, they both extend the previous work on the global effect in two ways. Firstly, more complex targets are used, thus increasing our knowledge of the properties of the visual channels which are requisite to saccade programming. Secondly, both studies present targets against a structured background. All previous studies of the global effect have looked at saccades to targets presented against a uniform background. This situation is clearly artificial and the dangers of following lines of research which lack ecological validity have been strongly emphasized in recent years.

A number of observations summarized in the previous sections are consistent with the view that the signal for target oriented saccades might reflect mainstream visual processing. This suggestion is supported by results we report here, particularly those of the Munich experiments (Chapter 3), in which it is shown that signals which lead to early segregation based on texture differences will also influence the grouping shown in the saccadic global effect. We believe that this is a finding of considerable importance since it also implies that the study of spatial integration in the signal for saccades may be able to shed light on one of the processes operating in early vision.

2. Durham Experiment (Experiment 1)

The general introduction has suggested that target elicited saccades are directed to a locus which is the centre of gravity of the target configuration. The concern in this experiment was to attempt to link this finding with work in the tradition of visual channels. A large body of psychophysical data may be interpreted by assuming that the visual signal is processed through a series of channels, each responding to a filtered representation of the retinal stimulation (Wilson & Bergen, 1979; Regan, 1982). The critical stimulus variable in this filtered representation which generates activity in the channel is stimulus contrast. For many purposes the channels are regarded as linear, although it is recognized that the concept of linearity may possess several interpretations. So, several results suggest that, in addition to linear processing, substantial nonlinear processing also takes place. Henning, Hertz, and Broadbent (1975) demonstrated interactions between a low frequency grating and a low frequency envelope of amplitude modulation produced by the combination of high frequency gratings. The latter contains no spectral low frequency component and thus such interaction implies significant nonlinear processing. Shapley and Gordon (1985) show that some even nonlinear function of contrast is used in segregating patterns from background. The following experiment will demonstrate nonlinear properties of information processing in saccade control.

2.1 Methods

Stimuli and procedure

The requirement was to generate stimuli that had both positive and negative contrast differences and also stimuli whose spatial frequency components were restricted, particularly in the low spatial frequency part of the spectrum. The

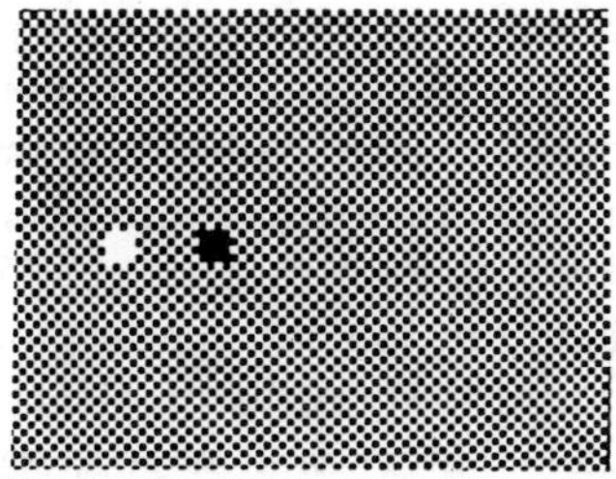

Fig. 1: Example of targets used in Experiment 1. Positive and negative contrast targets presented against the coarse checkerboard background. The figure is photographed from the VDU screen used in the experiment.

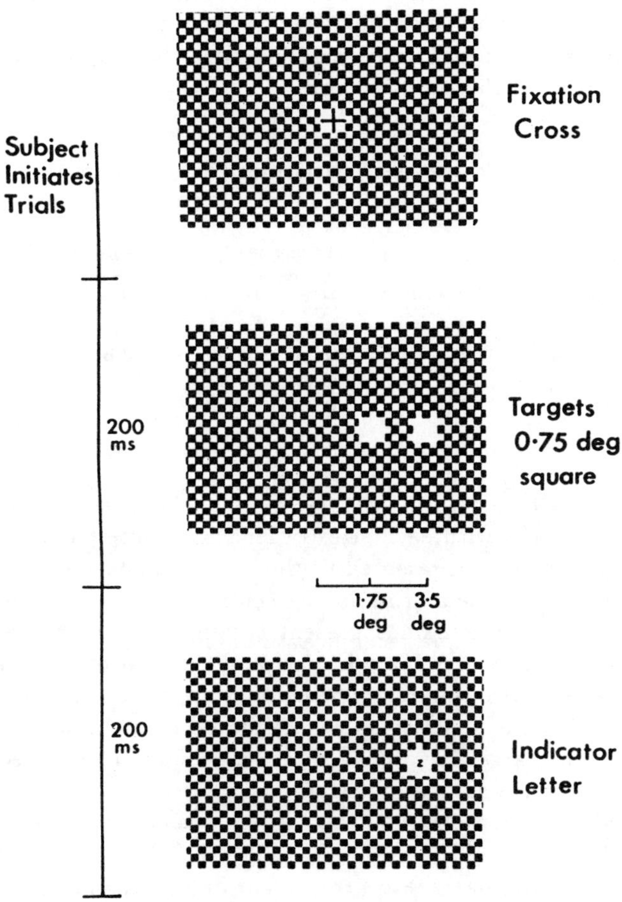

Fig. 2 : The stimulus sequence used in the Experiment 1. Targets etc. are not drawn to scale (see Figure 1).

realization of these requirements was achieved using a standard microcomputer-generated display with raster scan graphics. Figure 1 shows the type of display adopted. The screen was programmed with a checkerboard pattern which formed a background of intermediate luminance upon which both positive and negative contrast targets could be superimposed. Additionally, targets of the same space averaged luminance as the background could be generated by phase reversing the checks in the target region. Thus, the targets always had the same check size as the background. The stimuli were generated using a BBC B microcomputer and presented on a Phillips TP-200 monitor (30 cm screen, P31 phosphor) which was chosen because of its exceptionally stable and well focused display. The display (640 x 256 pixels) was viewed from a distance of 85 cm and subtended a visual angle of 10.5 ° (horizontal) x 7.5 ° (vertical). The space average luminance of the various targets was measured with a UDT 111 photometer and is shown in Table 1 together with the spatial frequency of the diagonal component of the checkerboard.

Tab. 1: Parameters of displays used in Experiment 1

	Target Luminance cd / sq m	Target Spatial frequency c p d
Small checks	13.4	15.2
Medium checks	13.7	7.6
Large checks	13.1	3.8
White targets	33.3	
Black targets	0.2	

Each subject was tested with the three sizes of checks shown in Table 1 and performed three blocks with each size (order was counterbalanced). Figure 2 shows the display sequence presented to the subject on each trial. Initially, the subject was asked to fixate a cross in the centre of the screen with a uniform check background which remained present throughout. When ready, the subject initiated the trial by pressing a button and the fixation cross was replaced by the target (one or two squares) which could appear either on the left or on the right). After 200 ms, the targets were replaced by an indicator letter which occupied one of the target positions on the same side. The subject's task was to indicate whether the indicator letter was a vowel or a consonant. In this way, the saccadic eye movement to the targets was elicited as an integral part of a visual task.

Trials were presented in blocks of 60. In each block one particular check size was used and 4 examples of each of fifteen target types occur in a randomly permuted order. The fifteen target types were as follows :

1 - 3.	Single squares at 1.75 deg	Black, White, Checked
4 - 6.	Single squares at 3.50 deg	Black, White, Checked
7 - 15.	Double squares	Black + Black, White + White
	(at 1.75 and 3.5 deg)	Black + White, White + Black
		White + Check, Black+ Check
		Check + White, Check+ Black
		Check + Check

Data will be presented from three subjects, two of the authors (JF and DB) and another laboratory worker. Two further subjects gave data which confirmed the general patterns, but the eye movement records were noisy and thus have not been included in the analysis. Eye movements were recorded from subjects JF and DB using a search coil technique based on that of Collewijn, van der Mark and Janssen (1975). Eye movements from subject RB were recorded using the fibre optic probe technique (Findlay, 1974). The eye movement signal was digitized with a 5 ms sampling rate.

Each subject carried out three blocks with each of the target check sizes. Thus for each target configuration, 12 saccades were recorded (six leftwards and six rightwards). Trials were excluded from the analysis for the following reasons (i) anticipatory saccades occurred with latency less than 100 ms; (ii) latency of the first saccade was above a criterion level (250 ms in amplitude analyses: 300 ms in latency analyses); (iii) blinks or other contaminating factors. Very few saccades were eliminated under criteria (i) and (iii) but criterion (ii) occurred quite frequently with fine grain checkerboard targets.

2.2 Results

Target detectability

A subsidiary test examined the subject's abilities to detect the checkerboard target at the test eccentricities. Subjects were presented with a display in which the target was exposed for 200 ms and asked to indicate on which side of the fixation point it occurred. Subjects JF and RB had no difficulty with this task but for subject DB the finest checkerboard target was close to threshold level when presented in the 3.5 ° position.

Saccade amplitudes

Table 2 shows saccade amplitudes for each subject and check size. The standard deviation of the amplitudes over a set of trials was typically 0.3 ° for the near single and double targets, rising to a slightly greater value (0.4 °) for single targets in the far position. Saccades to double targets, in general, showed no greater variability than those to single targets.

Saccades to single targets show small undershoots with some variability from block to block. As discussed in Findlay (1982), uncertainties about the accuracy of fixation during calibration can contribute to apparent variability in

Tab. 2: Saccadic amplitudes for each subject and check size

	B–	W–	C–	BB	BC	BW	CB	CC	CW	WB	WC	WW	–B	–C	–W
Small checks															
DB	1.65	1.56	1.66	2.37	1.61	2.39	2.88	1.83	3.06	2.29	1.67	2.36	2.99	n.a	2.91
JF	1.57	1.65	1.59	2.08	1.69	2.32	2.68	2.07	2.70	2.09	1.66	2.05	3.15	3.27	3.20
RB	1.44	1.50	1.46	1.83	1.49	1.92	2.28	1.78	2.07	1.92	1.53	1.66	2.50	2.53	2.38
Medium checks															
DB	1.57	1.43	1.63	2.45	1.62	2.42	2.40	1.49	2.23	2.22	1.61	2.25	2.17	2.79	2.87
JF	1.62	1.61	1.59	2.10	1.75	2.13	2.63	2.09	2.25	2.19	1.71	1.90	3.08	2.98	3.10
RB	1.35	1.32	1.31	1.84	1.62	1.84	2.04	1.42	1.73	1.92	1.63	1.74	2.46	2.62	2.50
Large checks															
DB	1.97	1.85	1.81	2.51	2.76	2.79	2.18	2.35	2.29	2.28	2.47	2.31	3.13	3.03	3.17
JF	1.36	1.41	1.42	1.57	1.92	1.63	1.83	1.57	1.62	1.81	1.86	1.66	2.80	2.73	2.64
RB	1.50	1.59	1.52	2.30	2.20	2.38	1.92	2.00	2.18	2.10	2.19	2.02	3.54	3.49	3.25

amplitude of small saccades. For this reason, the data were normalized by using the saccades to single targets as a reference. This normalization was carried out as follows to provide a figure for the global effect overshoot. For each block, denote the mean amplitude of all saccades to single targets in the near position (An) and the mean amplitude of all saccades in the far position (Af). For a target configuration resulting in a mean saccade amplitude of A, the global effect overshoot is calculated as (A - An)/(Af - An). This results in a very consistent pattern as shown in Figure 3.

In Figure 3, the data from positive contrast targets (white squares) and negative contrast targets (black squares) have been combined. As can be seen from the table, the sign of the contrast exerts very little effect, confirming the previous report by Zetzsche et al. (1984). Likewise, positive contrast and negative contrast targets gave very similar weightings in the centre of gravity combination when they were combined with checkerboards. When a square with a luminance difference was paired with a square without any overall luminance difference (phase reversed checkerboard), the result depended upon the check spacing. Stimuli with the finest check size showed only a small contribution to the centre of gravity calculation but targets with large check size appeared, at least, as effective as targets with overall luminance change.

As will be discussed in more detail in Chapter 4, these findings provide a consistent picture of the visual channels used in saccade elicitation. It is clear that a highly non-linear process is involved in which the spatial integration is performed on a signal preprocessed in such a way that the sign of the contrast is unimportant. The differential effect of the different checkerboard sizes shows that some filtering has already occurred. The check size that shows the greatest

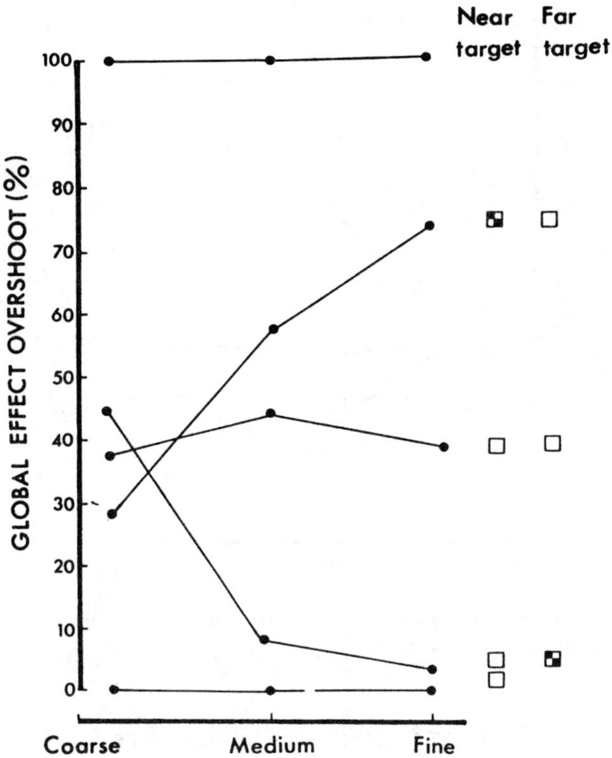

Fig. 3 : Figure summarising the results of the saccade amplitude measure. The amplitudes are normalised to the mean amplitudes for single targets (these are plotted as 0% and 100%). For double square targets, the data for positive and negative luminance contrast targets have been pooled.

salience has a principal spatial frequency which is close to the optimal for the location used (2 - 4 °) in the near periphery (Rovamo et al. 1978). This suggests that the channels involved in perception, at threshold, have access to the saccade control system.

A plot of the latencies of saccades to the different target types is presented in Figure 4 and shows some features of interest. When single checkerboard targets are used, decreasing the check size leads to a substantial and systematic increase in latency. This is reminiscent of similar spatial frequency dependent changes in latency when other measures are taken (reaction times, Vassilev & Mitov, 1976; visual evoked potentials, Parker & Salzen, 1977). Targets with luminance contrast, whether single or double, show saccade latencies of 160 - 180 ms (it seems unwise to attach any major importance to the small latency difference between conditions for these targets).

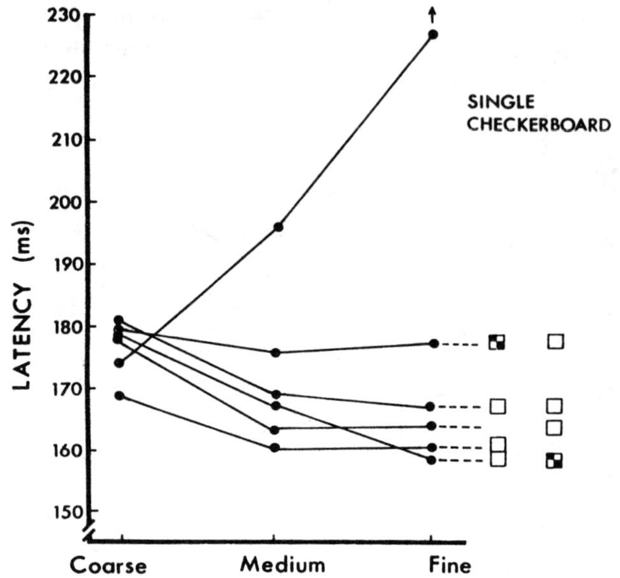

Fig. 4 : Data on saccade latencies for various types of targets. Results from positive and negative luminance targets have been pooled.

3. Munich experiments (Experiments 2 - 7)*

The aim of the following experiments was to systematically investigate the effect of presence of background texture on saccadic eye movements in a target/nontarget situation. It is evident that our natural visual environment is normally characterized by highly complex visual structure in which objects ("foreground") have first to be segregated from the background in order to become potential targets for eye movements. This was the rationale for using stimuli in which foreground/background segregation is a necessary prerequisite for saccadic programming. It seemed reasonable to hypothesize that under these conditions the salience of an individual target should be related to its structure difference to the background. In order to test this hypothesis we used stimuli in which the dissimilarity to the background could be varied systematically. Stimuli of this kind have already been used by other authors in the context of investigations on texture perception (e.g. Julesz & Bergen, 1983; Nothdurft, 1985). The results will demonstrate that texture discontinuities form an important determinant in saccade programming.

*A short version of the results have been published in Deubel et al., 1987.

3.1 Methods

Apparatus

The visual stimuli consisted in computer-generated half-tone images of 512 by 512 pixels, loaded into an image memory system (Kürzinger & Deubel, 1986). Since the total available image memory was 8 Mbytes, all the different images necessary for an individual session (up to 56) were then resident in hardware memory and could be arbitrarily presented in realtime. For stimulus presentation, a high resolution video display with a width of 30 cm was used. Frame frequency was set to 110 Hz. Background luminance of the screen and illuminance of a surrounding mask of 1.20 m by 1.20 m was adjusted to 10 cd/m^2.

In total, 5 naive subjects participated in the experiments. They were set at a viewing distance of 1 m from the display screen. Head movements were restricted by a forehead holder and a biteboard made from deep dental impressions. Eye movements were recorded monocularly by an infrared technique (Bach et al., 1983) with a resolution of 4 min of arc. The analogue signal was digitized at 500 Hz and stored on magnetic disk for off-line analysis.

The stimulus scene consisted of texture images composed of short line elements of specific luminance and orientation (Figure 5). For this purpose, the display, with a total width of 17 ° of visual angle, was filled with 32 times 32 line elements, resulting in an interelement distance of 0.53 °. Element length was 0.47 ° of visual angle. In order to avoid local energy variations, it was taken care that all elements were composed of the same number of pixels, independent of their orientation.

By definition, the scene consisted of "background," "target" and "distractor." Except for the reference experiment (c.f. Exp 2), the whole display was filled by texture ("background"). The luminance of the line elements forming the background was adjusted to 20 cd/m^2. Within the background texture, a bar-like "target" (T) and a "distractor" (D) were defined, forming vertically elongated areas in which line luminance or line orientation differed from the background structure. In the cases in which the objects were luminance-defined, element luminance was adjusted to 30 cd/m^2. In general, the "targets" were composed of 1 by 19 elements, equivalent to a height of 10.1 ° of visual angle. The "distractors" extended 4 by 13 elements, equivalent to a width of 2.1 ° and a height of 6.9 °. Also, a fixation cross (F) was present. The angular distance between the fixation cross and the target (F-T) was varied randomly between values of 7.4, 9.5 and 12.7 degrees. In the trials including the presence of a distractor, the distractor appeared at a distance of 2.9 ° from the target (D-T), and either with smaller or with larger eccentricity than the target. The data shown in the Result section mainly stem from trials in which the distractor eccentricity was smaller than the target eccentricity. Moreover, the data

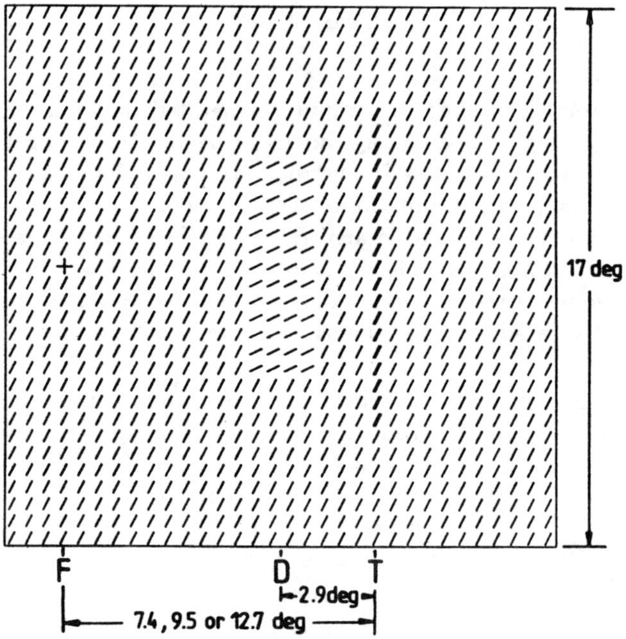

Fig. 5: Example for the stimulus scenes used in the experiments (from Experiment 4). The diagram also gives stimuli sizes and eccentricities in degree of visual angle. The scene is composed of background structure upon which the fixation cross F, target T and distractor D are superimposed. The luminance of the line elements forming the background was adjusted to 20 cd/m^2 Target and distractor form vertically elongated areas in which line luminance or line orientation differed from the background structure. In the cases in which these foreground objects were luminance-defined, element luminance was adjusted to 30 cd/m^2. The target is composed of 1 by 19 elements while the distractor extends 4 by 13 elements. The angular distance between the fixation cross and the target (F-T) was varied randomly from trial to trial between values of 7.4, 9.5 and 12.7 degrees. In the trials including the presence of a distractor, the distractor appeared at a distance of 2.9 ° from the target (D-T), and either with smaller or with larger eccentricity than the target.

shown in the amplitude histograms only include the saccadic responses to the targets presented at 9.5 degrees of eccentricity.

Procedure

Before the session, the subject was shown the stimulus scene and was informed about the target definition. The experimental sequence started with the presentation of a fixation cross on one side of a blank display. After a delay selected randomly between 600 and 1500 ms, the visual scene including background structure, target, and, in half of the trials, distractor appeared abruptly. The subject had to saccade to the target "as fast and precisely as possible" and then to keep fixation on an additional pixel within the target bar which was only visible foveally. After about 500 ms of fixation, the screen was blanked and the fixation cross reappeared, now on the other side of the display. After refixation, the next trial was started.

An additional pilot experiment (Exp 7) was aimed at testing the effect of spatial frequency discontinuities on saccadic amplitude computation. For this purpose, a stimulus scene was used in which the "background" consisted of a vertical sinusoidal grating with a spatial frequency of 1.5 c/° and 25% contrast. The subject had to saccade from a fixation cross to a small, high-contrast dark line embedded in the background. In half of the trials of each session, an additional distractor was present consisting in an area of the grating in which spatial frequency was higher than in the rest of the scene. Target and distractor eccentricities were chosen as in the previously described paradigm.

3.2 Results

Reference experiment

In Experiment 2, parameters of saccadic reactions to targets given without presence of background structure were investigated. Otherwise, the experimental procedure was as described in the Methods section. The results give a baseline for saccadic latency and accuracy.

Figure 6 displays stimulus scenes from the reference experiment (Exp 2) together with representative distributions of the amplitudes of the primary saccades (subject Th). In this and in the following plots, amplitude data are given as percentages of total target eccentricity. The diagram inset gives the mean saccadic latency (T), mean saccadic amplitudes (A, in percent) and the total number of trials (N) included in the data. The left part of the figure represents data from the case in which no distractor was present. As expected, this is a very easy task for the subjects to accomplish. As a consequence, the precision of the saccades is high yielding standard deviations of 5% or less for the tested subjects. As usual, a slight undershoot to the target position can be observed; mean amplitudes are generally slightly smaller than 100%. Mean latencies range from 180 to 240 ms for different subjects.

The right part of Figure 6 shows the stimulus scene and the distribution of saccadic amplitudes under the condition when the target and distractor were simultaneously presented, which was given in the other half of the trials in each experimental session. Here, the saccadic responses clearly show spatial averaging. The distribution is shifted considerably towards the distractor leading to a reduced saccadic amplitude. Generally, the amplitude histograms remain unimodal. Also, it was found that the additional presentation of a distractor had no significant effect on mean saccadic latencies. Note again that all diagrams (except for Figure 7c) only include data from trials in which the distractor appeared between the fixation mark and target. It should be mentioned that for

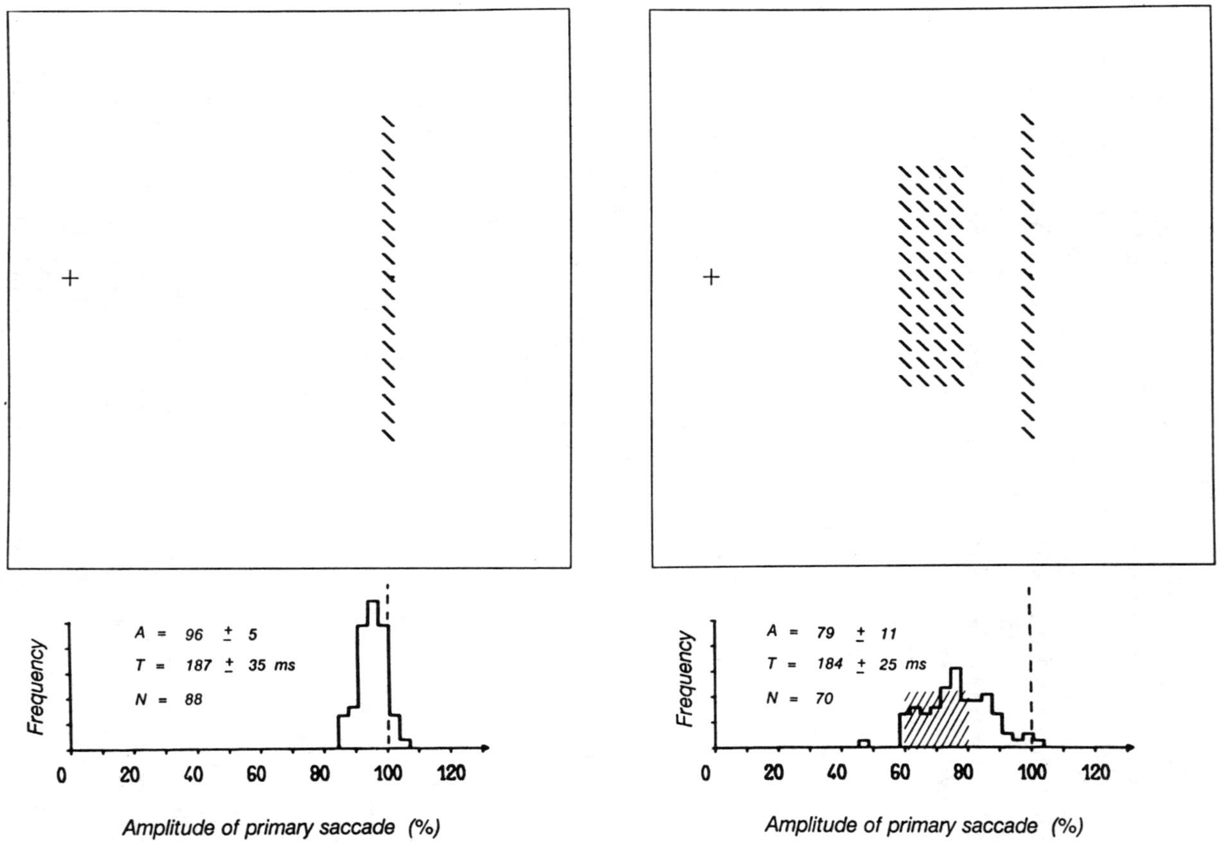

Fig. 6: Stimulus scenes and saccadic amplitude distributions from the reference experiment (Exp. 2). The subject has to saccade horizontally from the fixation cross to the elongated target bar which is composed of short line elements. Left: Single target situation. Right: An additional distractor is present. The hatched area in the amplitude histogram denotes the distractor position. The insets in the diagrams present mean saccadic amplitudes A in percent of total target eccentricity, mean latency T of primary saccades and the number N of trials included in the data.

the cases in which the distractor eccentricity was larger than target eccentricity, the amount of distraction was in general smaller.

Luminance versus texture (Experiment 3)

In the following experiments a background structure was present in which the bar-like target was embedded. Again, in half of the cases, an additional distractor was also embedded in the scene. Target and distractor were defined by their difference to the background structure; more specifically, either by a luminance or orientation difference, yielding four different combinations of target/distractor qualities.

In the first of these experiments, target and distractor were defined by luminance difference. Figure 7 displays examples for the stimuli and the resulting saccadic amplitude histograms. Figure 7a represents data from trials in which no additional distractor was present (single target situation). Although this situation looks considerably more complex due to the background structure, the subjects obviously had no problem in performing the task. This is reflected in the maintained high saccadic accuracy yielding low standard deviations in the cases without the presence of a distractor. Also, the size of saccadic undershoot remains unchanged. Some additional information processing, however, is reflected in the slightly higher saccadic latencies. For this subject, mean saccadic latency increased from 187 ms in the condition without background to 216 ms in the situation in which background structure was present.

Another important finding is that the additional presence of a distractor led to averaging responses, directing the eye to locations between the target and distractor. This is demonstrated in Figure 7b and c; showing stimuli and data for cases in which the distractor was presented at a smaller and larger eccentricity than the target, respectively. It can be seen that the distractor presentation yielded reduced mean saccadic amplitudes (86%) in the first case and increased amplitudes (110%) in the latter case. It can be concluded that the effective saccadic goal is constituted from some spatial center of gravity of the target and distractor, which is largely determined independent of the presence or absence of a background structure. Also, it should be mentioned that within the range of the resulting saccadic latencies, no significant latency-dependent effects on the amplitudes of the saccades were observed.

In the experiment described previously, the target was defined by a first-order statistical difference (=luminance difference) to the background structure. Here the question arises as to whether the saccadic system can perform equally well with targets defined by second-order statistical differences (=orientation differences) of their elements. This was investigated by using the paradigm displayed in Figure 8. Here, target (and distractor) were equiluminant and displayed with an orientation difference of 90 ° with respect to the background elements. The left part of Figure 8 represents stimulus and data from single target trials. The

Figure 7

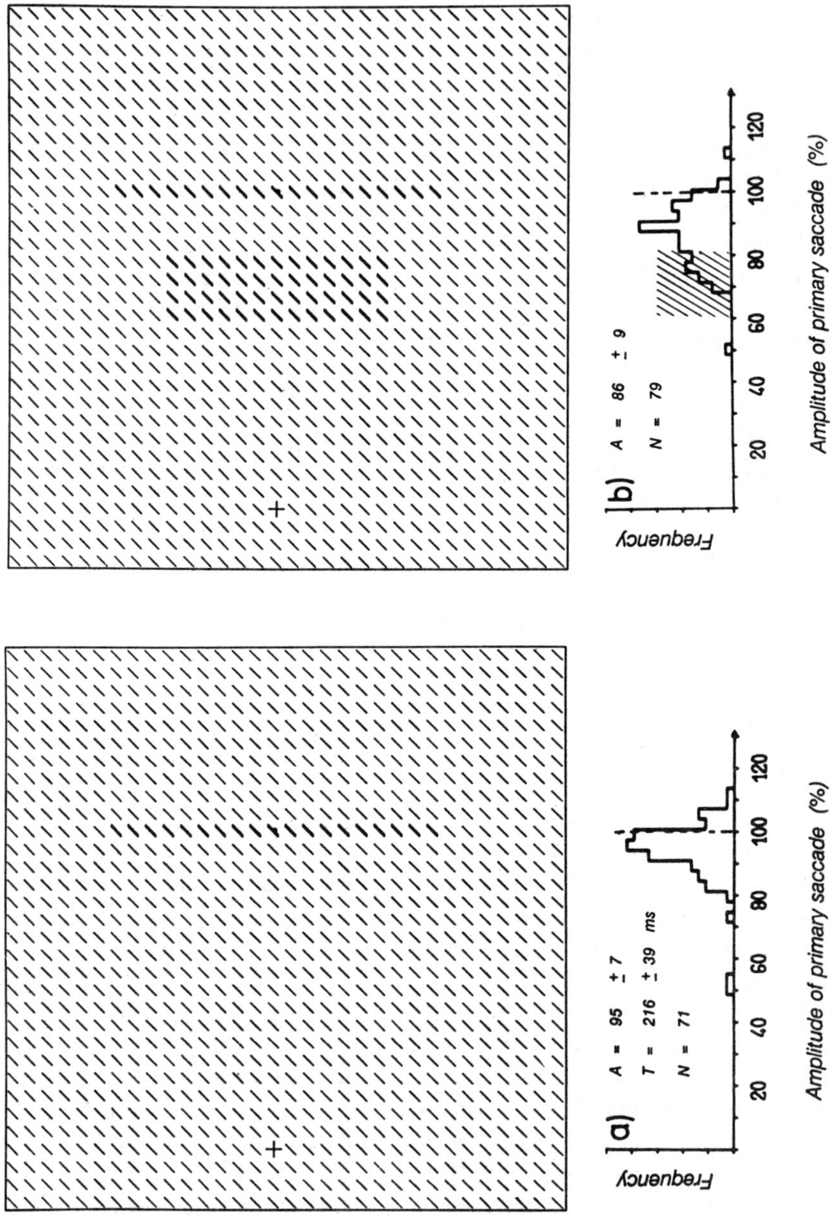

a)
A = 95 ± 7
T = 216 ± 39 ms
N = 71
Frequency
20
40
60
80
100
120
Amplitude of primary saccade (%)
b)
A = 86 ± 9
N = 79
Frequency
20
40
60
80
100
120
Amplitude of primary saccade (%)

Figure 7 continued

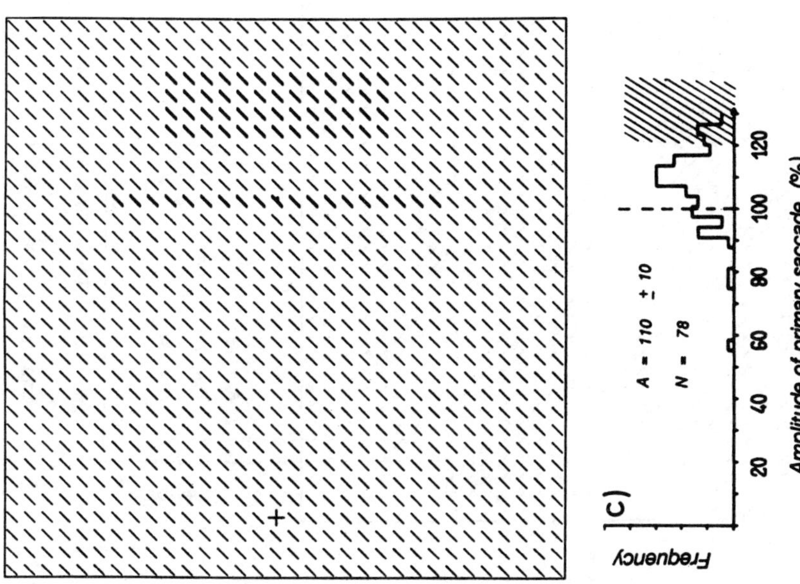

Fig. 7: Stimulus scenes and resulting saccade amplitude data from Experiment 3. In this experiment, target and distractor differ from the background structure in the higher luminance of their elements. Fig. 7a: Single target situation. Fig. 7b and 7c: An additional distractor is present at smaller and larger retinal eccentricities than the target, respectively.

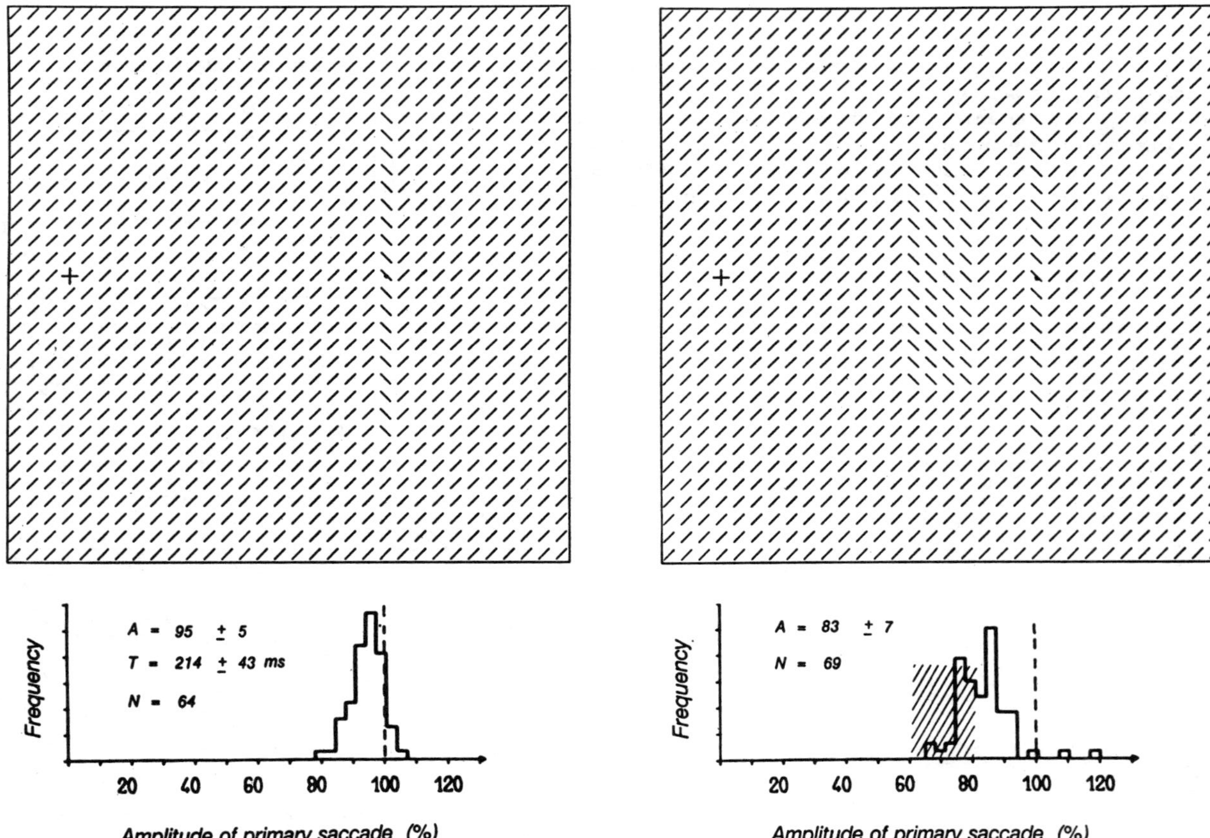

Fig. 8: Stimulus scenes and resulting saccade amplitude data from experiments in which target and distractor differ from the background structure in the orientation of their elements (Experiment 3).

data demonstrate that the performance of the saccadic system with targets defined only by texture differences is virtually identical to the performance with luminance-defined stimuli. Also in this case, movement precision is high and the data show low standard deviations. The right part of the figure shows the effect of the presence of the distractor. As can be seen from the shift of the amplitude histogram and the reduced mean saccade amplitude, presentation of a texture-defined distractor induces averaging responses directed to a location between target and distractor.

The data have demonstrated an interaction in saccadic programming producing a global effect due to spatially separated stimuli defined by their luminance or, for the second case, by their element orientation. The important question arises if this averaging response is still present when the simultaneously presented stimuli are defined by differing visual qualities. This was investigated using scenes as displayed in Figure 9. The left part of Figure 9 shows a visual scene in which the target is luminance-defined while the distractor is texure-defined. In the right part of Figure 9, these relations are reversed. The saccade data from these experimental sessions (not shown here in detail) clearly revealed that the global effect is still present when the target and distractor differ qualitatively.

This is demonstrated in Table 3, summarizing the amount of distraction for the different combinations of target and distractor qualities for two subjects. The largest effect was induced in the case in which no background was present. All other combinations of texture- and luminance-defined stimuli, however, also yield highly significant averaging effects.

Tab. 3: Percentage amount of distraction for the different combinations of target and distractor definitions, given for two subjects (Th and Ma).

Target	Tex	Lum	Lum	Tex	no
Distractor	Lum	Lum	Tex	Tex	background
Th	14.5	16.4	20.1	24.6	25
Ma	5.3	8.3	13.75	11	15.1

Figure 10 shows the mean latencies of the primary saccades for luminance-defined targets, texture-defined targets, and for the case without background for five subjects. It can be seen that latencies increase by 20-40 ms due to the background. The longest latencies occur for the case of luminance-defined stimuli.

Orientation difference dependency

Experiment 4 was aimed to quantitatively relate the amount of distraction to the orientation difference of the distractor elements with respect to the background. During the experimental sessions, the orientation differences were selected randomly from values between 0 and 65 °.

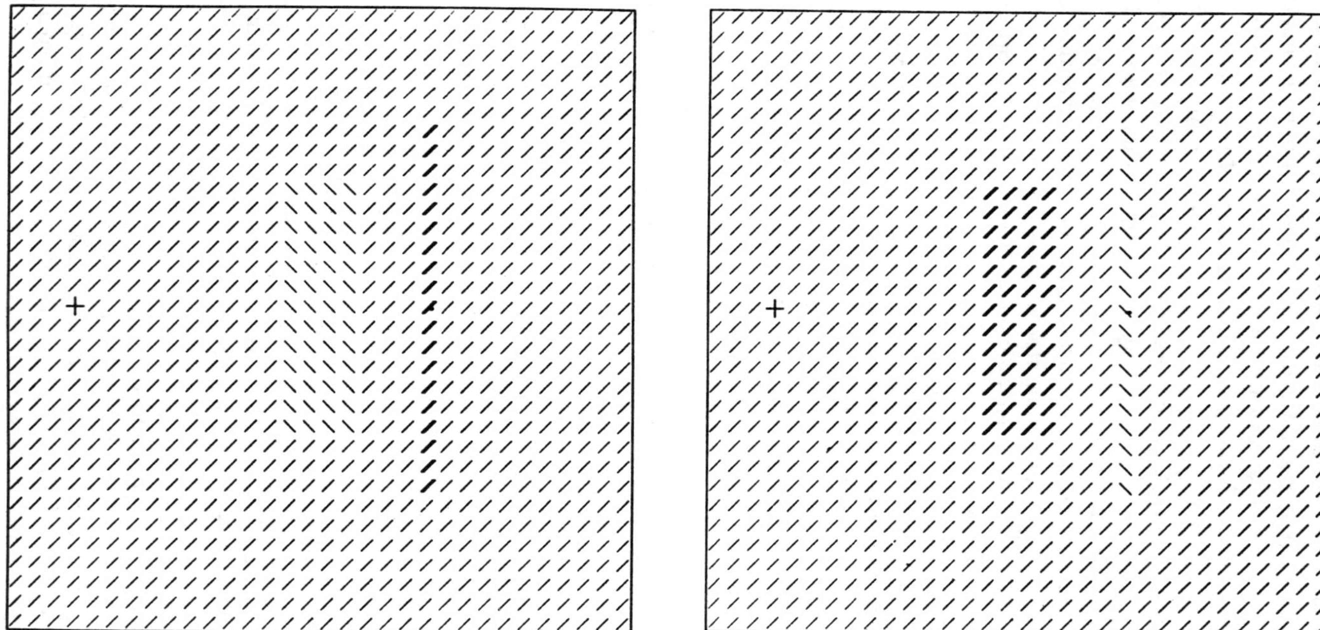

Fig. 9: Stimulus scenes from experiments in which target and distractor are defined by **differing** visual qualities (Experiment 3). Left scene: target is luminance-defined, distractor is texture-defined. Right scene: target is texture-**defined**, distractor is luminance-defined.

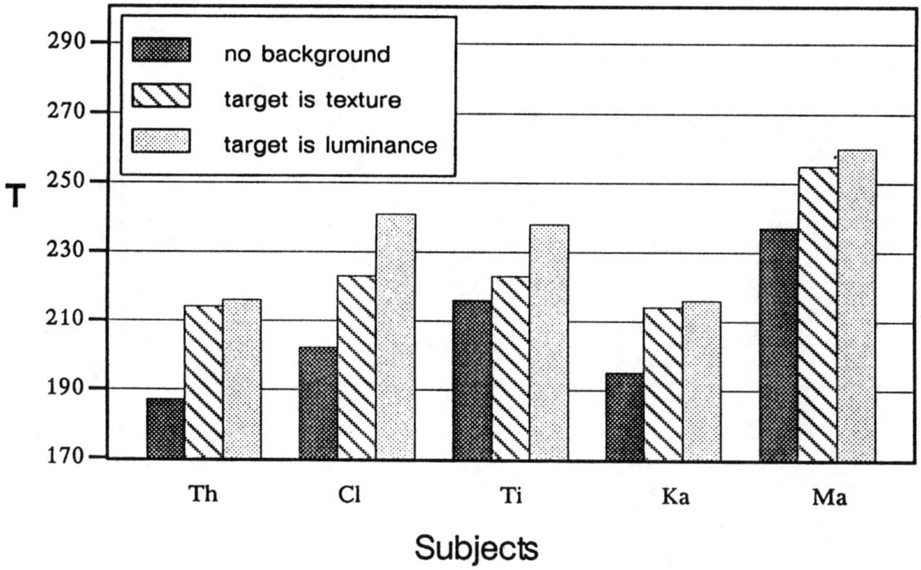

Fig. 10: Mean latencies of primary saccades for the different experimental situations in Experiment 3, given for five subjects. Data stem from experiments in which no background is present, or in which the target differs from the background in its luminance or texture, respectively.

Figure 11 sketches characteristic examples of the visual scenes and the resulting amplitude distributions. It can be seen that the amount of distraction was immediately related to the orientation difference. Figure 12 summarizes the results for three subjects, presenting the percentage of distraction as a function of orientation difference. It becomes evident that the saccades were only affected by distractors with orientation differences larger than about 12 °. Obviously, the effect saturates at orientation differences larger than 40 °.

Other types of background/distractor dissimilarities

Experiment 5 was designed to investigate whether distraction is limited to texture stimuli defined by orientation differences or is also present for other cases of background/distractor dissimilarity. For this purpose, stimulus elements were designed which allowed variable degrees of dissimilarity by changing the inner (positional) bindings of each element. In this experiment, the targets were luminance-defined. Figure 13 displays various elements used for background and distractor, respectively. The data demonstrate increasing distraction with increasing structure "distance" of the distractor from the texture of circles used as background (Figure 13).

Figure 11

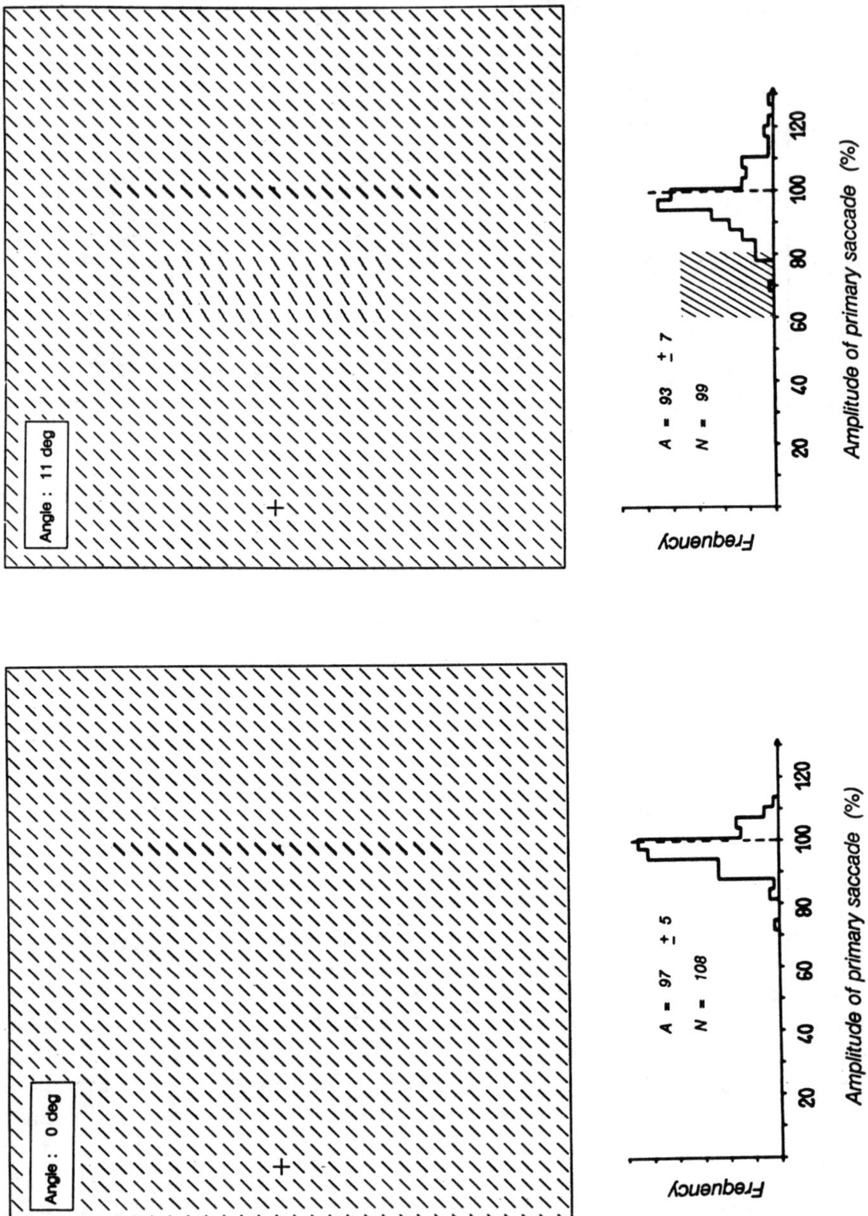
Angle : 11 deg
A = 93 ± 7
N = 99
Frequency
20 40 60 80 100 120
Amplitude of primary saccade (%)
Angle : 0 deg
A = 97 ± 5
N = 108
Frequency
20 40 60 80 100 120
Amplitude of primary saccade (%)

Figure 11 continued

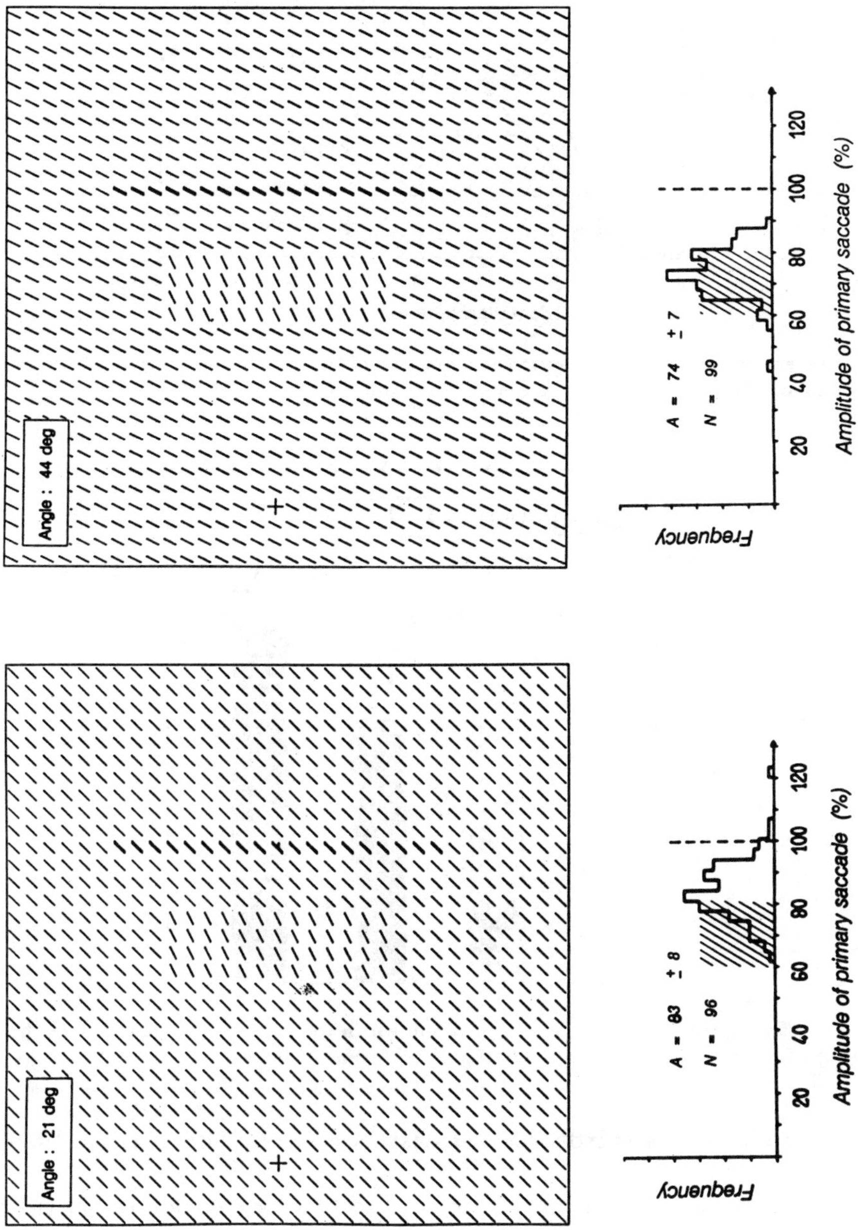

Fig. 11: Stimulus scenes and resulting saccade amplitude distributions in Experiment 4 (Subject Ti). In this experiment the target was luminance-defined. The distracting effect of various orientation differences (0,11, 21 and 44 °) of the distractor elements with respect to the background structure was determined.

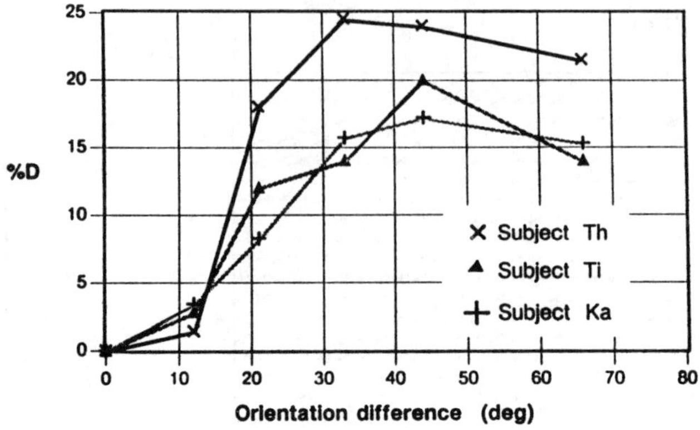

Fig. 12: Means of percentage distraction as a function of the orientation difference between background and distractor elements, given for three subjects

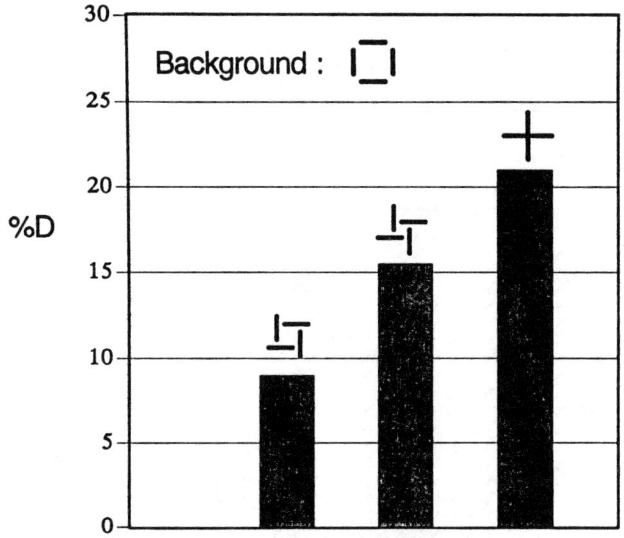

Fig. 13: Percentage distraction in Experiment 5 in which the distractor is characterized by increasing structure dissimilarity to the background. Means of three subjects.

Second-order versus third-order statistics defining the texture borders

The experiments described in the previous section have demonstrated that texture elements defined by differences in their second-order statistics (=orientation) can act as target and as distractors for saccadic eye movements. It seemed interesting to test whether preattentive discriminability is a necessary prerequisite for the observed behaviour. Therefore, in this experiment (Experiment 6) stimuli were used which had identical first- and second-order statistics, only differing in their third order statistics. A sketch of the stimuli is displayed in Figure 14 which also gives the percentage distraction for both cases. Here again, the target was luminance-defined. The averaging effect is clearly visible for the distractor which differs from the background in its second-order statistics (left diagram). For the third-order stimulus, the amount of distraction is significantly decreased (right diagram).

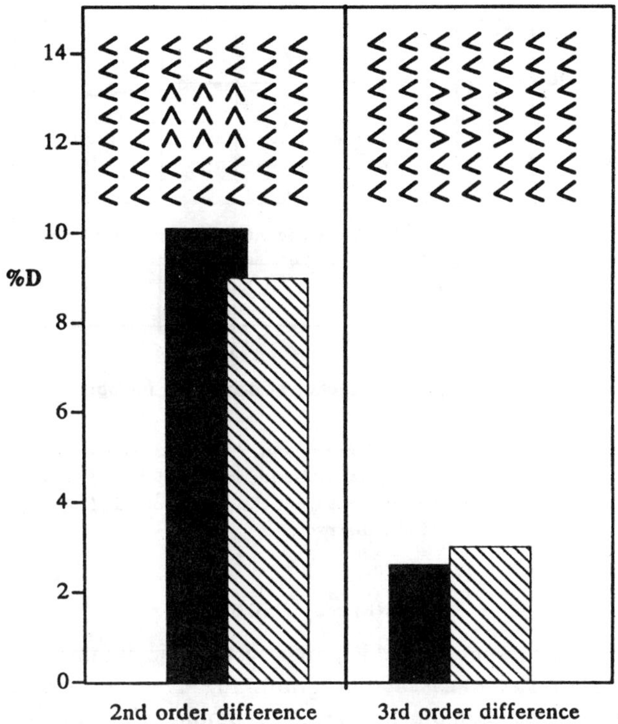

Fig. 14: Sketches of the stimuli used in Experiment 6 and resulting amount of saccadic distraction. Left scene: The distractor differs from background in its second order statistics or, more specifically, in the orientation of the elements forming the micropattern. Right scene: First and second-order statistics of background and distractor are identical (same luminance and element orientation); foreground and background structures differ only in their third-order statistics. Percentage saccade deviation due to the distractors are given for two subjects.

Targets defined by discontinuities in spatial frequency

The question arises as to what kind of inhomogeneities, other than texture borders, can serve as distractor or target. In order to test if spatial frequency gradients are also effective, a pilot experiment (Experiment 7) was performed in which the background consisted of a sine-wave grating of specific spatial frequency. The subject had to saccade to a high-contrast bar. The distractor was constituted by an area in which spatial frequency differed from the background.

Figure 15 shows the percentage of distraction as a function of the spatial frequency of the distractor. The background had 1.5 c/°. It can be seen that the amount of distraction increased monotonically with increasing spatial frequency difference. Saturation occurred at a difference of about 2 octaves.

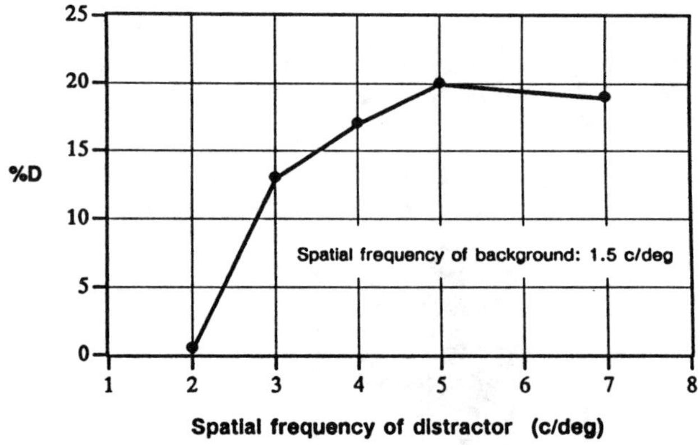

Fig. 15: Percentage of distraction in Experiment 7. In this experiment, the background consisted in a sine wave grating with a spatial frequency of 1.5 c/°. The distractor is defined by an area with a spatial frequency different from the background. The data are shown as a function of the spatial frequency of the distractor.

4. General Discussion

The experiments presented in this paper systematically introduce a novel aspect in the investigation of saccade programming. Due to the presence of background structure, target definition is more complex than in the conventional case with a homogeneous background. In our experiments, the subject had to direct her/his eyes to a specific area within the visual field which was constituted by its textural difference to the background structure. In this situation, saccadic performance demands the segregation of foreground objects from the background which means that the evaluation of texture borders is a necessary prerequisite for saccadic programming. The data, in fact, demonstrate that visual regions defined by texture properties can perfectly form saccadic targets with no significant deterioration or restraint on oculomotor performance. As detailed in the section on oculomotor performance, the saccadic system seems to handle the presence or absence of background structure equally well. These results have considerable importance for the study of early visual processing and we believe that they show how several research traditions in this area may be integrated.

Oculomotor performance with structured backgrounds

The majority of studies of saccadic eye movements have measured the properties of saccades to small targets presented against uniform backgrounds. In this section we discuss whether the introduction of a structured background affects the process of saccade generation.

In general, the data show that the presence of background structure seems to have little effect on the production of saccades. This is reflected by the fact that the high precision of the saccadic response to single targets is maintained. Some minor differences in saccadic performance can be observed however. So, the presence of a background appears to produce a small but consistent increase in the latency of target elicited saccades. The mean latencies in Experiment 1 (Durham) were about 170 ms (with a suggestion that latency could be increased for the coarse check backgrounds). This compares with a latency of about 150 ms for similar studies (Findlay 1982; Deubel et al., 1982, etc.) using homogeneous backgrounds. As detailed in Figure 10, comparable latency increases amounting to 20-40 ms were found in the Munich experiments. It is noteworthy that the targets defined by luminance differences actually led to longer latencies than texture-defined targets, which is an indication for the high salience of texture targets. It should be noted that for the Munich studies, latencies were longer in general. This might be attributable to the variable warning signal and also to the fact that, in the experimental paradigm, the fixation cross remained on with the presentation of the stimulus scene. This is equivalent to the "overlap" condition of Saslow (1967) in which, even for single dot stimuli, latencies of 200 ms or more can be expected. There are further differences in the methodology adapted in the two laboratories which may account for deviations in the results. In the Munich experiments (Exp. 2-7), target and background structure were presented together following prior fixation against a blank field. In the Durham experiment (Exp. 1), the structured background was continuously present during the fixation period prior to the sudden appearance of the targets. Thus, in the latter case, the local transient activation due to the onset of the targets within the stationary field may act as a highly effective trigger for the saccade. Finally, the trials in the Durham experiments were self-initiated, whereas in the Munich experiments, the target appeared with a variable delay following a warning signal.

Global processing and spatial integration

Our principal finding is the prevalence of the global integration effect which appeared irrespective of the presence or absence of background, and of the exact testing conditions. Therefore, in the experiment without background structure (Figure 6), the presentation of an additional visual stimulus led to a saccade directed to an intermediate position between the target and the distractor. For the cases including background structure the experimental data clearly demonstrate that areas with a texture differing from the background can also act as distractors for saccadic eye movements. As can be seen from Figures 3, 7, 8 and 11, the presentation of luminance-defined as well as texture-defined distractors embedded in a background structure led to distinct shifts of the mean saccade landing position while the distribution of the saccadic amplitudes essentially remained unaffected. Thus, the signal for saccades appears to integrate visual stimulation in an automatic and systematic way which does not differentiate between target and distractor (Ottes et al., 1985).

Global processing demonstrates clearly some form of spatial integration. Findlay (1982) argued that this must arise because of the convergence of visual signals into a spatially integrative channel and suggested a hypothetical correlate for such a channel might be a cell with a large receptive field. As detailed in a subsequent section, cells with large receptive fields are indeed found in the superior colliculus and frontal eye fields, two brain centres involved in the control of saccadic eye movements. While it is clear that convergence must occur at some level to give the requisite spatial integration, there is a danger of conceiving of this integration as a simple process.

Our results demonstrate that this is not the case. Firstly, the additivity of positive and negative contrasts (Exp. 1) shows that the integration involves some nonlinear processing. This experimental result is a confirmation of the findings of Deubel and Hauske (1988) that saccadic amplitudes to combinations of spatially separated dark and bright target lines are essentially directed to a centre of gravity determined by the absolute contrast values. Secondly, it seems very unlikely that any centre of gravity calculation involving simple weighting of crude spatial information on the pattern elements could provide an appropriate signal for the texture-defined stimuli of Experiments 3-6. The results suggest rather that spatial averaging as observed in the global effect occurs on a representation of the visual signal which is already the result of complex visual preprocessing. Specifying the signal presented to the spatial integration stage has already involved extraction of orientation specific information and comparison of this information across neighbouring spatial regions. Obviously, the "primal sketch" for saccade control consists of objects already segregated from the background structure. In this signal, surprisingly, texture and luminance changes appear to exert very similar influences as reflected in the data on latencies and amount of distraction (Figures 7 and 8).

Also for the experimental situation presented in this work, the amount of distraction depends on specific visual properties of background and distractor. The fact that in Experiment 4 the weight of the distractor is found to be closely related to the orientation difference between background and foreground elements (Figure 12) suggests that the salience of a stimulus in saccade amplitude computation is a direct function of its dissimilarity to the background. Very similar conclusions can be drawn from our finding that local changes in spatial frequency also attract the eye (Figure 15). In this case, the salience of the distractor as reflected in its weight is a direct function of the spatial frequency difference between distractor and background.

The global effect in saccadic eye movement control demonstrates the existence of a signal which is extracted from the target configuration and which, in some way, groups the targets together. The existence of a signal grouping targets together in an holistic way was originally one of the postulates of the Gestalt School (Wertheimer, 1923). Whilst it has attracted much attention, efforts to capture this simple perceptual insight in terms of a more atomistic approach to early visual perception have not proved very successful. Ginsburg (1975; Ginsburg & Evans, 1979) attempted to assign the low spatial frequency channels a role in the Gestalt grouping process. They demonstrated, for example, that some visual illusions could be "seen" when the relevant visual stimulus was subject to low pass filtering. However, a damaging finding is that visual illusions survive when presented in ways which remove low spatial frequency components (Carlson, Moeller, & Anderson, 1984). Thus, it is apparent that some nonlinear processing is involved in the grouping operation. This conclusion was reached by Julesz and Schumer (1981) who described the suggested process as "enigmatic." It is important, therefore, to know more about the nonlinear properties of the grouping signal concerned with saccadic eye movements.

The signal directing saccadic eye movements has the requisite nonlinear grouping property. Two other properties can be specified from our results. Firstly, the signal is dependent in a specifiable, albeit complex, way upon the properties of the visual stimulation. Thus, the weight of a distractor depends upon the visual properties of target background and distractor. The results of Experiment 4 suggest that the salience of a stimulus in saccade amplitude computation is a direct function of its dissimilarity to the background. On the other hand, in no case is the similarity of target and distractor a necessary precondition for the averaging effect. So, in Experiment 1, dark and light stimuli, in Experiment 3, luminance-defined and texture-defined stimuli are grouped together. Thus, the grouping effect obeys many, but not all, of the "laws" advocated by the Gestaltists (Wertheimer, 1923).

Our results are consistent with the view that the role of spatial frequency channels relates to the formation of a primal sketch quite similar to that of

Marr (1982) which forms an early stage of visual processing. In Marr's view, this sketch was a symbolic, or categorized, representation. Some support for this comes from the finding that beyond a difference in texton orientation of about 40 degrees, regions segregated by texture show an effect on the centre of gravity weighting which is independent of the angular difference in texton orientation (Figure 12). However, it is possible that this finding represents a ceiling effect. From the results for texton orientation differences of less than 40 degrees, it would appear that the "edges" extracted by preattentive processing are associated with a "strength" or "activation level" since the salience in the centre of gravity weighting varies systematically.

We should finally note the similarity of these ideas to those reached independently by Kröse (1986, 1987), who found that the salience of an object to become a target for a saccade is related to its dissimilarity to background structure. Another relevant theoretical model of early visual perception (Watt, 1987) is making heavy reliance on early grouping processes.

Texture processing and preattentive vision

Since the data reveal a continuous effect of target/background dissimilarity, the experimental approach proposed in this paper may offer a novel methodological means to investigate complex processing of visual signals. So, it is tempting to compare our results with data from experiments studying texture perception by means of conventional psychophysical approaches.

A large body of work on texture discrimination has been presented by Julesz (for reviews see Julesz & Bergen, 1983; Julesz, 1986). In his texton theory it is stated that preattentive vision is immediately able to detect texture gradients defined as differences in textons or in the density of textons. Discriminability of different texture areas is determined by the salience of the texture gradient which is related to the ratio of shared and unshared features. A clear equivalence to Julesz's findings is given by those of our experiments in which the texton "blob" and the texton "crossing," presented with various dissimilarity, are combined as background and distractor (Figure 13). As predicted by Julesz's theory, the salience of the texture border as reflected in the amount of distraction increases with increasing structure difference.

In earlier work, Julesz stated that the discriminability between areas of different textures largely depends upon the statistical properties of the element structure. According to this hypothesis, only textures consisting of micropatterns differing in their first order statistics (luminance) and/or second order statistics (orientation) can be immediately discriminated by preattentive vision. Textures which agree in their first and second order statistics and differ only in third or higher order are not available to preattentive discrimination. For these patterns, the evaluation of texture borders includes laborious element-by-element comparison, involving scanning eye movements. Although this rule has experienced some retrenchment (Caelli & Julesz, 1978), it still holds for the majority of cases. The relation of the order of element statistics and stimulus salience is exactly reflected in the experimental results given in Figure 14. Obviously, stimuli that agree in their first and second order statistics are not considered in the processing of sensory information for saccade control, leading to saccades unaffected by distractor presence.

In a psychophysical approach, Nothdurft (1985) quantitatively determined the discriminability of textures composed of oriented line elements very similar to the stimuli presented in Figure 11. Texture orientation difference and line length were systematically varied. The results from these experiments indicated that texture discriminability is closely related to the orientation difference of related texture areas. The result is now quantitatively confirmed by the saccade data from our Experiments 4 (Figure 11). Our data demonstrate that, at least for the line length chosen in these experiments, texture borders with angular element differences smaller than 10 ° have no distracting effect on the saccade which is functionally an indication of the existence of a threshold for orientation difference being effective. For elements with angles between 10 ° and 30-40 °, the salience of the distractor is a direct function of the orientation difference with larger angular distance yielding increasing distraction. For angles above 40 °, the distraction effect saturates.

A number of interesting implications follow. So the data represent another indication that processing of afferent signals is very much identical for perception and oculomotor processing (Zetzsche et al., 1984). Further, the conformity between Nothdurft's data and the results presented in this paper suggests that texture discrimination in the visual periphery is not essentially different from the foveal capabilities. Finally, the observation that there is no differential response for angles above 40 ° implies that the internal representation of angular difference is not coding visual angles continuously. Rather the S-shaped curves of Figure 12 suggest a representation which might be closely related to orientation selective channels postulated for visual processing (e.g. Campbell & Kulikowski, 1966). Within this concept, object and background would be classified as different when their orientations fell into different filters. In fact, for these orientation selective mechanisms, angular bandwidths close to those suggested in our results have been found. Such a channel concept may also take account of the data presented in Figure 15 demonstrating that the distractor becomes effective when the spatial frequency difference is higher than about 1 octave, which is again in conformity with the bandwidths of spatial frequency channels assumed in visual processing.

Neural mechanisms

Much research in low level vision is motivated in part by the hope of establishing neurophysiological correlates of the hypothesized processes. In the case of visually elicited saccadic eye movements, two interrelated questions can be addressed. Firstly, which neural pathways convey the information from the visual system to the oculomotor system. Secondly, what are the properties of individual cells involved in the response. We believe that our results have some relevance for both questions.

Information from the retina can reach the oculomotor centres by at least three different possible routes namely, (a) retina - superior colliculus - brainstem; (b) retina - LGN - visual cortex - superior colliculus - brainstem; (c) retina - LGN - visual cortex - frontal eye fields - oculomotor centres. Lesion studies with animals have shown that none of the three visual cortex centres, superior colliculus and frontal eye fields are indispensable for the production of target elicited saccades and eliminate such saccades totally. For target elicited saccade suppression two separate pathways must be blocked (Mohler & Wurtz, 1977; Schiller, True, & Conway, 1980). Human patients with damage to the visual cortical areas are able to make saccades to targets with reasonable accuracy even in regions of the visual field for which a cortical route is unavailable (Pöppel, Held, & Frost, 1973; Perenin & Jeannerod, 1975; Zihl, 1980; Barbur, Forsyth, & Findlay, 1988). Animal studies consistently find that collicular lesions increase the latency of visually elicited saccades and this has led to the suggestion that the most rapid target elicited saccades are made through the collicular pathway (Fischer, 1987).

Another aspect of the superior colliculus which has attracted the attention of eye movement researchers has been the presence of cells with very large visual receptive fields in this structure. Thus, the global averaging seen in the global effect might perhaps reflect the "primitive" properties of this pathways. In fact, McIlwain (1976) suggested that such large field cells could play a key role in the sensorimotor transformation occurring during the programming of a visually elicited saccade. Specifically, the suggestion was that large field activation could act as a "spotlight" to "illuminate" and hence recruit the appropriate population of premotor units in a motor map within the colliculus. Superficially, it would seem that cells with large receptive fields should provide the appropriate substrate for the spatial integration shown in the global effect. The potential for such connectionist modelling has recently been explored in more detail (van Gisbergen, van Opstal, & Tax, 1987; Findlay, 1988), and these modelling studies have shown that without further assumptions, the global effect is not predicted. Another finding which is at variance with the suggestion that the direct retino-collicular pathway produces the global effect comes from study of a hemianopic patient who was able to make saccades to targets in his blind visual hemifield (Barbur, Forsyth, & Findlay, 1988). This patient did not invariably produce a global effect when two targets were presented simultaneously in his blind hemifield.

The results presented in this paper strongly support the viewpoint that cortical pathways are involved in visually elicited saccades. The direct retino-collicular pathway is generally assumed not to exhibit properties selective to form aspects such as orientation (Wurtz & Albano, 1980). The properties of collicular cells are rather non-specific, showing most sensitivity to coarse, transient stimulation with large receptive fields (Goldberg & Wurtz, 1972; Sparks, 1986). The results of Experiments 3-6, however, show that the spatial signal for saccades is sensitive to the discrimination of texture areas defined by local orientation differences among small elements. It is, therefore, unlikely that the information about the locus of texture-defined targets is conveyed by the direct retino-collicular pathways. Retinal ganglion cells and cells of the lateral geniculate nucleus (LGN) are most sensitive to differences in luminance and show no marked orientation selectivity. Thus, these structures may suffice to detect object borders which are defined by a discontinuity in first order statistics (equivalent to a luminance change). Striate cortex cells, on the other hand, show marked sensitivity to line orientation (Hubel & Wiesel, 1962). Thus, the striate cortex might detect differences in the 2nd order statistics, such as texture orientations as used in our experiments. In fact Nothdurft and Li (1985) suggested that responses of striate cortex cells in the cat represent texture features defined by element orientation. Textures which are identical in their 1st and 2nd order statistics, differing only in 3rd or higher order, then would not evoke differential responses in either LGN or striate cortex cells. Such textures cannot be immediately discriminated by preattentive vision and, accordingly, do not attract the eye in a saccade task (Figure 14). In our view, this provides a promising way of analyzing cortical/subcortical interactions in sensorimotor processing.

5. Conclusions

It is evident that our natural visual environment is normally characterized by the presence of highly complex visual structure in which the segregation of objects from a background is a necessary precondition for object recognition. In order to strengthen the ecological validity of our study, we systematically investigated saccadic performance in an experimental situation which we consider as being closer to the ecological reality (for a related approach see also Deubel & Zetzsche, 1983). Our data demonstrate that the sensorimotor system can perfectly handle this highly complex task. This result and the fact that global averaging also occurs in a situation which includes prominent background structure shows that saccade computation occurs on a non-linearily preprocessed version of the visual information in which foreground objects are already segregated from the background. In that, our results also indicate that eye movements do not only disclose properties of motor programming but may also serve as an elegant probe for investigating elements of visual processing.

The data strongly suggest that area boundaries defined by discontinuities in luminance, structure orientation, spatial frequency or even more complex textural properties exhibit considerable salience for eye movements. Clearly, this is in conformance with their high behavioural significance, since it is the border of visual objects that carry essential information on the things that surround us.

Acknowledgements

This investigation was supported by the Deutsche Forschungsgemeinschaft (Ha 872/1) and by the European Science Foundation (ESF TW/86/15). Author H.D. is indebted to Katrin Junglaß for her never impatient typing and retyping of parts of the manuscript.

References

Bach, M., Bouis, D., & Fischer, B., *An accurate infrared oculometer*, Journal of Neuroscience Methods **9** (1983), 9-14.

Barbur, J.L., Forsyth, P.M., & Findlay, J.M., *Human saccadic eye movements in the absence of the geniculo-calcarine projection*, Brain (1988) (to appear).

Becker, W., & Jürgens, R., *An analysis of the saccadic system by means of double step stimuli*, Vision Research **19** (1979), 967-983.

Caelli, T., & Julesz, B., *On perceptual analyzers underlying visual texture discrimination : Part I*, Biological Cybernetics **28** (1978), 167-175.

Campbell, F.W., & Kulikowski, J.J., *Orientation selectivity of the human visual system*, Journal of Physiology **187** (1966), 437-445.

Carlson, C.R., Moeller, J.R., & Anderson, C.H., *Visual illusions without low spatial frequencies*, Vision Research **24** (1984), 1407-1413.

Coeffé, C., & O'Reagan, J.K., *Reducing the influence of non-target stimuli on saccade accuracy: predictability and latency effects*, Vision Research **27** (1987), 227-240.

Collewijn, H., van der Mark, F., & Jansen, T.C., *Precise recordings of human eye movements*, Vision Research **15** (1975), 447-450.

Coren, S., & Hoenig, P., *Effect of non-target stimuli on the length of voluntary saccades*, Perceptual and Motor Skills **34** (1972), 499-508.

Deubel, H., "Wechselwirkung von Sensorik und Motorik bei sakkadischen Augenbewegungen: Eine kybernetische Beschreibung des visuellen Systems," Unpublished doctoral dissertation, Technical University of Munich, 1984.

Deubel, H., *Adaptivity of gain and direction in oblique saccades*, in "J.K. O'Regan & A. Lévy- Schoen (Eds.), Eye movements : from physiology to cognition," Elsevier, North Holland, Amsterdam, 1986, pp. 181-190.

Deubel, H., & Hauske, G., *The programming of visually guided saccades*, in "H. Marko, G. Hauske & A. Struppler (Eds.), Processing structures for perception and action," Verlag Chemie, Weinheim, 1988, pp. 119-132.

Deubel, H., Jacobs A.M., & Kürzinger, G., *Texture gradients affect saccadic eye movements*, in "G. Lüer & U. Lass (Eds.), Fourth European Conference on Eye Movements, Volume 1: Proceedings," C.J. Hogrefe Inc., Toronto, 1987, pp. 125-126.

Deubel, H., & Wolf, W., *The programming of correction saccades by retinal feedback*, Investigative Ophthalmology and Visual Science **22** (1982), p. 86, Suppl.

Deubel. H., Wolf, W., & Hauske, G., *Corrective saccades : the effect of shifting the saccade goal*, Vision Research **22** (1982), 353-364.

Deubel, H., Wolf, W., & Hauske, G., *The evaluation of the oculomotor error signal*, in "A.G. Gale & F.W. Johnson (Eds.), Theoretical and applied aspects of eye movement research," North-Holland, Amsterdam, 1984, pp. 55-62.

Deubel, H., & Zetzsche, C., *Goal-directed saccades in complex visual environment: comparison of pre- and post-saccadic visual information determines the correction saccade*, Perception **12** (1983), A30-A31.

Ferman, L., Collewijn, H., & van den Berg, A.V., *A direct test of Listing's Law II: Human ocular torsion measured in dynamic conditions*, Vision Research **27** (1987), 939-951.

Fischer, B., *The preparation of visually guided saccades*, Review of Physiology, Biochemistry, and Pharmacology **106** (1987), 1-35.

Findlay, J.M., *A simple apparatus for recording microsaccades during visual fixation*, Quarterly Journal of Experimental Psychology **26** (1974), 167-170.

Findlay, J.M., *Local and global influences on saccadic eye movements*, in "D.F. Fisher, R.A. Monty & J.W. Senders (Eds.), Eye movements, cognition and visual perception," Erlbaum, Hillsdale, N.J., 1981.

Findlay, J.M., *Global processing for saccadic eye movements*, Vision Research **22** (1982), 1033- 1045.

Findlay, J.M., *Eye movements and visual cognition*, L'Année psychologique **85** (1985), 101-136.

Findlay, J.M., *Visual computation and saccadic eye movements*, Spatial Vision (1988) (to appear).

Findlay, J.M., & Crawford, T.J., *The visual control of saccadic eye movements : evidence for limited plasticity*, in "R. Groner, C. Menz, D.F. Fisher & R.A. Monty (Eds.), Eye movements and psychological processes: International views," Erlbaum, Hillsdale, N.J., 1983, pp. 115-127.

Findlay, J.M., & Harris, L.R., *Small saccades to double stepped targets moving in two dimensions*, in "A.G. Gale & F.W. Johnson (Eds.), Theoretical and applied aspects of oculomotor research," Elsevier, Amsterdam, 1984, pp. 71-77.

Fuchs, A.F., Kaneko, C.R.S, & Scudder, C.A., *Brainstem control of saccadic eye movements*, Annual Review of Neuroscience **8** (1985), 307-337.

Ginsburg, A.P., *Is the illusory triangle physical or imaginary*, Nature **257** (1975), 219-220.

Ginsburg, A.P. & Evans, P.W., *Predicting visual illusion from filtered images based on biological data*, Journal of the Optical Society of America **69** (1979), p. 1443.

Goldberg, M.E., & Wurtz, R.H., *Activity of superior colliculus cells in behaving monkey I. Visual receptive fields of single neurons*, Journal of Neurophysiology **35** (1972), 542-559.

Henning, G.B., Hertz, B.G., & Broadbent, D.E., *Some experiments bearing on the hypothesis that the visual system analyses spatial patterns in independent bands of spatial frequency*, Vision Research **15** (1975), 887-897.

Hubel, D.H., & Wiesel, T.N., *Receptive fields, binocular interaction and functional architecture in the cat's visual cortex*, Journal of Physiology **160** (1962), 106-154.

Jacobs, A.M., *On localization and saccade programming*, Vision Research **27** (1987), 1953-1966.

Julesz, B., *Texton gradients : the texton theory revisited*, Biological Cybernetics **54** (1986), 245-251.

Julesz, B., & Bergen, J.R., *Textons, the fundamental elements in preattentive vision and perception of textures*, Bell System Technical Journal **62** (1983), 1619-1645.

Julesz, B., & Schumer, R.A., *Early visual perception*, Annual Review of Psychology **32** (1981), 575-627.

Koenderink, J.J., & van Doorn, A., *Visual detection of spatial contrast: influence of location in the visual field, target extent and illuminance level*, Biological Cybernetics **30** (1978), 157-167.

Kröse, B., *A description of visual structure*, "Proefschrift," Department of Industrial Design Engineering, Delft University of Technology, 1986.

Kröse, B., *Preattentive or attentive saccade programming*, Investigative Ophthalmology and Visual Science **28** (1987), p. 314, Suppl.

Kürzinger, G., & Deubel, H., *A versatile digital image presentation system for research in visual psychophysics*, Perception **15** (1986), p. A30.

McIlwain, J.T., *Large receptive fields and spatial transformations in the visual system*, in "R. Porter (Ed.), International review of physiology, Volume 10: Neurophysiology II," 1976, pp. 223-248.

Marr, D., *Early processing of visual information*, Philosophical Transactions of the Royal Society of London **275B** (1976), 483-524.

Marr, D., "Vision," W.H. Freeman, San Francisco, 1982.

Marr, D., & Hildreth, E., *Theory of edge detection*, Proceedings of the Royal Society of London **207B** (1980), 187-217.

Menz, C., & Groner, R., *Saccadic programming with multiple targets under different task conditions*, in "J.K. O'Regan & A. Lévy-Schoen (Eds.), Eye Movements: from physiology to cognition," North-Holland, Amsterdam, 1987.

Mohler, C.W., & Wurtz, R.H., *Role of striate cortex and superior colliculus in visual guidance of saccadic eye movements in monkeys*, Journal of Neurophysiology **40** (1977), 74-94.

Nothdurft, C., *Orientation sensitivity and texture segmentation in patterns with different line orientations*, Vision Research **25** (1985), 551-560.

Nothdurft, C., & Li, C.Y., *Texture discrimination: representation of orientation and luminance differences in cells of the cat striate cortex*, Vision Research **25** (1985), 99-113.

Ottes, F.P., van Gisbergen, J.A.M., & Eggermont, J.J., *Latency dependence of colour-based target vs nontarget information by the saccadic system*, Vision Research **25** (1985), 849-862.

Parker, D.M., & Salzen, E., *Latency changes in the human visual evoked response to sinusoidal gratings*, Vision Research **17** (1977), 1201-1204.

Perenin, M.-T., & Jeannerod, M., *Residual vision in cortically blind hemifields*, Neuropsychologia **13** (1975), 1-7.

Pöppel, E., Held, R., & Frost, D., *Residual visual function after brain wounds involving central visual pathways in man*, Nature **243** (1973), 295-296.

Regan, D., *Visual information channeling in normal and disordered vision*, Psychological Review **89** (1982), 407-444.

Rovamo, J., Virsu, V., & Näsänen, R., *Cortical magnification factor predicts the photopic contrast sensitivity of peripheral vision*, Investigative Ophthalmology and Visual Science **23** (1978), 666-670.

Robinson, D.A., *The mechanics of human saccadic eye movements*, Journal of Physiology (Lond.) **174** (1964), 245-264.

Robinson, D.A., *The use of matrices in analyzing the three-dimensional behaviour of the vestibulo - ocular reflex*, Biological Cybernetics **46** (1982), 53-66.

Saslow, M.G., *Effects of components of displacement step stimuli upon latency for saccadic eye movement*, Journal of the optical Society of America **57** (1967), 1030-1033.

Schiller, P.H., True, S.D., & Conway, J.L., *Deficits in eye movements flowing frontal eye field and superior colliculus ablations*, Journal of Neurophysiology **44** (1980), 1175-1189.

Shapley, R., & Gordon, J., *Nonlinearity in the perception of form*, Perception and Psychophysics **37** (1985), 84-88.

Smit, A.C., van Gisbergen, J.A.M., & Cools, A.R., *A parametric analysis of human saccades in different experimental paradigms*, Vision Research **27** (1987), 1745-1762.

Sparks, D.L., *Translation of sensory signals into commands for control of saccadic eye movements: role of primate superior colliculus*, Physiological Reviews **66** (1986), 118-171.

van Gisbergen, J.A.M, van Opstal, J.J., & Tax, A.A.M., *Collicular ensemble coding of saccades based on vector stimulation*, Neuroscience **21** (1987), 541-555.

Vassilev, A., & Mitov, D., Vision Research **16** (1976), 89-92.

Watt, R.J., *Scanning from coarse to fine spatial scales in the visual system after the onset of a stimulus*, Journal of the Optical Society of America **A4** (1987), 2006-2021.

Wertheimer, M., *Untersuchungen zu Lehre von der Gestalt II*, Psychologische Forschung **4** (1923), 301-350.

Westheimer, G., *Eye movement responses to a horizontally moving visual stimulus*, Archives Ophthalmology **52** (1954), 932-941.

Wheeless, L., Boynton, R., & Cohen, G., *Eye movement responses to step and pulse-step stimuli*, Journal of the Optical Society of America **56** (1966), 956-960.

Wilson, H.R., & Bergen, J.R., *A four mechanism model for spatial vision*, Vision Research **19** (1979), 19-32.

Wurtz, R.H., & Albano, J.E., *Visual-motor function of the primate superior colliculus*, Annual Review of Neuroscience **3** (1980), 189-226.

Young, L.R., & Stark, L., *A sampled-data model for eye tracking movements*, Quarterly Progress Report, Research Lab of Electronics., M.I.T. **66** (1962), 370-384.

Zetzsche, C., Kürzinger, G., Deubel, H., & Elsner, T., *Similar mechanisms of visual processing in perception and oculomotor control*, Perception **13** (1984), p. A16.

Zihl, J., *"Blindsight": Improvement of visually guided eye movements by systematic practice in patients with cerebral blindness*, Neuropsychologia **18** (1980), 71-77.

VESTIBULAR NYSTAGMUS AS A MANIFESTATION OF A STRATEGY OF HEAD-EYE COORDINATION

ROBERTO SCHMID AND DANIELA ZAMBARBIERI

Dipartimento di Informatica e Sistemistica,
Universita' di Pavia

INTRODUCTION

Since the pioneering works of the last century (see Jeannerod, 1981, for a historical review), vestibular nystagmus has been the objective response, most frequently used in the investigation of the vestibular system. Countless papers have been published describing nystagmus characteristics in normal subjects and their modifications in pathological situations. Nevertheless, very few of these papers have considered the fundamental question regarding this oculomotor response. Why is it that the stimulation of the vestibular system in the dark provokes a pattern of eye movement consisting of alternating slow and fast components? At present, we may presume to know how vestibular nystagmus is produced, what peripheral and central mechanisms are involved, and how they adapt during plastic processes. We still don't know *why* nystagmus occurs.

The vestibulo-ocular reflex (VOR) has developed in order to make the eyes a stable platform for vision. When we rotate the head in one direction in a normal visual surround while fixating a stationary object, the eyes rotate in the opposite direction and the image of the external world remains stationary on the retina. But, when head rotation is produced in the dark or, more generally, in the absence of a visual reference, there is apparently no need for this compensatory eye movement. Nevertheless, it takes place, although interrupted by saccades in the opposite direction (*slow* and *fast* phase of vestibular nystagmus).

One might consider the slow phase of nystagmus as a reflex response which, as such, occurs either in the light or in darkness. Fast phase saccades would have the function of resetting the system by bringing the eyes back to the primary position as they approach their extreme deviation in the orbit.

This interpretation of nystagmus contrasts with a considerable body of experimental evidence. First of all, it is not true that the compensatory VOR response cannot be suppressed. Apart from the possibility of reducing VOR gain during long-term adaptive processes (for a review see Berthoz & Melvill Jones, 1985), on-line VOR inhibition during a saccadic response was reported by many authors (Jürgens et al., 1981; Laurutis & Robinson, 1986; Tomlinson & Bahra, 1986; Guitton & Volle, 1987; Pelisson et al., 1988). Secondly, even an eye inspection of nystagmus will show that fast phase saccades interrupt the slow phase long before the mechanical limit of eye rotation in the orbit. Thirdly, it is not true that fast phase saccades always bring the eyes back to the primary position.

A deviation of the nystagmic response in the anticompensatory direction, with a pattern of modulation related to stimulus velocity, was first pointed out by Melvill Jones in 1964. It was suggested that the functional role of the predominance of the anticompensatory oculomotor response during rapid head rotation would be "to have the eyes automatically thrown out in advance of the head when turning the head towards a point of interest, the quicker to pick up the intended target."

The predominant direction of gaze during slow head rotation in the dark was later investigated by Mishkin and Melvill Jones (1966) who reached the conclusion that "the phase advanced waveform of averaged eye position seen during slow sinusoidal head rotation is probably essentially driven by the attendant semicircular canal stimulation." It was, therefore, suggested that "the vestibular signal may also be capable of exercising quantitative control over the saccadic mode of eye movement."

An attempt to formalize these concepts was made by Barnes and Benson (1973), Schmid and Lardini (1976), and Chun and Robinson (1978) who proposed three mathematical models for the generation of the fast phase of vestibular nystagmus. A strict correlation between the strategies of eye-head coordination in the orientation of gaze and the characteristics of vestibular nystagmus was clearly stated, particularly in Chun and Robinson's paper. Nevertheless, due to the lack of systematic investigation, the dominant view on vestibular nystagmus is still that the slow phase deviates the eyes from the central position and the fast phase resets them.

The aim of this paper is to present a general theory on sensorimotor control in which the nystagmic response is seen as a manifestation of a strategy of eye-head coordination. Some experimental results obtained during fast and slow orientation head movements in the dark are reported. It is then shown that the eye movement evoked by passive rotatory stimulations in the dark (vestibular nystagmus) reflects the same motor coordination strategy as observed during active head rotation. Finally, a mathematical model is proposed which assigns a precise functional significance to nystagmus slow and fast phase, and predicts nystagmus characteristics in a rigorous, quantitative way.

Methods

The experimental results reported in this paper were obtained in our laboratory by using the following apparatus

- A rotatory chair driven by a DC motor. Chair movement was controlled by an IBM Personal Computer on which several profiles of movement were programmed.
- A circular frame, 1.6 m in diameter, supporting light-emitting diodes (LEDs) and loudspeakers which were used as target sources. LEDs and loudspeakers were placed at equal intervals (10 °) at positions seen by the subject with angles from -70 to 70 degrees. The switch on and off of LEDs or loudspeakers was controlled by the computer.

Eye movement was recorded using a conventional electro-oculographic technique (EOG). Two silver-silver chloride electrodes were placed on the skin at the external canthus of each orbit. The EOG signals were amplified by a DC differential amplifier and passed through a low-pass filter with a 125 Hz corner frequency. Head rotation was recorded by means of a rotatory variable difference transformer (Schaevitz R30D), attached to the top of a light helmet mounted on the subject's head. The transmission of head rotation to the transducer was obtained through a bellows coupling with two universal joints which provided very little resistance to vertical and lateral head movements. Eye and head signals were A/D converted at 250 Hz and stored on a floppy disk for subsequent data processing. Gaze, defined as absolute eye position in space, was computed via software by adding the EOG signal, giving eye position in the orbit, to the head signal. Signal analysis was done by using an interactive program developed in the laboratory. Three experimental conditions were considered.

A Vestibular stimulation in the dark. Subjects were seated on the rotatory chair with the head blocked. Three types of test were performed: post-rotational (sudden stop of the chair after a period of rotation at constant velocity), sinusoidal (chair oscillation at different frequencies), and per-rotational (constant acceleration of the chair up to a given velocity and then rotation at constant velocity).

B Target fixation in free head condition. Subjects were seated at the center of the circular frame with the trunk fixed to the chair. Visual targets (LEDs) were presented in a random sequence and subjects were asked to fixate at the presented target.

C Voluntary head rotation in the dark. Subjects were asked to rotate their head from right to left or from left to right at different velocities, while keeping their trunk still.

Ten subjects with no history of visual, vestibular or oculomotor disorders participated in the experiments, which were carried out on different days.

VESTIBULAR NYSTAGMUS MUST HAVE A FUNCTIONAL SIGNIFICANCE. HOW TO FIND IT?

As previously mentioned in the introduction, the VOR has the function of producing eye movements that compensate head movements to maintain stable vision. Thus, the presence of a stationary visual surround seems to be a necessary condition for the VOR response to make sense. When the head movement is produced in the dark or to pursue a moving visual target, the VOR response becomes useless or even detrimental. Hence, no functional significance can be found for vestibular nystagmus if we assume that the vestibular afferent signal is used by the oculomotor control system only to produce compensatory eye movements. On the other hand, there must be a functional significance since vestibular nystagmus takes place in spite of the proved ability of the central nervous system (CNS) to suppress the VOR (Haddad & Robinson, 1977; Jürgens et al., 1981; Laurutis & Robinson, 1986; Tomlinson & Bahra, 1986; Guitton & Volle, 1987; Pelisson et al., 1988).

What goal is the CNS pursuing when eye movements are controlled in a way that produces a nystagmic response? The best way to find an answer to this question is to imagine that we were inside the CNS and to ask what interpretation we should give to the vestibular afferent signal during a stimulation that is known to produce nystagmus. As a reference point in our interpretation and when deciding what oculomotor action is to be made, we can only consider the patterns of discharge received during head movements performed to satisfy the needs of everyday life.

Let us consider the vestibular stimulation provoked during a classic post-rotational test (see Methods) and the corresponding vestibular afferent signal. Since the chair stop will never be instantaneous, head velocity ($\dot{H}$) and acceleration ($\ddot{H}$) should follow the profiles shown schematically in Figure 1A. With a good braking system, the chair will stop in about 300-400 ms with a deceleration reaching a maximum after about 100 ms from the beginning of the maneuver. In the first 300-400 ms, the semicircular canals (SCC), to which a time constant of about 6 s can be assigned in man, behave as a perfect integrator of head acceleration. Thus, the discharge frequency (f) of primary vestibular neurons (Figure 1B) will increase up to a maximum reached after 300-400 ms, and then decline slowly with the same time constant as that of the SCC. The resting discharge will be re-established in about 15-20 s.

In what natural condition does the CNS receive from the SCC a similar pattern of discharge, at least, in the first 300-400 ms?

If we consider a rapid orientation head movement towards a visual (or auditory) target, profiles like those shown in Figure 1C can be recorded for head position, velocity, and acceleration, respectively. The head movement is accomplished in about 500-600 ms with a peak velocity reached at the midpoint

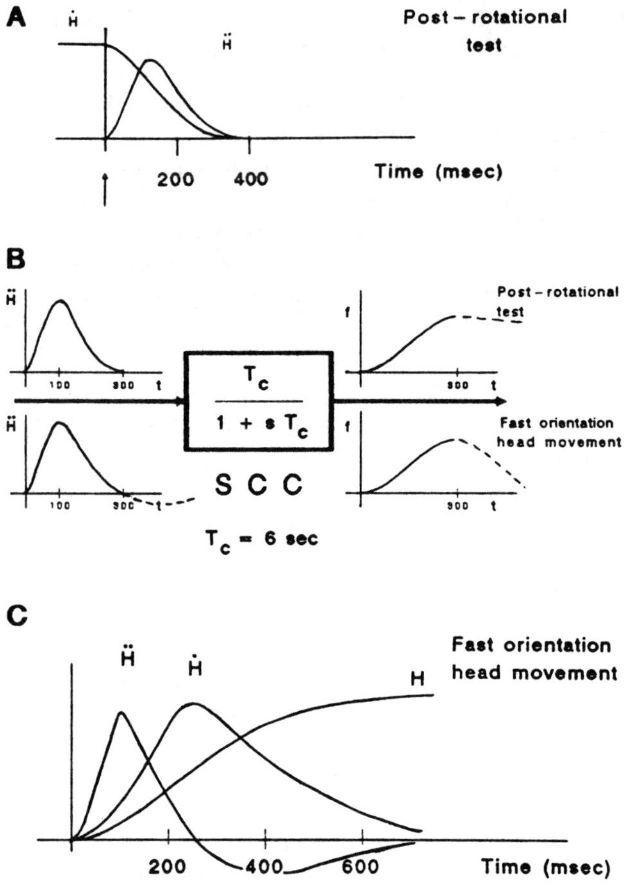

Fig. 1 - **A**: profiles of head velocity ($\dot{H}$) and acceleration ($\ddot{H}$) during a post-rotational test. **B**: predicted time course of the discharge frequency (f) in primary vestibular neurons following the onset of a post-rotational stimulus and during a fast orientation head movement. **C**: profiles of head position (H), velocity ($\dot{H}$) and acceleration ($\ddot{H}$) during a fast head movement.

of this temporal range, when the head starts decelerating. Head acceleration reaches a maximum after about 100 ms from the beginning of the movement. What is important to note is that the acceleration profile during the first 300 ms is exactly the same as that produced by a post-rotational stimulus. In this time interval, the pattern of discharge of primary vestibular neurons would appear to be the same as before. Hence, in the first 300 ms, the two situations are almost indistinguishable for the CNS, at least, as far as vestibular information is concerned.

The question now is whether, in some natural condition of head orientation, the CNS uses the vestibular afferent signal received within the first 300 ms to program some kind of motor strategy for eye-head coordination. If this is the case, the same motor strategy is likely to be activated at the onset of a post-rotatory stimulation and the beginning of the post-rotatory nystagmus may be explained in the same way.

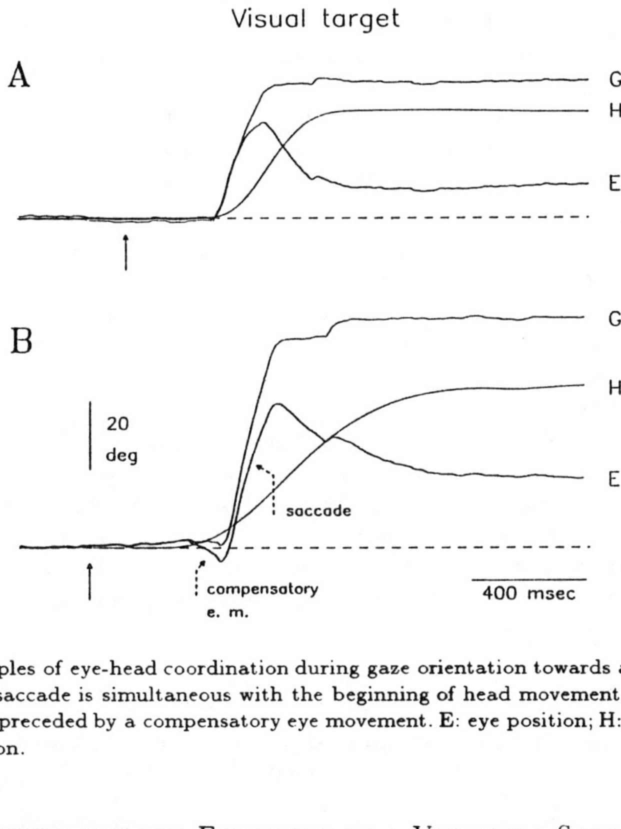

Fig. 2: Examples of eye-head coordination during gaze orientation towards a visual target. In **A** the eye saccade is simultaneous with the beginning of head movement, whereas in **B** the saccade is preceded by a compensatory eye movement. **E**: eye position; **H**: head position; G: gaze position.

Evidence for the Existence of a Vestibulo-Saccadic Pathway

It is well known (Morasso et al., 1973) that when a subject is presented with an eccentric visual target in a free head condition, target fixation is accomplished through a coordinated eye-head movement of the type shown in Figure 2A. By anticipating the head movement by a few ms the eyes make a saccade to the target. Gaze fixation is then maintained during the following head movement by a compensatory eye movement moving in the opposite direction to the head. Since the eyes make a saccade before the head starts to move, any role of the vestibular system in programming this saccade can be excluded. Nevertheless, Barnes (1979) has demonstrated that when target eccentricity exceeds 30-40°, the saccade normally follows the beginning of head movement by about 100 ms, during which time the eyes move in a compensatory direction (Figure 2B). Barnes suggested the existence of two different strategies in eye-head coordination; one pertaining to small target eccentricities, the other to large eccentricities. He further suggested that the second strategy may use vestibular information to program the saccadic eye movement. It might be inferred that the first strategy is adopted when the eyes can easily reach the target also with no head movement, the second strategy when both eye and head movements are needed to orient the gaze to the target.

Similar patterns of eye-head coordination, as observed when the second strategy is adopted, were recorded by Barnes (1979) during passive head rotations on the trunk (head rotated on the fixed body by an external device) and by Roucoux et al. (1981) during body rotation in toto, both in the dark and reproducing the pattern of a natural orientation head movement. The absence of an external target, the passiveness of the head movement, and, in the latter condition, the absence of proprioceptive signals from the neck muscles support the assumption that in these conditions, at least, the saccadic eye movement is driven by vestibular afferent signals.

If this is the case, within the first 300 ms of a rapid orientation head movement in the dark, the CNS would use the vestibular afferent signal to program a motor strategy of eye-head coordination. Some neurophysiological evidence for the existence of a vestibulo-saccadic pathway (VSP) has been recently provided (Whittington et al., 1984; Shimazu et al., 1986). Whether this pathway represents a subcortical reflex mechanism or involves higher neural levels is still a matter of speculation.

Functional Significance and Characteristics of the Vestibulo-Saccadic Pathway

What could be the functional significance of a vestibular input to the saccadic system? The most reasonable interpretation is that given by Melvill Jones in early 1964. The head takes several hundred milliseconds to reach an intended position. This time is far too long in many circumstances of everyday life. It is better to estimate from the vestibular signal where the head is moving to and "throw the eyes" close to this position by a fast saccadic movement. This strategy also makes sense when the head moves towards a point of interest in the dark. Actually, it is not known, a priori, whether a visible object is really present in that position. Only if the head movement is repeated many times in the dark, always in the absence of a final visible target, might the CNS be induced to leave off this strategy by reducing progressively the oculomotor response. A progressive suppression of nystagmus (VOR habituation) was actually observed in these conditions (Schmid & Jeannerod, 1985).

In order to carry out this strategy, a kind of predictor must exist in the VSP. It must receive a head velocity signal from the vestibular system and compute an estimate of the head movement amplitude. A low-pass filter with a time constant of 600 ms, as in the Chun and Robinson model (1978), or a pure integrator of the vestibular output, as in the Laurutis and Robinson model (1986), cannot work as a predictor, since knowledge of the final head position would be made available only at the end of the head movement.

What kind of signal processing is likely to occur in the VSP in order to obtain an early estimate of the amplitude of the head movement?

No precise identification of the VSP on the anatomical plane is, as yet, available, and no electrophysiological data are available that can be used to determine the VSP transfer function.

A simple hypothesis on the VSP signal processing is suggested by the finding that in natural orientation head movements there is a linear relationship between the amplitude of head rotation and its peak velocity (Zangemeister et al., 1981). An estimate of the former can thus be obtained from the latter. Zangemeister et al. showed that peak head velocity was reached after about 200 ms from the beginning of the head movement. During this time, the frequency discharge of primary vestibular neurons very precisely reproduces the profile of head velocity. The predictor could, then, be a simple mechanism that starts to detect the output of the vestibular receptors after about 200 ms from the onset of their discharge, provided that the level of discharge is high enough to indicate the occurrence of a fast head movement (Figure 3). The detected signal is then sent to the saccadic mechanism after multiplication by a gain factor representing the ratio between amplitude and peak velocity in fast orientation head movements (gain factor σ of 0.3-0.4). Dimensionally, the output of this mechanism would be a position reference signal, homogeneous to all other possible inputs to the saccadic mechanism.

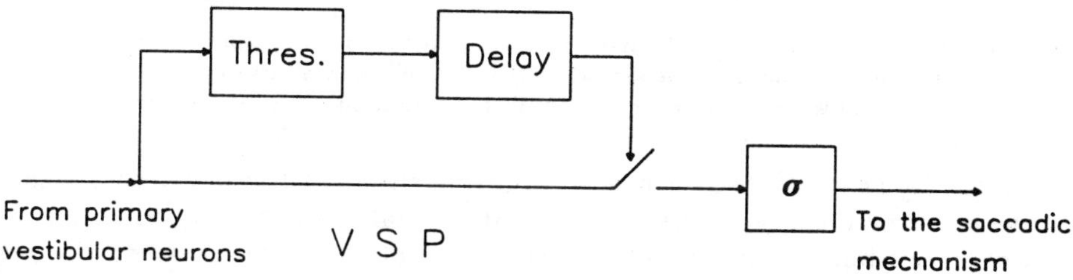

Fig. 3: Hypothetical model of the "predictor" in the vestibulo-saccadic pathway (VSP). The gain σ represents the ratio between amplitude and peak velocity in fast orientation head movements.

However, other studies indicate that in many orientation head movements, the time of peak head velocity may be significantly delayed with respect to the value of 200 ms (Guitton et al., 1984; Laurutis & Robinson, 1986). We suggest that, also in these conditions, the value of head velocity at 200 ms can still be used to quickly orient the eyes in the direction of head movement.

After this first gaze orienting saccade, the saccadic mechanism undergoes a temporary inhibition. The head movement is compensated by the VOR, and gaze remains stationary. At the end of inhibition, the head movement can be completed or not. In the former case, no further saccade will be made (Figure 4A). In the latter case, a new saccade is made in the direction of the head movement (Figure 4B). We suggest that the amplitude of the new saccade depends on the residual head velocity, and therefore, on the vestibular output at that time.

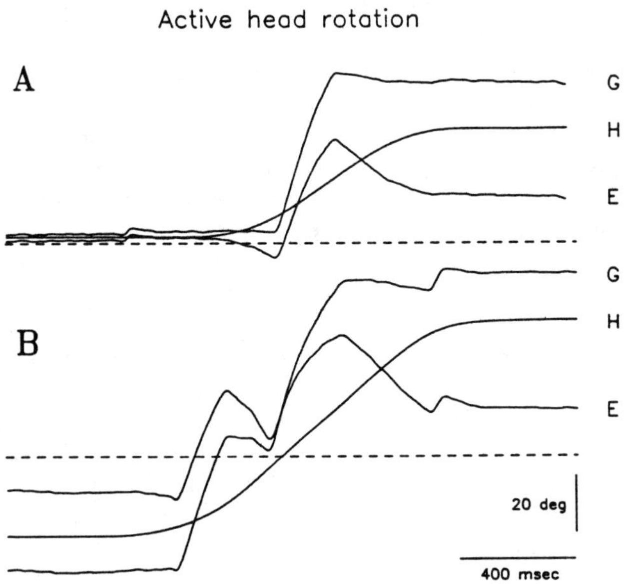

Fig. 4: Examples of eye-head coordination in which the final gaze position is reached with only one saccade (**A**) and multiple saccades (**B**). The subject was asked to make voluntary head movements in the dark. E: eye position; H: head position; G: gaze position.

From the point of view of neural circuitry, the model in Figure 3 appears to be extremely simple. The head velocity signal, available at the output of primary vestibular neurons, only needs to be scaled by a factor σ, which may well be a synaptic gain. The process is started by removing the inhibition in the main pathway and terminates when the primary vestibular neurons return to a resting condition.

More complex signal processing cannot be excluded. Barnes and Benson (1973) proposed that the predictor is a lead-lag element. The signal sent to the saccadic mechanism is, therefore, a linear combination of head velocity and acceleration. Since acceleration is taken into account, better performances can be obtained in terms of early prediction. Nevertheless, for the same reason, this predictor would be much more sensitive to high frequency disturbances.

In whatever way the function of estimating the amplitude of the ongoing head movement is performed, the nature of this function and the need to integrate its results with other sensory information would suggest the involvement of high level strucures. A vestibular projection to the posterior parietal cortex, especially to area 7, has been demonstrated (Kawano et al., 1984). This area is considered as an associative area, dealing with gaze orientation towards targets and with programming spatially directed movements.

Eye-Head Coordination during Voluntarily Controlled Head Movements in the Dark

In the previous section, eye-head coordination was examined during fast orientation head movement in the dark. The head velocity profile was similar to that observed during gaze orientation towards a real target. In this section, eye-head coordination was examined when the subjects were asked to move their head from left to right or from right to left at different voluntarily controlled velocities (see Methods, condition C).

The head movement shown in Figure 5A started from 45 ° left and terminated, after about 2.5 s, at 30 ° right. During the central part of the movement, an almost constant head velocity was maintained at about 50 °/s. The eyes started to move in the compensatory direction and the first saccade in the direction of head movement occured after about 250 ms. The remaining part of the eye response consisted of a series of saccades separated by compensatory eye movements. When head velocity was kept constant, the amplitude of the saccades was also nearly constant.

An example of faster head movement is shown in Figure 5B (from 40 ° left to 40 ° right in about 1.6 s). The amplitude of the first two saccades presents the same linear relation with head velocity as found for the saccades in Figure 5A. The last two saccades show a clear saturation effect.

A head movement from left to right followed, after a pause of about 1.5 s, by a movement in the opposite direction is shown in Figure 6A, whereas an almost sinusoidal voluntary head movement is shown in Figure 6B. The eye response in the latter case is the composition of elementary responses (A-B, B-C, C-D). Each of them corresponds to the head movement in one direction. The resulting profile of eye movement is very similar to that of vestibular nystagmus recorded

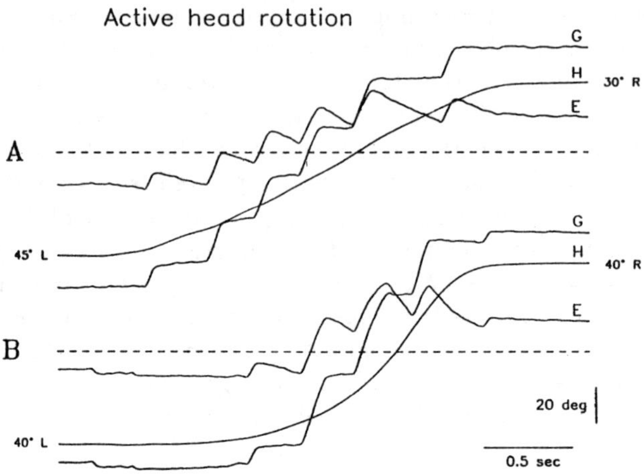

Fig. 5. Two examples of eye-head coordination during voluntarily controlled head movements in the dark. The subject was asked to make voluntary head movements in the dark. E: eye position; H: head position; G: gaze position.

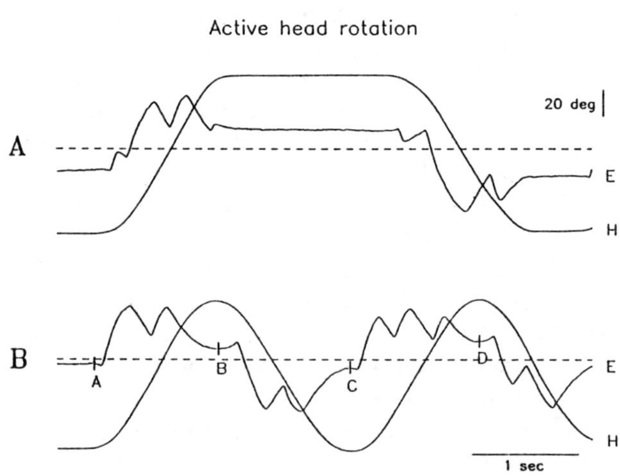

Fig. 6 Eye-head coordination during two active head rotations in the opposite direction (**A**) and during an active sinusoidal head oscillation (**B**) in the dark.

at the same frequency during passive sinusoidal head rotation in the dark (see the last record in Figure 10A).

DIFFERENT STRATEGIES OF EYE-HEAD COORDINATION

The results reported in this paper and in many others (Barnes, 1976, 1979; Barnes & Prosser, 1981; Berthoz, 1985; Bizzi et al., 1972; Gresty & Ell, 1982; Morasso et al., 1977; Roucoux et al., 1981) suggest the existence of different strategies of eye-head coordination. To perform the task of orienting gaze in an intended direction, the CNS uses the available motor subsystems (eye in head, head on trunk, and trunk on body) in a variety of coordination strategies. In each situation, the most appropriate strategy is selected according to what the subject intends or is instructed to do, taking into account the incoming sensory information and the actual state of the system. The task division among the cooperating subsystems is centrally programmed in such a way that the peculiar characteristics of each subsystem (dynamics and range of operation) are used to best advantage. Once the strategy has been selected and an appropriate reference signal has been sent to the controlled subsystems, a number of reflex mechanisms are brought into play in order to ensure that the goal of the overall system is reached, regardless of any disturbances or any imperfect calibration in some subsystems. Such reflex mechanisms are fed back with reafferent signals from sensory receptors or with efference copies of the motor commands.

As suggested by Morasso et al. (1977), the highly practised motor tasks are likely to be coded by programs which can be quickly loaded and executed whenever needed. New programs can be compiled when the subject is faced with new motor tasks. After a period of training, the CNS can develop new modes of eye-head-trunk coordination and perform unusual motor tasks under voluntary control. The normally cooperating subsystems can even be decoupled and behave individually in ways opposite to their usual mode of operation during cooperative actions.

The concepts of "correlation storage" and "neural store" introduced by Held (1961) and Reason (1978), respectively, can be extended and integrated with that of a "library of tasks and motor programs" suggested by Morasso et al. (1977).

If we look at the most frequently observed patterns of eye-head coordination, two broad classes of motor programs can be delineated. The first corresponds to the task of *orienting the gaze* towards a point of interest by using the eyes and the head with equal dignity. This strategy requires the central reconstruction of an absolute reference signal representing the intended gaze direction (Chun & Robinson, 1978). If a real target is present, this can be done by comparing the incoming sensory information (providing the relative position of the target in space), with proprioceptive and efference copy information (providing the state of the system). In the absence of a real target, the gaze reference signal can be produced voluntarily. The intended gaze is compared with the actual gaze position and appropriate motor commands are sent to the eye and head motor systems, which are activated in parallel. The VOR has the function of automatically stabilizing gaze direction after a saccade. The sharing of total gaze displacement between the eyes and head is centrally determined. One reasonable hypothesis is that the balance is determined according to the amplitude of the initial gaze error and taking into account the initial positions of the eyes and the head. For small gaze errors and with the eyes close to the primary position, the CNS can even decide not to move the head.

A model of eye-head coordination in this condition is shown in Figure 7. It is assumed that the intended gaze direction G_D is compared with the estimate ($\hat{H}$) of the actual head position in order to obtain the desired position E_D of the eyes in the head. Obviously, E_D cannot exceed the mechanical limits of eye rotation in the orbit. After a possible limitation, E_D is compared with the estimated actual position $\hat{E}$ of the eyes in the head, and an appropriate input signal is sent to the saccadic mechanism. The reference signal R_H to the head motor system is the intended gaze direction G_D multiplied by a factor α, which represents the centrally programmed ratio between head and eye displacement at steady state. It is also assumed that the estimates of the actual position of the head and of the eyes in the head ($\hat{H}$ and $\hat{E}$, respectively) are obtained from corollary discharge signals of the relevant motor commands. In order to obtain an efference copy (estimate) of the output variable, a corollary discharge signal has to be passed through an internal model of the plant. Due to the negligible dynamics of the eye plant, the internal model of it could be reduced to a simple gain factor. A reasonable internal model of the head plant might be a low-pass filter with a time constant of about 500 ms.

The second class of eye-head coordination strategies relates to the task of *orienting the head* to a point of interest or to that of *exploring the visual surround* by a smooth voluntary rotation of the head. To perform these tasks, the head is likely to play the role of master and the eyes that of slaves, since the eyes appear to be driven by the head movement. The CNS controls the head movement and lets the eyes cooperate with it through some automatic or quasi-automatic mechanism. The head starts first and the eyes make a reflex compensatory movement. As soon as an estimate of where the head is moving to is made, the eyes make a saccade that bring the gaze to this position. The amplitude of the saccade represent the intended head deviation.

This strategy, which may be appropriately referred to as a strategy of *head-eye coordination*, seems to be the one most frequently adopted during head orientation in the dark when the point of interest is not determined by the appearence of a real target, as in the experiments described in the previous section. In order to interpret the results of these experiments, we can still

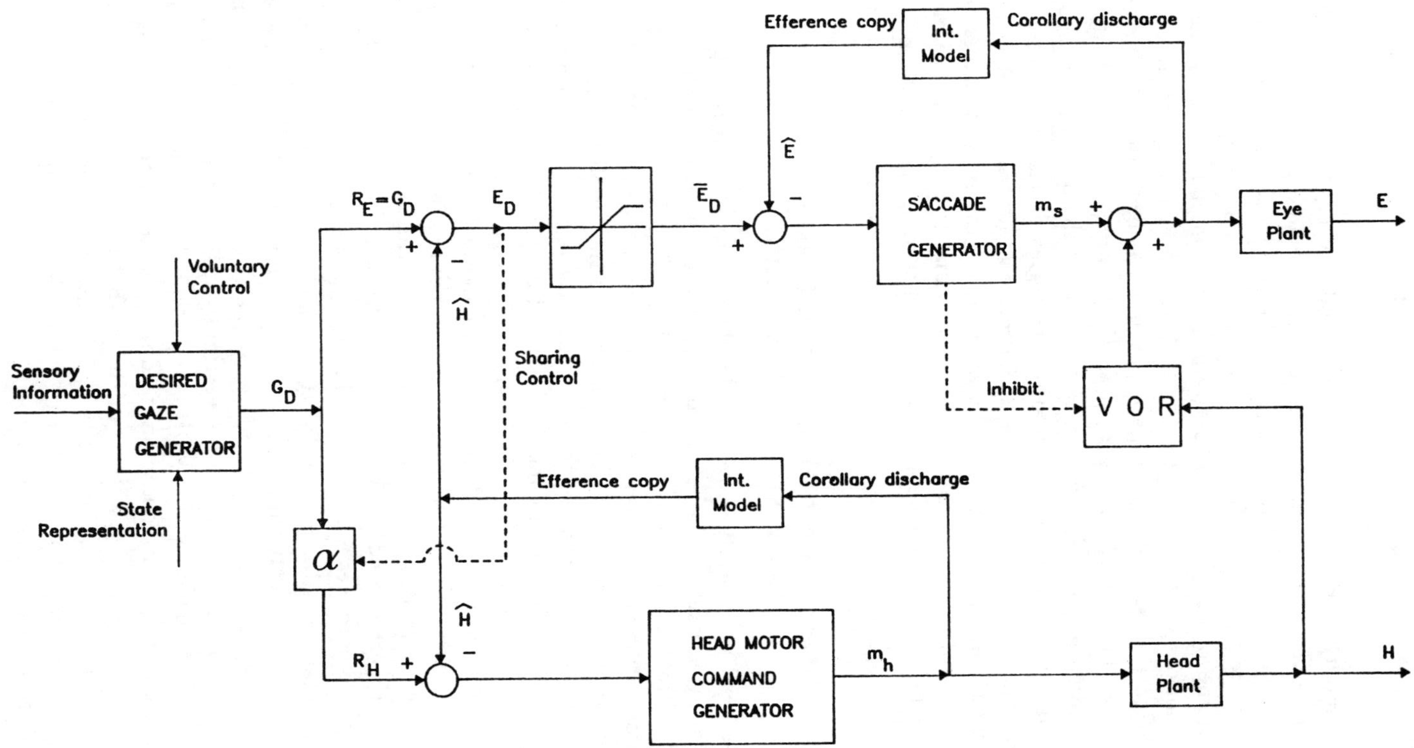

Fig. 7: Model of eye-head coordination in which the motor command signals to the eyes and head are computed from the intended gaze direction G_D.

consider the model in Figure 7 and assume that the input R_H to the head motor system is the head-voluntary-control signal, whereas the input to the saccadic mechanism is an estimate $\Delta_s H$ of the head displacement obtained from vestibular reafference. When this estimate is made available after 200-300 ms from the onset of the head movement, the intended gaze generator will produce an output G_D equal to $G_o + \Delta_s H$, in which $G_o = H_o + E_o$ is the initial gaze direction. Since gaze has not changed, due to the VOR compensatory action, a gaze error $G_E = \Delta_s H$ will arise from the comparison between the intended gaze G_D and the estimate $\hat{G}$ of the actual gaze.

The two classes of eye-head coordination strategies described above correspond to the modes termed by Barnes and Prosser (1981) as "target acquisition" and "visual search." In the visual search mode "the subject makes head movements in the direction of the target location and the saccadic eye movement is generated as a reflex response to the head-turning movement."

Passive Head Movement in Darkness and Vestibular Nystagmus

When the head is passively moved in the dark, a motor program of head-eye coordination is likely to be automatically executed. Also in the case of passive body rotations in toto, which exclude any role of neck proprioceptors, feedback information on head movement is still available to the CNS through the vestibular receptors. It can be used to estimate the amplitude $\Delta_s H$ of the ongoing head rotation, in exactly the same way as during active head movements in the dark. What is missing in this condition is the motor command to the head muscles. Therefore, the efference copy signal $\hat{H}$ would appear to be permanently equal to zero. Hence, if the model of head-eye coordination proposed at the end of the previous section also applies in this case, the only changes being those relating to the passive nature of the head movement, then the scheme in Figure 8 needs to be considered for a proper interpretation of the relevant oculomotor response (vestibular nystagmus).

The input signal is head angular velocity $\dot{H}$ which is passed through a block describing SCC dynamics. A value of 6 s can be assumed for the time constant T_c of SCC. The signal, F1, corresponding to the discharge frequency of primary vestibular neurons enters both the vestibulo-ocular reflex (VOR) and the vestibulo-saccadic pathway (VSP). VOR is represented in the lower part of the figure and contains the positive internal feedback loop suggested by Robinson (1977). Due to the presence of this loop, the VOR time constant is 3-4 times greater than T_c. According to the results by Laurutis and Robinson (1986) and by Pelisson et al. (1988), it is assumed in the model (dashed line) that VOR is inhibited during a saccadic eye movement.

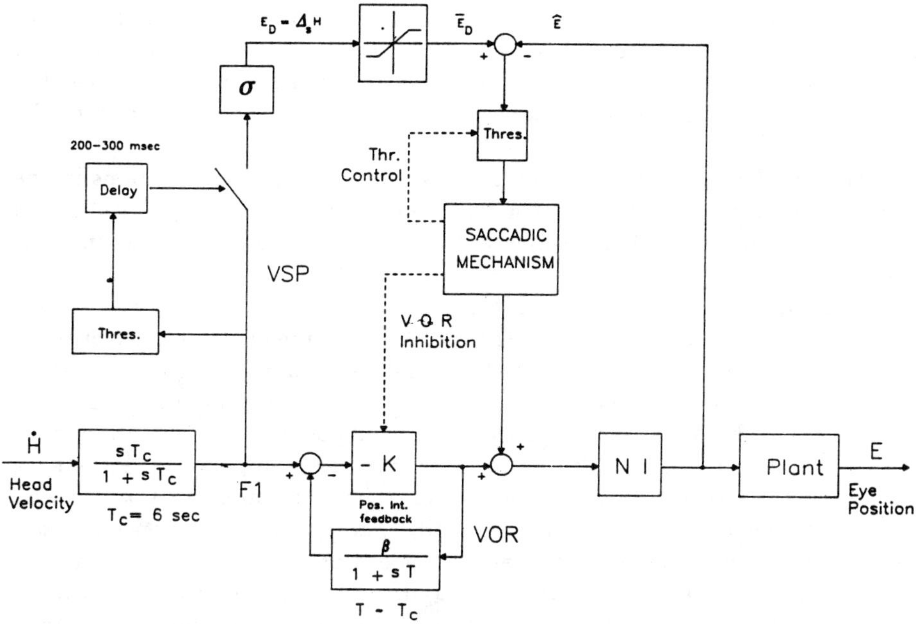

Fig. 8: Model of head-eye coordination during passive head rotation in the dark.

The predictor of head angular rotation in the VSP has been described by the model shown in Figure 3. Its output $\Delta_s H$ passes through a limiter and it is compared with the estimated actual position $\hat{E}$ of the eyes in the head. Finally, a threshold control on the input to the saccadic mechanism has been introduced to describe its temporary inhibition after each saccade.

Let us now use the model shown in Figure 8 to predict the oculomotor response evoked by a passive head rotation in the dark. The beginning of the eye response is always a compensatory movement, the minimum duration of which is the delay of the mechanism for VSP activation. A significant increase with respect to this minimum value occurs when the vestibular discharge takes time to reach threshold. Once the VSP has been activated, the output of the vestibular receptors, appropriately scaled and limited (Guitton et al., 1984), is sent to the saccadic mechanism as a reference signal. A first saccade is produced in the anticompensatory direction with an amplitude that depends on both the value of the vestibular output at the time of VSP activation and the eye position relative to the head at that time. After this first saccade, the saccadic mechanism is temporarily inhibited and a slow compensatory movement can take place. As soon as the saccadic mechanism is enabled again, a second saccade is produced which brings the eyes to the position indicated by the vestibular input to the saccadic mechanism at that time, and so on. A nystagmic pattern of eye movement is then predicted. The saccades in the anticompensatory direction would appear to correspond to the so-called nystagmus fast phase, whereas the intersaccadic compensatory eye movement would appear to correspond to the slow phase.

With regard to particular patterns of passive vestibular stimulations in the dark (see Methods, condition A), the model in Figure 8 is able to predict certain specific features observed experimentally in the eye response recorded in these conditions.

The predominance of the anticompensatory phase in post-rotational nystagmus has been described by Melvill Jones (1964). At the onset of the vestibular stimulation (when the chair on which the subject was rotating at a constant velocity stops), the eyes first make a short compensatory movement. Then, a large saccade takes the eyes far beyond the central position. The remaining part of the response consists of alternating slow and fast components. For strong vestibular stimulations, during the first 2-3 s, the fast components take the eyes close to their extreme position in the orbit. The nystagmic response remains deviated from the baseline in the anticompensatory direction and returns to it after about 15-20 s. Thereafter, nystagmus develops close to the primary position of the eyes with the slow components deviating the eyes from it and the fast components bringing the eyes back to it. A reversal in the direction of nystagmus normally occurs, in man, after about 40-50 s from the onset of the stimulus. The origin of nystagmus reversal is not yet clear. For the purpose of the following discussion, it is worth noting that the return of the response to the baseline appears to be dominated by a time constant close to that of the SCC, whereas the time required for nystagmus reversal depends on the 3-4 times greater VOR time constant. The typical features of a post-rotational response are schematically represented in Figure 9A.

The predominance of the anticompensatory phase depends on the intensity of the stimulus and increases with it. The first 15 s of a post-rotational nystagmus recorded in our laboratory in response to a velocity step of 100 °/s are shown in Figure 9B.

These characteristics of post-rotational response can easily be explained by the model shown in Figure 8 in which the saccadic system is driven by a signal proportional to the discharge frequency of primary vestibular neurons. In a post rotational test, the signal denoted in the model by F1 reaches a maximum in about 1 s and then declines with the time constant of the SCC (see the schematic diagram in Figure 1B). As long as this signal is not zero a predominance of the anticompensatory phase is predictable. After about 20 s, F1 returns to zero and the input to the saccadic mechanism becomes $-\hat{E}$. Then, the fast phase will bring the eyes back to baseline after the deviation produced by the VOR in the compensatory direction.

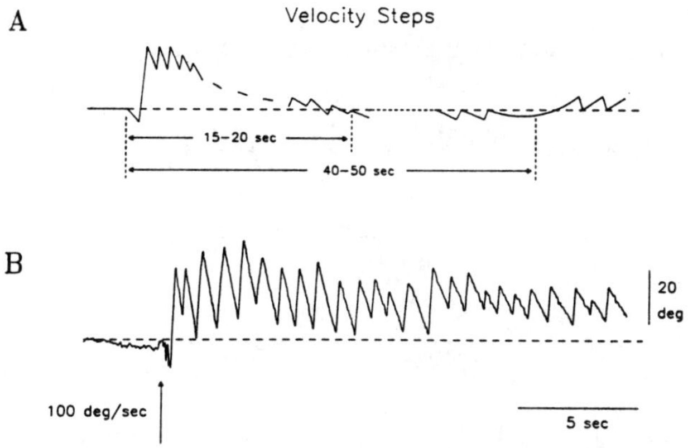

Fig. 9 - A: Schematic representation of the typical features of a post-rotational nystagmus. **B**: Beginning of the post-rotational response to a velocity step of 100 °/s.

The predominance of the anticompensatory phase of nystagmus during sinusoidal oscillations in the dark has been described by Mishkin and Melvill Jones (1966) in man and by Furman et al. (1981) in the monkey. As shown in our records of Figure 10A (responses of one subject to sinusoidal stimulations of the same peak velocity, 100 °/s, and frequencies from 0.02 to 0.5 Hz), and Figure 11A (responses of the same subject to sinusoidal oscillations of the same frequency, 0.08 Hz, and peak velocities from 50 to 200 °/s), nystagmus appears to be sinusoidally modulated with the following characteristics:

(1) the frequency of modulation is the same as the frequency of the stimulus;
(2) it is the fast phase that deviates the eyes from the central position and the slow phase that brings the eyes back towards it;
(3) for the same frequency, the amplitude of nystagmus modulation increases with peak head velocity (Figure 11A);
(4) for large peak head velocities (see the last record in Figure 11A), a saturation in the fast phase eye deviation occurs for a long interval during each period of stimulation;
(5) at low frequencies, the envelope of nystagmus is phase advanced with respect to head velocity, and becomes in phase at high frequencies (bars in Figure 10A indicate the zero crossing of chair velocity).

These general characteristics of the nystagmic response evoked by sinusoidal head rotations in the dark can be predicted by the model shown in Figure 8, in which the reference signal for eye position in the orbit is the sinusoidal output of SCC, multiplied by a gain factor and passed through a limiter. The envelope of nystagmus should, therefore, correspond to this signal.

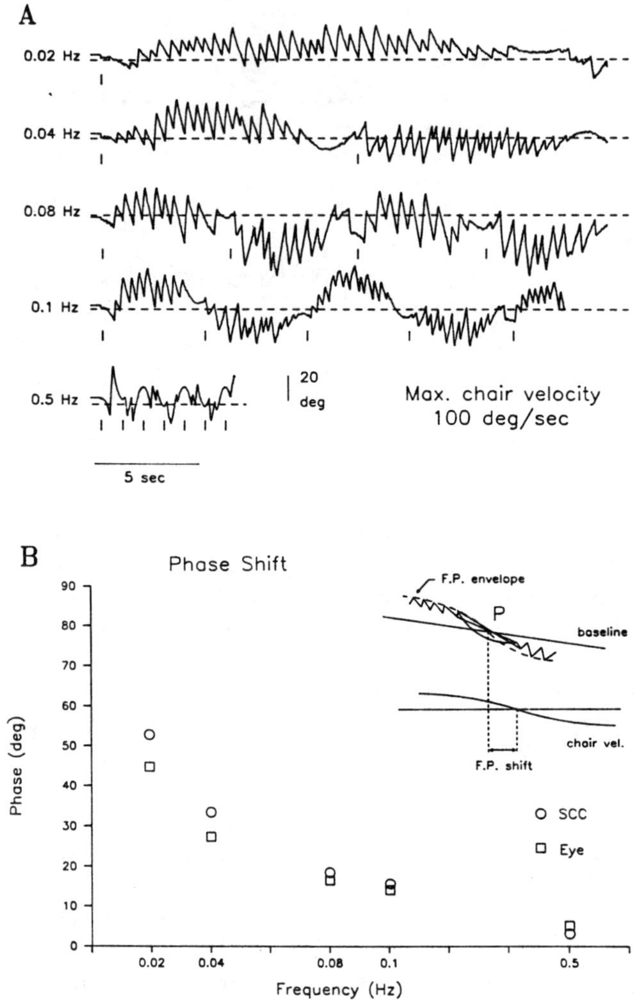

Fig. 10 - **A**: Responses of one subject to passive sinusoidal head oscillations in the dark with the same peak velocity (100 °/s) and different frequencies (from 0.02 to 0.5 Hz) **B**: Open squares, phase shift between the envelope of nystagmus and chair velocity computed from the responses in **A** by estimating the zero points P of the envelope as shown schematically in the inset; open circles, phase shift of the output of the vestibular receptors computed from the model of the SCC used in Fig.8 with T_c=6 s

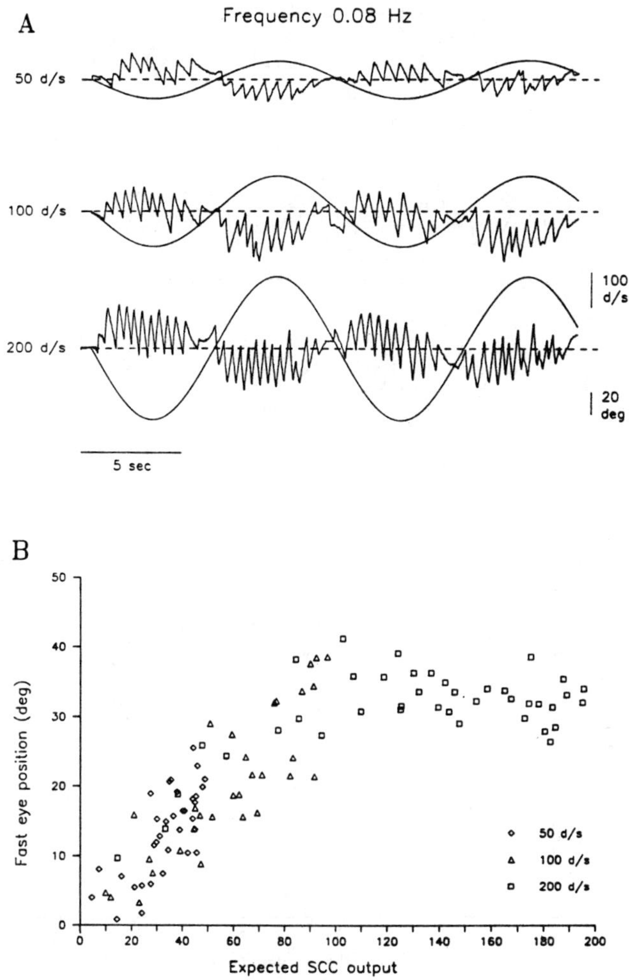

Fig. 11 - A: Responses of one subject to passive sinusoidal oscillations of the same frequency (0.08 Hz) and different peak velocities (from 50 to 200 °/s). **B**: Eye position at the end of each fast phase plotted against the expected output of SCC at the beginning of the same phase.

The phase shift between the nystagmus envelope and chair velocity obtained from the responses in Figure 10A is plotted versus frequency in Figure 10B (open squares). The phase shift was computed by estimating the zero points P of the envelope as shown schematically in the inset. In this way, errors due to the fact that the envelope is defined only by a discrete number of points and may present a saturation, and errors due to a shift of the baseline can both

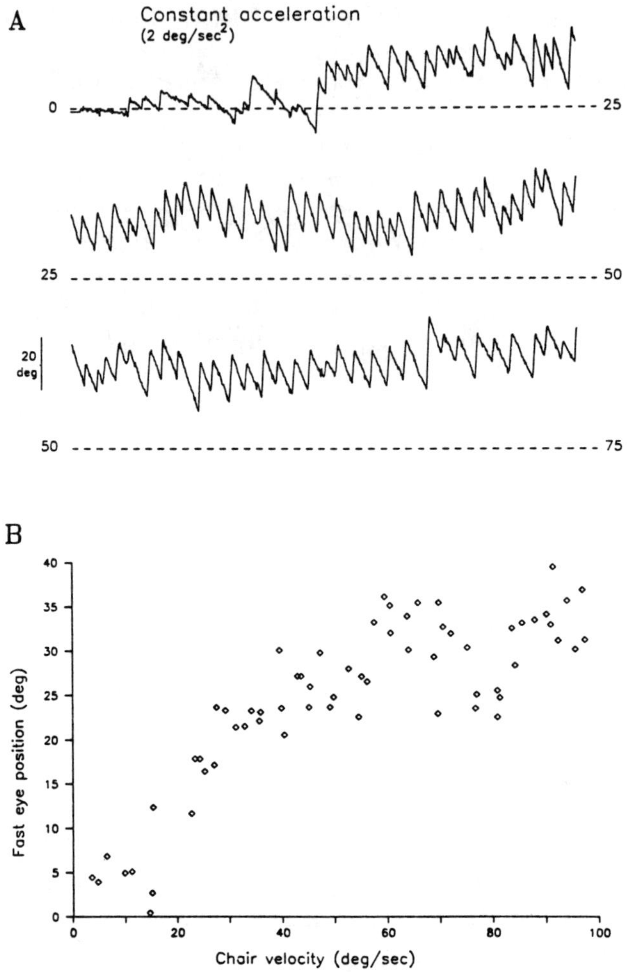

Fig. 12 - A: Nystagmic response recorded during a constant acceleration test of 2 °/s^2 from 0 to 150 °/s. **B**: Relationship between eye position at the end of each fast phase and chair velocity at the beginning of the same phase.

be avoided. Open circles in the same figure give the phase shift of the output of the vestibular receptors computed from the model of SCC used in Figure 8 with $T_c = 6$ s.

The eye position at the end of each fast phase computed from the responses in Figure 11A is plotted in Figure 11B against the output of SCC at the beginning of the same phase as computed from the model of SCC in Figure 8.

A linear scale with arbitrary units was used for the abscissa. There is a linear relationship up to an eye deviation of 35-40 ° and then a clear saturation. The non-linearity resulting from the data in Figure 11B is likely to correspond to the non-linear characteristic introduced in the VSP of the model in Fig. 8.

One way to fully explore this characteristic is to perform a constant acceleration (per-rotational) test in which chair velocity is increased linearly from 0 to a maximum. The nystagmic response recorded during a constant acceleration test of 2 $^{\circ}/s^2$ from 0 to 150 °/s is shown in Figure 12A. The subject was the same as in the previous tests. The amplitude of eye deviation in the anticompensatory direction increases linearly with chair velocity up to a maximum of about 40 °, which is reached when chair velocity approaches 80 °/s. Thereafter, the deviation remains constant, and the response is made of slow phases deviating the eyes towards the central position and fast phases bringing the eyes to a deviated position of about 40 °.

The relationship obtained from this response between eye position at the end of each fast phase and chair velocity at the beginning of the same phase is shown in Figure 12B. The same non-linear characteristic as derived from sinusoidal responses is obtained.

CONCLUSION

The presence of an oculomotor response during passive head rotations in the dark (vestibular nystagmus), owing to the CNS's ability to suppress a response when the environmental situation makes it useless or inappropriate, has been a puzzle for many people working in oculomotor research. In most of the papers dealing with vestibular nystagmus, the question of why vestibular nystagmus occurs was simply ignored, and attention was focused on defining this or that characteristic of nystagmus. Indeed, no reasonable explaination can be found if one assumes that vestibular afference is used in oculomotor control only to produce compensatory eye movements through the vestibulo-ocular reflex (VOR). In the absence of vision, there is apparently no need to stabilize the gaze.

However, if we look carefully into the literature we can find a few papers in which the belief that the fast phase of nystagmus is related to a strategy of orienting the gaze toward a point of interest is clearly stated (Melvill Jones, 1964; Mishkin & Melvill Jones, 1966; Barnes, 1976). Some attempt has been made to formalize this concept by means of mathematical models (Barnes & Benson, 1973; Schmid & Lardini, 1976; Chun & Robinson, 1978).

The results of recent studies on eye-head coordination have suggested the existence of several strategies in the use of eyes and head to perform a task of gaze orientation (Barnes, 1976, 1979; Barnes & Prosser, 1981; Berthoz, 1985; Bizzi et al., 1972; Gresty & Ell, 1982; Morasso et al., 1977; Roucoux et al., 1981). The most appropriate strategy is selected according to the environmental conditions, the nature of the incoming sensory information, the state of the system and the subject's voluntary control (Morasso et al., 1977). To execute some of these strategies, the CNS is likely to use the vestibular information to program the amplitude of the eye orienting saccades. These strategies have been referred to in this paper as strategies of "head-eye coordination," since the head seems to play the role of master and the eyes that of slaves.

A head-eye coordination strategy implies the existence of a vestibulo-saccadic pathway (VSP), i.e. a second means of using vestibular information in oculomotor control. This pathway, which might involve high level neural structures, has the main function of predicting where the head is moving to and sending an appropriate motor command to the saccadic system to bring the gaze quickly to this position. A hypothetical model of the predictor, based on the linear relationship existing between amplitude and peak velocity in fast orientation head movements, has been proposed in this paper.

A strategy of head-eye coordination, which also makes sense in darkness, could be activated by passive vestibular stimulations in a quasi-automatic way. This is likely to occur when the passive stimulation evokes a pattern of discharge in primary vestibular neurons that starts with a shape qualitatively not too different from those induced by active orientation head movements. If this is the case, vestibular nystagmus is the manifestation of this strategy at the oculomotor level.

To test this hypothesis, we first constructed a model of head-eye coordination during voluntary head orientation in the dark, then we adapted the model to the case of passive stimulations of the semicircular canals and, finally, we examined whether it was able to predict the main characteristics of vestibular nystagmus recorded during the usual rotatory tests in the dark.

Although a more systematic analysis needs to be carried out, in particular to define the type of signal processing occurring in the vestibulo-saccadic pathway, the preliminary results reported in this paper suggest that vestibular nystagmus is actually the manifestation of a strategy of head-eye coordination.

In our model, the fast phase of nystagmus no longer has the passive function of resetting the system after eye deviation has occurred in a reflex way during the slow phase, but it is rather seen as the active part of the response. Moreover, the eye position at the end of nystagmus fast phases is seen corresponding to the discrete representation of a signal strictly correlated to the output of the semicircular canals. Thus, in the investigation of the vestibular function, the fast phase of nystagmus deserves much more attention than it has received so far. In particular, the discrimination between peripheral and central vestibular disorders in clinical examination of nystagmus would probably be easier if the analysis of nystagmus were carried out by considering both the slow and the fast phase, and comparing these two components.

Acknowledgement

Work supported by Ministero della Pubblica Istruzione (M.P.I.), Rome, Italy.

References

Barnes, G.R., "Vestibulo-ocular responses to head turning movements and their functional significance during visual target acquisition, Ph. D. Thesis," University of Surrey, Guildford, U.K., 1976.

Barnes, G.R., *Vestibulo-ocular function during co-ordinated head and eye movements to acquire visual targets*, Journal of Physiology **287** (1979), 127-147.

Barnes, G.R., & Benson, A.J., *A model for the prediction of the nystagmic response to angular and linear acceleration stimuli*, in "The use of nystagmography in aviation medicine (NATO AGARD CCP-128, A 23)," 1973, pp. 1-13.

Barnes, G.R., & Prosser, A.J., *Vestibular influence upon head-eye coordination*, in "B. Cohen (Ed.), Vestibular and oculomotor physiology (Annual of the New York Academy of Sciences)," 1981, pp. 560-570.

Berthoz, A., *Adaptive mechanisms in eye-head coordination*, in "A. Berthoz & G. Melvill Jones (Eds.), Adaptive mechanisms in gaze control, reviews of oculomotor research," Elsevier Science Publishers B. V., 1985, pp. 177-201.

Berthoz. A., & Melvill Jones, G. (Eds.), "Adaptive mechanisms in gaze control," Elsevier Science Publishers B. V., 1985.

Bizzi, E., Kalil, R.E., & Morasso, P., *Two modes of active eye-head coordination in monkeys*, Brain Research **40** (1972), 45-48.

Chun, K.S., & Robinson, D.A., *A model of quick phase generation in the vestibuloocular reflex*, Biological Cybernetics **28** (1978), 209-221.

Furman, J.M., O'Leary, D.P., & Wolfe, J.W., *Modulation of mean eye position during vestibular induced eye movements of the rhesus monkey*, Acta Otolaryngologica (Stockholm) **97** (1984), 627-632.

Gresty, M.A., & Ell, J.J., *Normal modes of head and eye coordination*, in "G. Lennerstrand, D.S. Zee, & E.L. Keller (Eds.), Functional basis of ocular motility disorders," Pergamon, Oxford, 1982, pp. 391-406.

Guitton, D., Douglas, R.M., & Volle, M., *Eye-head coordination in cats*, Journal of Neurophysiology **52** (1984), 1030-1050.

Guitton, D., & Volle, M., *Gaze control in humans: eye-head coordination during orienting movements to targets within and beyond the oculomotor range*, Journal of Neurophysiology **58** (1987), 427-459.

Haddad, G.M., & Robinson, D.A., *Cancellation of the vestibuloocular reflex during active and passive head movements in the normal cat*, Society Neuroscience Abstracts **3** (1977), p. 155.

Held, R., *Exposure history as a factor of mantaining stability of perception and coordination*, Journal of Nervous and Mental Disease **132** (1961), 26-32.

Jeannerod, M., *La decouverte de la fonction vestibulaire*, Acta Oto - Rhino - Laryngologica Belgica **35 Suppl. III** (1981), 975-1006.

Jürgens, R., Becker, W., & Rieger, P., *Different effects involved in the interaction of saccades and the vestibulo-ocular reflex*, in "B. Cohen (Ed.), Vestibular and oculomotor physiology (Annual of the New York Academy of Sciences)," 1981, pp. 744-754.

Kawano, K., Sasaki, M., & Yamashita, M., *Response properties of neurons in posterior parietal cortex of the monkey during visual vestibular stimulation. I. Visual tracking neurons*, Journal of Neurophysiology **51** (1984), 340-351.

Laurutis, V.P., & Robinson, D.A., *The vestibulo-ocular reflex during human saccadic eye movements*, Journal of Physiology **373** (1986), 209-233.

Melvill Jones, G., *Predominance of anticompensatory oculomotor response during rapid head movement*, Aerospace Medicine **35** (1964), 965-968.

Mishkin, S., & Melvill Jones, G., *Predominant direction of gaze during slow head rotation*, Aviation, Space and Environmental Medicine **37** (1966), 897-900.

Morasso, P., Bizzi, E., & Dichgans, J., *Adjustment of saccade characteristics during head movements*, Experimental Brain Research **16** (1973), 492-500.

Morasso, P., Sandini, G., Tagliasco, V., & Zaccaria, R., *Control strategies in the eye-head coordination system*, IEEE Transaction, SCM-7 (1977), 639-651.

Pelisson, D., Prablanc, C., & Urquizar, C., *Vestibulo-ocular reflex (VOR) inhibition and gaze saccadic control characteristics during eye-head orientation in man*, Journal of Neurophysiology (1988) (to appear).

Reason, J.T., *Motion sickness: a neural mismatch model*, Journal of Royal Society of Medicine **71** (1978), 819-829.

Robinson, D.A., *Vestibular and optokinetic symbiosis: an example of explaining by modelling*, in "R. Baker & A. Berthoz (Eds.), Control of gaze by brain stem neurons," Elsevier/North Holland Biomedical Press, Amsterdam, New York, 1977, pp. 49-58.

Roucoux, A., Crommelinck, M., Guerit, J.M., & Meulders, M., *Two modes of eye-head coordination and the role of the vestibulo-ocular reflex in these two strategies*, in "A.F. Fuchs & W. Becker (Eds.), Progress in oculomotor research," Elsevier/North Holland, Amsterdam, 1981, pp. 309-315.

Schmid, R., & Jeannerod, M., *Vestibular habituation an adaptive process?*, in "A. Berthoz & G. Melvill Jones (Eds.), Adaptive mechanisms in gaze control, reviews of oculomotor research," Elsevier Science Publishers, 1985, pp. 113-122.

Schmid, R., & Lardini, F., *On the predominance of anti-compensatory eye movements in vestibular nystagmus*, Biological Cybernetics **23** (1976), 135-148.

Shimazu, H., Ohki, Y., & Suzuki, I., *Excitatory input to burst neurons from the horizontal semicircular canal in the cat*, in "Proceedings of Developments in Oculomotor Research Congress (WP-26)," 1986.

Tomlinson, R.D., & Bahra, P.S., *Combined eye-head gaze shifts in the primate. II. Interactions between saccades and the vestibuloocular reflex*, Journal of Neurophysiology **56** (1986), 1558-1570.

Whittington, D.A., Lestienne, F., & Bizzi, E., *Behavior of preoculomotor burst neurons during eye-head coordination*, Experimental Brain Research **55** (1984), 215-222.

Zangemeister, W.H., Jones, A., & Stark, L., *Dynamics of head movement trajectories: main sequence relationship*, Experimental Neurology **71** (1981), 76-91.

SACCADES TO DOUBLE AND SINGLE STEP STIMULI IN PATIENTS WITH CEREBRAL LESIONS

HESSEL FRANSSEN [1] AND DIRK FREDERIK STEGEMAN [2]

[1] Department of Clinical Neurophysiology,
University of Utrecht
[2] Department of Clinical Neurophysiology,
Institute of Neurology, University of Nijmegen

INTRODUCTION

The reaction time of a visually evoked saccade, defined as the time interval between the appearance of the target and the onset of the saccade, is about 250 ms in humans. Such a long interval suggests that, before a saccade is executed, substantial processing has taken place in the brain. The model of the saccadic system by Becker and Jürgens (1979) describes these processes in a system-analytical way The model is partially based on experiments with double step stimuli of the pulse-undershoot type (Figure 1). With this type of stimulus a visual target steps from a fixation point at 0 ° to, for instance, 20 ° on the left or right (first step) Less than 200 ms later, the target steps back to 10 ° on the same side (second step). In order to foveate the target, the first step usually triggers the preparation for a saccade. As, however, the second step occurs before the onset of this saccade, a saccade of 20 ° will be too large since the second step brings the target back to 10 °. In certain conditions the saccadic system is able to modify the preparation of the saccade so that it will foveate the target at 10 °. This depends on the time interval (D) between the occurrence of the second step and the onset of the saccade. Within one subject D varies from one saccade to another due to variation of the saccadic reaction time. It has been shown that the larger the value of D, the more time is available for the saccadic system to modify the preparation of the saccade. When D is less than about 80 ms (modification time = Dm) the preparation is too far advanced to be modified. Therefore, the saccade will be directed to the target at 20 ° (Figure 1 upper). When D is larger than about 200 ms, the preparation of the saccade can be completely modified. The saccade will be directed to the target at 10 ° (Figure 1 lower). With values of D between 80 ms (Dm) and 200 ms, the amplitude of the saccade decreases with increasing D (Figure 1 middle). The interval between D = Dm = 80 ms and D = 200 ms is called the transition time (Tw). Saccades in this interval are directed *between* the targets at 20 ° and 10 ° ("averaging"). By collecting a large number of saccadic responses to double step stimuli within one subject, Becker and Jürgens obtained a scatter diagram as shown in Figure 1. They fitted the scatter diagram with 3 straight

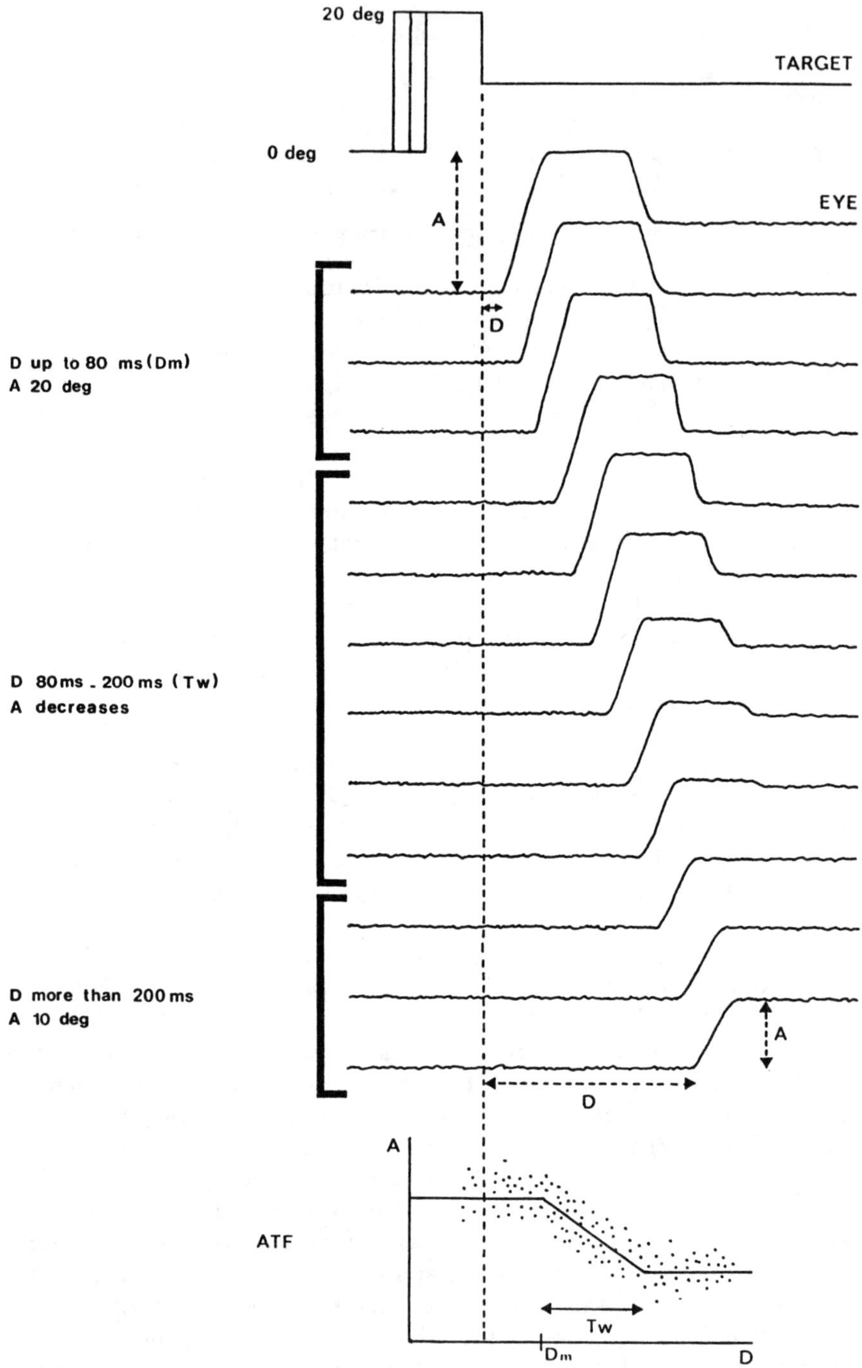

Fig. 1: Saccades (EYE = eye position) in response to a pulse undershoot stimulus (TARGET = target position) and the resulting ATF. The saccadic responses are arranged in such a way that D (interval between second step and onset of saccade) increases, going from upper to lower. A = amplitude of the first saccade.

lines: a first horizontal segment representing saccades of about 20 ° for which D < Dm, an oblique segment representing saccades during the transition time and a second horizontal segment representing saccades of about 10 ° for which D > (Dm + Tw). The three straight lines expressing the relation between amplitude and D are known as the amplitude transition function (ATF).

Becker and Jürgens proposed that the saccadic system can be described as a chain of four processing elements each with a time delay. *The afferent element* (delay Ta) signals the retinal error of a target to a central decision and computing structure consisting of the decision and averaging elements. *The decision element* (variable delay Td) decides whether or not a saccade has to be made. *The averaging element* (delay Tw) consists of a time window and an averager. The time window, when initiated by the decision element, feeds the retinal error signal into the averager during a period Tw which equals the transition time in the ATF. At the end of this period an average of the retinal error signal has been calculated which then initiates the *efferent element* (delay Te) needed to signal the calculated amplitude and direction of a saccade to efferent mechanisms. In other words the saccadic reaction time equals the sum of the delays of these four elements: reaction time = Ta + Td + Tw + Te. The advantage of averaging is that the ensuing saccade will be less dependent upon random fluctuations of the retinal error signal. Moreover, Becker and Jürgens proposed that Dm = Ta + Te.

It is not known through which structures the decision and averaging processes are performed.

The aim of this study is to test the above mentioned hypotheses proposed by Becker and Jürgens and to establish whether the cerebral cortex, thalamus or superior colliculus are involved in the decision and averaging processes. For these purposes, saccades to double step and single step stimuli were investigated in normal subjects and patients with focal cerebral lesions.

SUBJECTS

Twenty-two patients (mean age 54.6 years, range 31-74) and 10 normal subjects (mean age 42.3 years, range 19-66) were investigated.

The patients were alert and co-operative. They had no signs of brainstem or cerebellar dysfunction, hemianopia or visual neglect. One patient (C17) had a homonymous quadrantanopia.

The patient group consisted of 17 patients with a cortical lesion (C1-C17), 3 patients with a thalamic lesion (T1-T3), one patient with lesions in both superior colliculi (S) and one patient with bilateral corona radiata lesions (R). The lesions were ascertained by means of CT-scanning. The patients were scanned from the foramen magnum to the vertex with 10 mm slices parallel to a slice through the pineal body and foramina of Monro. One patient (C16) did not have a visible lesion on CT-scanning but had, clinically and electroencephalographically, a parietal deficit. The interval between CT-scanning and the recording of eye movements was less than one week. The clinical data of the patients is given in Table 1.

Tab. 1: Clinical data on the patient group. Side: l = left, r = right. Site: f = frontal, t = temporal, p = parietal, o = occipital. Perimetry: 1 log-unit r = 1 log unit decrease of retinal threshold in the right visual field of both eyes.

			LESION					
PATIENT	AGE (years)	DURATION OF SYMPTOMS (days)	SIDE	SITE	DISPLACEMENT ON CT-SCAN	VOLUME (cm^3)	NATURE	PERIMETRY
C1	71	390	l	ftp	yes	150	tumor	1-1.8 log unit r
C2	62	373	r	ftp	yes	148	tumor	1 log unit l
C3	54	43	r	o	no	6	tumor	normal
C4	68	22	l	f	no	49	tumor	normal
C5	57	17	r	fpo	yes	177	tumor	normal
C6	60	20	r	fp	yes	133	tumor	normal
C7	40	186	l	t	no	12	infarct	normal
C8	54	570	l	fp	yes	127	tumor	normal
C9	41	9	r	f	no	90	tumor	normal
C10	57	11	l	f	no	41	tumor	normal
C11	49	6	l	f	no	53	infarct	normal
C12	74	255	l	p	no	82	tumor	not performed
C13	56	40	l	ft	yes	166	tumor	not performed
C14	35	24	l	f	no	8	tumor	normal
C15	46	49	l	f	no	33	infarct	normal
C16	31	4	r	p	CT-scan normal			normal
C17	67	369	r	po	no	35	hemorrhage	>2 log unit l
T1	54	20	l		no	17	infarct	normal
T2	56	9	r		no	2	infarct	normal
T3	48	14	l		no	3	infarct	normal
S	53	189	l, r		no	1	infarct	normal
R	68	11	l, r		no	2	hemorrhage	not performed

The lesions of patients C1-C17 were mapped according to the method described by Mazzocchi and Vignolo (1978). On a template of the lateral surface of the left cerebral hemisphere with outlines of the ventricular system and skull (scale 1:1) as made by New and Scott (1975), parallel lines were drawn 10 mm apart in such a way that one of the lines ran through the pineal body and foramina of Monro. The cerebral cortical surface was cut along this line by the CT-scan slice through the pineal body and foramina of Monro. The other parallel lines similarly represented the other CT-scan slices. From every CT-scan slice the anterior and posterior cortical ends of the lesion were determined and projected as points on the line of the template corresponding with the slice. Subsequently, the points on the template were connected by a smooth line. The resulting contour map yielded the site and extent of the cortical region involved in the lesion. The subcortical extension of the lesions was assessed with the aid of the atlas of Nieuwenhuys et al. (1978).

The lesions in patients T1 to T3 were all located on the CT-scan slice through the foramina of Monro and the pineal body. The lesion extended to the slice 10 mm more dorsally involving the internal capsule in patient T1 only. With the aid of the atlas of Nieuwenhuys et al. (1978) and that of Van Buren and Borke (1972) a drawing was made of the right thalamus and its nuclei at the level of the CT-scan slice through the foramina of Monro and the pineal body. The lesions of patients T1 to T3 were projected on a copy of this drawing.

METHODS

Eye movements were recorded in a quiet, dark room. The targets consisted of light emitting diodes (LEDs), placed in a horizontal array at eye level in a cylindrical screen 150 cm in front of the subject. The distance between the LEDs was 10 °. Each LED subtended a visual angle of 0.15 °. The luminance of a LED was 4 log units above mean foveal threshold and its rise time was 10 μs. The LEDs were controlled by a semi-automatic stimulator.

After the subject was seated, four AgAgCl electrodes (Beckmann) were fixed on the nasal and temporal epicanthi of both eyes in order to separately record the horizontal movements of each eye by means of electrooculography (EOG). The head of the subject was stabilized by a forehead holder. Prior to the investigation, the subjects were dark adapted for 10 minutes. The only instruction given to the subjects was to follow the lights with the eyes as rapidly as possible. They were repeatedly encouraged. None of the subjects had knowledge of the properties of eye movements.

The EOG signal was amplified and filtered using a bandpass between 0 and 50 Hz (-3 dB).

Description of an experiment

Each subject took part in one experiment consisting of:

(1) Twelve series of double step stimuli. Before each series, the EOG was calibrated by 5 single step stimuli of 10 ° to each side. One series consisted of 10 pulse undershoot stimuli to the right (i.e. first step from 0 ° to 20 ° on the right, second step from 20 ° on the right to 10 ° on the right) and 10 pulse undershoot stimuli to the left. In each series, 6 double step stimuli of the staircase type were added in order to increase stimulus unpredictability. They were not analyzed. Within one series, the time interval between the first and second step was fixed (200, 150, 100 or 50 ms). A total amount of 240 pulse undershoot stimuli was given.

(2) One series consisting of 25 single step stimuli of 10 ° to each side (i.e. the target stepped from 0 to 10 °) and 25 single step stimuli of 20 ° (the target stepped from 0 to 20 °) to each side. A total amount of 100 single step stimuli was given.

The time interval between stimuli varied pseudo-randomly between 2 and 10 s. The sequence of stimulus type within one series varied randomly. Visual stimulation was binocular in all cases.

Data analysis

All data was analyzed with a VAX 11/785 computer (Digital Equipment Corporation).

Double step stimuli. From each saccadic response to a pulse undershoot stimulus were determined: (1) the time interval (D) between the second step and the onset of the first saccade after the stimulus, (2) the amplitude (A) of that saccade. The values of A and D of each saccade were plotted in a scatter diagram, each dot representing one response. Within one subject, separate scatter diagrams were obtained from pulse undershoot stimuli to the left and right. The scatter diagram was fitted with the 3 straight lines after Becker and Jürgens' model (Figure 2). The fit was performed by a least-squares fit algorithm (Marquardt, 1963) of the CURFIT procedure described by Bevington (1969). After rejection of data for which D $<$ -90 ms or D $>$ 500 ms or A $<$ 3 ° or A $>$ 25 ° the CURFIT procedure was started. When, by manipulation of the 3 parameters described below, the "goodness of fit" (= the mean squared difference between the data points and the fit line at corresponding values of D) could not be improved further by more than a factor of 10^{-6}, the search was stopped. Subsequently, all data lying beyond 2.5 times the standard deviation (SD) from the fit line was rejected after which the fit procedure was started again, resulting in the final fit. The 3 parameters which were manipulated by

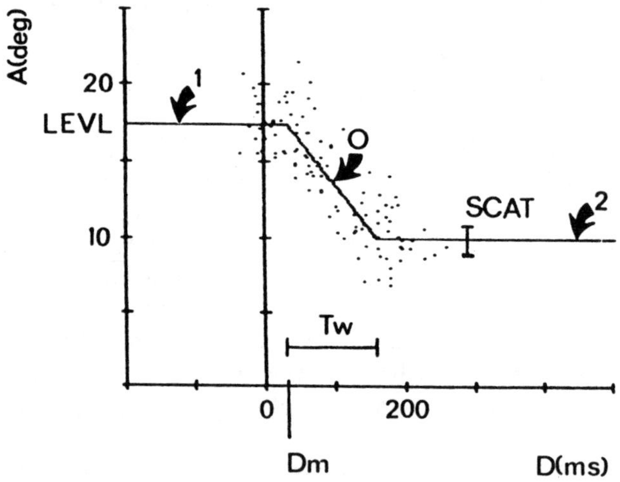

Fig. 2: A scatter diagram in response to pulse undershoot stimuli and the fit resulting in the ATF. 1 = first horizontal segment. 0= oblique segment. 2 = second horizontal segment. Abscissa: D, each subdivision = 100 ms. Ordinate: A, each subdivision = 5 °. The vertical line represents D = 0 ms. Dm = value of D at the intersection of the first horizontal and oblique segment. Tw =time interval between Dm and the intersection of the oblique and second horizontal segment. SCAT = standard deviation of the difference between the data points and the fit line. LEVL = level of the first horizontal segment.

the CURFIT procedure in order to obtain the best fit were: Dm, the slope of the oblique segment and the level (in °) of the first horizontal segment. The level of the second horizontal segment was fixed and determined by the mean amplitude of the first saccadic responses to the single step calibration stimuli of 10 °, obtained separately from saccades to each side. After the final fit, each scatter diagram was characterized by the following *ATF-parameters* (Figure 2):

- Dm (ms): value of D at the intersection of the first horizontal and oblique segment.
- Tw (ms): time interval between Dm and the intersection of the oblique and second horizontal segment.
- SCAT (°): standard deviation of the differences between the data points and the fit line.
- LEVL (°): level of the first horizontal segment.

Single step stimuli. From each response to a single step stimulus were measured: (1) the reaction time (the time interval between the moment of the stimulus and the onset of the first saccade after the stimulus), (2) the amplitude of this saccade. In each subject the following parameters were determined:

- RT (ms): mean reaction time.
- AMP20 (°): mean amplitude of saccades to 20 °.
- varAMP20 (°): variation (= SD) of amplitudes of saccades to 20 °.

In the normal subjects, each parameter was determined separately from saccades directed to the left and right. In the patients, each parameter was determined separately from saccades directed contralaterally with respect to the lesion and from saccades directed ipsilaterally to the lesion. For each parameter the difference left minus right (in normals) or contralateral minus ipsilateral (in patients) was determined.

Results

As the saccadic responses of the left and right eye were not essentially different, only the responses of the right eye were further analyzed.

In the group of normal subjects, no significant difference was found between the values of any parameter for saccades directed to the left and the value of the same parameter for saccades directed to the right. Therefore, the values of each parameter were pooled in order to determine the mean and SD (Table 2) in normal subjects. The values of the individual ATF parameters in the patients are given in Table 3. An ATF parameter was considered abnormal when lying outside the normal mean ± 2 SD.

Tab. 2: Normative values derived from the control group. The middle column gives the mean and SD for the parameters themselves. The right column gives the mean and SD for the left-right difference of these parameters.

	l, r $\bar{x}$ (SD)	l-r difference $\bar{x}$ (SD)
Dm (ms)	36.70 (19.68)	-0.80 (26.08)
Tw (ms)	114.60 (35.68)	-4.00 (40.17)
SCAT (deg)	1.92 (0.30)	-0.17 (0.47)
LEVL (deg)	18.07 (1.25)	-0.64 (1.81)

Tab. 3: Values for ATF parameters in the patient group. Contra, ipsi, left and right refer to values obtained from saccades directed contralaterally to the lesion, ipsilaterally to the lesion, to the left or to the right. The underlined numbers indicate abnormal values. * = abnormally large left-right difference.

	Dm (ms)		Tw (ms)		SCAT (deg)		LEVL (deg)	
PATIENT	CONTRA	IPSI	CONTRA	IPSI	CONTRA	IPSI	CONTRA	IPSI
C1	81	52	67	125	1.9	1.7	17.0	17.9
C2	48	62	106	114	2.6	2.4	16.1	16.0
C3	96	80	104	172	2.4 *	4.4	16.3	17.1
C4	26	45	137	142	1.6	1.5	19.2	16.3
C5	13	21	226	277	3.2	2.9	18.7	19.5
C6	53	49	87	121	1.8 *	3.6	17.5	19.2
C7	33	52	129	62	1.8	2.0	18.9	18.4
C8	18	8	249	302	1.4	2.0	16.0	17.7
C9	89 *	24	47 *	181	1.8 *	3.1	18.1	17.8
C10	6 *	89	494 *	384	3.0	3.4	16.4	15.4
C11	29	3	225	184	2.4	2.5	17.1	20.0
C12	73	52	180	145	2.3	1.5	16.8	16.7
C13	14	41	156	99	2.4	1.9	17.7	16.4
C14	35	42	125	121	1.9	1.7	17.4	16.6
C15	31 *	94	164 *	51	1.6	1.5	18.2	15.7
C16	70	39	110	107	2.3	1.8	18.0	20.3
C17	26	46	474 *	97	3.4 *	1.5	17.9	18.1
T1	59 *	1	44 *	206	1.6	1.8	12.8 *	16.6
T2	26	0	233	280	2.7 *	1.7	18.1	20.2
T3	93	81	42	62	2.4	1.6	19.0	18.4
	LEFT	RIGHT	LEFT	RIGHT	LEFT	RIGHT	LEFT	RIGHT
S	44	45	148	179	2.0	2.1	18.2	19.5
R	89	97	48	56	1.8	1.9	17.5	18.4

Cortical lesions

One or more ATF parameters were abnormal in 11 out of the 17 patients (Table 3). Examples of abnormal ATFs are given in Figure 3. The deficits consisted of increased values for Dm, Tw, SCAT, decreased values for LEVL or increased contralateral - ipsilateral differences. Tw was the only parameter of which deficits might be related to the side of the lesion. Seven patients showed abnormalies of Tw (Table 3). In 4 patients (C9, C10, C15, C17), the difference between Tw for contralaterally directed and Tw for ipsilaterally directed saccades was abnormally large. In 3 of these patients, Tw was larger for contralaterally directed saccades. In another patient (C11), Tw was abnormally large for contralaterally directed saccades. In two more patients (C5, C8), Tw

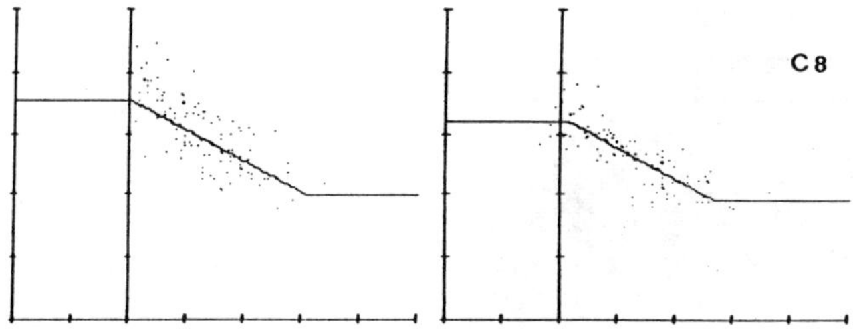

Fig. 3: Examples of ATFs in patients. The ATFs from leftward saccades are depicted on the left half, the ATFs from rightward saccades on the right half of the figure. For further explanation see Figure 2. In the ATFs of patient C8 (upper) Tw is increased bilaterally. In the ATFs of patient C9 (middle) Tw is relatively increased for rightward saccades while Dm is increased for leftward saccades. The ATFs of patient S (lower) are essentially normal.

was increased for contralaterally as well as ipsilaterally directed saccades. Thus, when the Tw deficit was asymmetrical, it usually consisted of an increase of Tw for contralaterally directed saccades.

When the cortical lesions of the patients with abnormal ATFs were superimposed, a maximal overlap of 7 lesions was seen in the region of the frontal eye field while, with one exception, in patients with normal ATFs, this region was spared (Figure 4). Lesions affecting the frontal eye field but also those affecting the inferior parietal lobule or the optic radiation were associated with ATF deficits or abnormalities of SCAT (Table 4). Abnormal values for Dm and/or Tw which are so important in the Becker and Jürgens model were particularly associated with frontal eye field lesions and, to a lesser degree, with inferior parietal lobule and optic radiation lesions (Table 4).

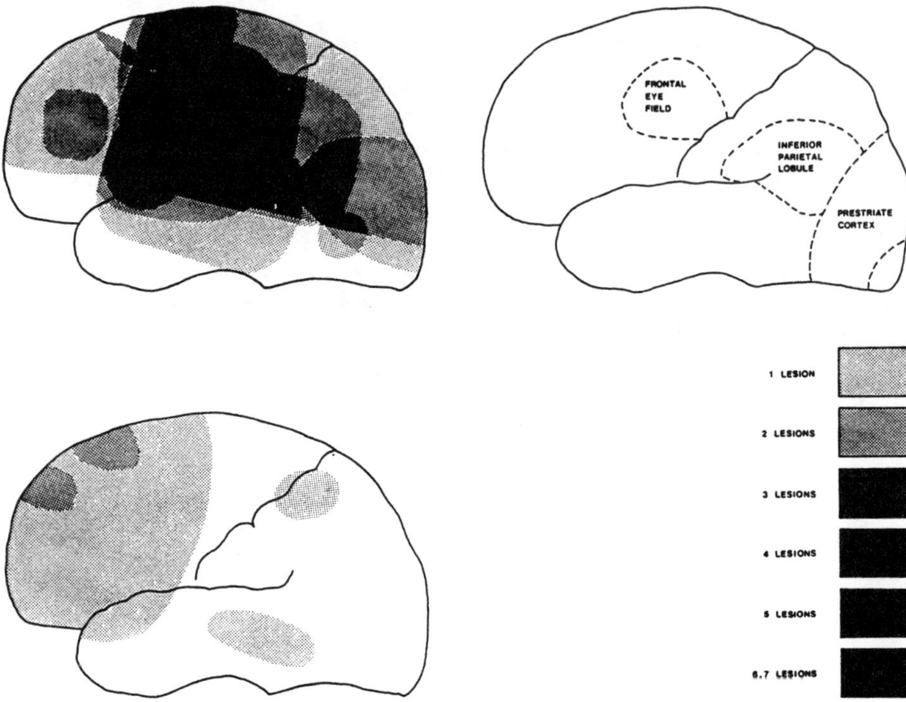

Fig. 4: Left: Superimposition of the maps of cortical lesions on the lateral surface of the brain. Left, upper: lesions, associated with abnormal ATFs. Note that the largest degree of overlap occurs in and near the frontal eye field. Left, lower: lesions, associated with normal ATFs. Note that all lesions but one are located outside the frontal eye field. The different grey tones indicate different degrees of overlap. Right, upper: the position of lateral cortical visuomotor areas. Right, lower: the significance of different grey tones.

Tab. 4: Relation between saccadic deficits and involvement of (sub)cortical structures in patients C1-C17. For every structure and group of parameters, the percentage of lesions associated with normality of all parameters ("normal"), abnormality of one or more parameters ("abnormal") and specific abnormalities are indicated. The numbers in brackets refer to the actual number of lesions.

ATF PARAMETERS		FRONTAL EYE FIELD	INFERIOR PARIETAL LOBULE	PRESTRIATE CORTEX	SUPPLE-MENTARY MOTOR AREA	OPTIC RADIATION	INTERNAL CAPSULE	BASAL GANGLIA
Normal	(6)	17% (1)	0% (0)	0% (0)	33% (2)	0% (0)	17% (1)	33% (2)
Abnormal	(11)	73% (8)	55% (6)	27% (3)	27% (3)	45% (5)	36% (4)	55% (6)
Abnormal Dm / Tw	(9)	67% (6)	44% (4)	33% (3)	33% (3)	44% (4)	33% (3)	44% (4)
Abnormal SCAT	(7)	71% (5)	57% (4)	43% (3)	43% (3)	57% (4)	29% (2)	43% (3)

Thalamic lesions

The ATF was abnormal in all 3 patients. No consistent abnormality was seen although the Tw deficit was different from that observed in patients with cortical lesions. In 2 patients Tw was either decreased for contralaterally directed saccades or increased for ipsilaterally directed saccades. The lesions associated with ATF deficits overlapped in the pulvinar and lateral posterior nucleus (Figure 5). Both nuclei are known to be involved in saccadic behavior.

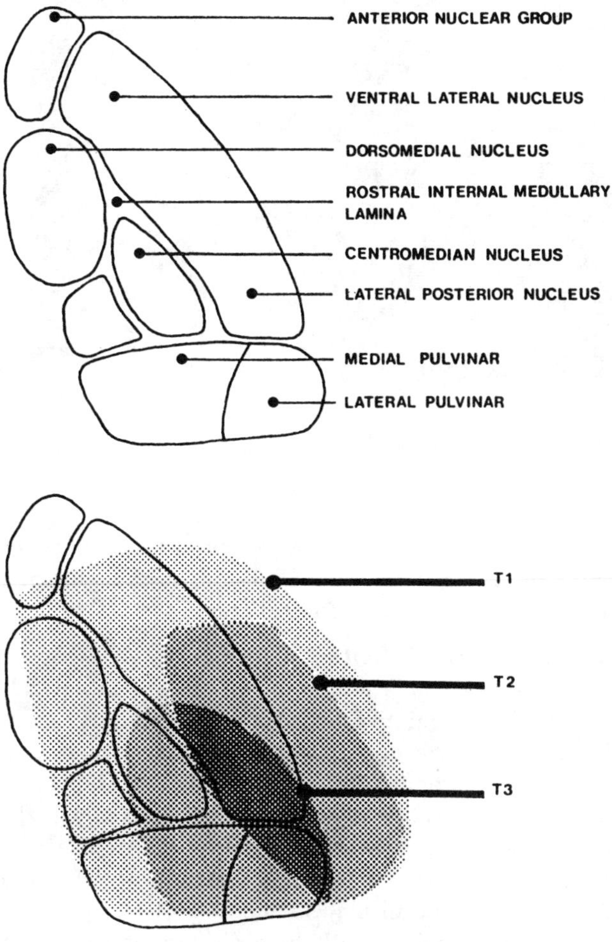

Fig. 5: Upper: the thalamic nuclei at the level of the CT-scan slice through the foramina of Monro and pineal body. Lower: overlap of the lesions in patients T1, T2 and T3 at this level. The different grey tones indicate different degrees of overlap (see Figure 4 right, lower).

Collicular lesions

A remarkable finding was that patient S, with bilateral superior colliculus lesions (Figure 6), had normal ATF parameters (Table 3, Figure 3). This is particularly interesting since the superior colliculus is regarded as being very important in the computation of the amplitude and direction of saccades.

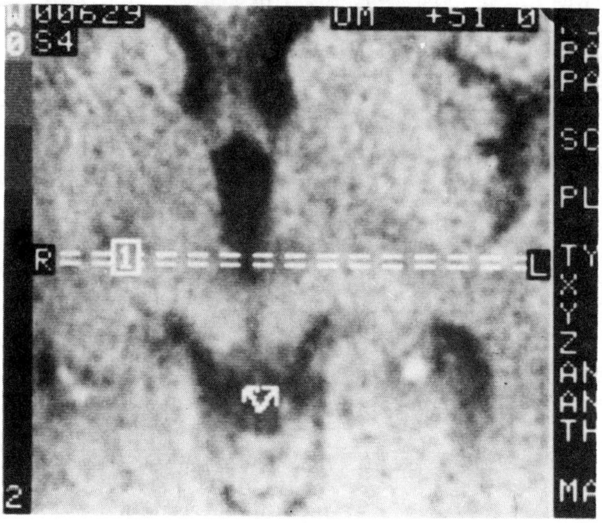

Fig. 6: CT-scan slice showing the superior colliculus infarctions (white arrows) in patient S.

Corona radiata lesions

In patient R, increased values for Dm were found for ipsilaterally as well as contralaterally directed saccades. The small lesions in this patient were located in the vicinity of the superior occipitofrontal tracts.

Bilateral versus unilateral deficits

Out of the 20 patients with unilateral lesions, 6 showed unilateral ATF abnormalities while 8 showed bilateral ATF abnormalities. Six patients with bilateral deficits showed a deficit of the same parameter for contralaterally as well as for ipsilaterally directed saccades. The patients with thalamic lesions all had bilateral deficits. The volumes of lesions in patients with bilateral ATF deficits were not significantly larger than the volumes of lesions in patients with unilateral ATF deficits (Mann-Whitney U-test). There was no relation between the occurrence of ATF deficits and displacement on CT-scan (Fisher-Yates test). Thus, many unilateral cortical and all thalamic lesions were associated with bilateral ATF abnormalities. The statistical evidence indicates that the occurrence of bilateral deficits was not due to large lesions affecting the opposite hemisphere.

Saccadic deficits and clinical data other than location of the lesion

There was no statistical evidence that the volumes of the lesions differed between patients with ATF deficits (tested for each group of deficits shown in Table 4) and those without deficits. This is also the case for duration of symptoms and ages of patients (Mann-Whitney U-test).

No relation was found between the occurrence of ATF deficits and abnormal perimetry (Fisher-Yates test).

Correlations between saccadic parameters

It was investigated whether correlations existed between Dm, Tw, SCAT, LEVL, RT, AMP20 and varAMP20.

The value of SCAT may be related with varAMP20 as both parameters express the variation in saccadic gain. Positive correlations existed between SCAT and varAMP20 ($r = 0.63$; $p < 0.0001$).

During the determination of the ATF the values for LEVL, Dm and the slope of the oblique segment were manipulated by the fit-procedure, in order to obtain the best fit. For this reason, it is to be expected that these parameters are related to each other. A negative correlation was found between Dm and Tw ($r = -0.57$; $p < 0.0003$). There was also a negative correlation between Dm and LEVL ($r = -0.35$; $p < 0.03$) and a positive correlation between Tw and LEVL ($r = 0.86$; $p < 0.001$). These findings suggest that Dm, Tw and LEVL are related to each other due to methodological factors. Therefore, it was investigated if LEVL was correlated with AMP20. Both parameters are indicators of saccadic gain, the latter being independent of the fit-procedure. A positive correlation existed between LEVL and AMP20 ($r = 0.35$, $p < 0.04$). This suggests that LEVL is, at least, determined partially by a physiological factor, i.e. the saccadic gain. Therefore, the interdependency of Dm and Tw may also be the result of physiological factors.

According to Becker and Jürgens' model (1979), the reaction time of a saccade is composed of several delays consisting of Dm, Tw and Td. If Dm or Tw are increased, then the saccadic reaction time should be increased as well. A positive correlation is therefore to be expected between Dm or Tw and RT. A positive correlation indeed existed between Tw and RT ($r = 0.35$; $p < 0.04$). No correlation existed between Dm and RT.

Becker and Jürgens supposed that the advantage of averaging is to ensure that the amplitude of a saccade is not determined by short-lived and random variations of the retinal error signal. Thus, if the position of a target is averaged during a longer time interval, the ensuing saccade might be more accurate. If this is true, a large value for Tw should result in smaller variations in saccadic amplitudes or a larger saccadic gain. Tw should then be negatively correlated with parameters, reflecting the variation of saccadic amplitudes (varAMP20 and SCAT) while it should be positively correlated with parameters reflecting the saccadic gain (AMP20 and LEVL). Indeed positive correlations were found between Tw and the gain-parameters LEVL ($r = 0.86$; $p < 0.001$) and AMP20 ($r = 0.35$; $p < 0.04$). It must, however, be stressed that the relation between Tw and LEVL is also determined by the methodological factors mentioned above. Contrary to what would be expected, positive correlations existed between Tw and the parameters reflecting the variation in saccadic amplitude. Tw was positively correlated with SCAT ($r = 0.65$; $p < 0.0001$) and varAMP20 ($r = 0.38$; $p < 0.02$).

Discussion

Binocular or monocular visual stimulation?

The question might be raised as to why binocular visual stimulation was used instead of monocular stimulation. The patients who were investigated had retrochiasmal lesions involving the cerebral cortex, thalamus or superior colliculus. These areas are reached by visual afferents from the contralateral hemifields of both eyes, the fibers from the left and right eye being more or less intermingled (Brodal, 1981). This intermingling is the least complete in the lateral geniculate body in which the layers receiving fibers from the contralateral hemifields are separated for each eye. It is more complete in the striate cortex in which the oculuar dominance columns receiving fibers from each eye are located adjacent to each other (Brodal, 1981). The inferior pulvinar receives a weak retinal projection from the contralateral hemifields of both eyes terminating in separate areas for each eye which lie close to each other (Campos-Ortega et al., 1970). Considering these findings it is theoretically possible that retrochiasmal lesions cause incongruous homonymous hemianopic field defects. Slightly incongruous field defects have been described in patients with a lesion in the anterior part of the optic radiation (Burde et al., 1985). However, none of our patients had a lesion in the inferior pulvinar or lateral geniculate body. Moreover, in the 3 patients with abnormal computerized perimetry, the homonymous hemianopic field defects were completely congruous. For these reasons it was not considered necessary to use monocular visual stimulation.

The Becker and Jürgens model

Becker and Jürgens (1979) proposed that, in the ATF obtained from pulse undershoot stimuli, Dm equals the sum of afferent and efferent delays (Dm = Ta + Te). Therefore, Dm is expected to be relatively fixed within one subject. However, there is evidence that Dm can vary considerably within one subject as indicated by experiments using double step stimuli with a large stimulus separation. The ATF obtained in these experiments was characterized by 2 horizontal segments only, without an oblique segment in between (Ottes et al. 1984). In this type of ATF, the transition between the 2 horizontal segments occurs abruptly at a value of D of about 140 ms and not gradually, as predicted by the Becker and Jürgens model. In these ATFs, Dm is 140 ms while Tw equals zero. When the same subject is tested with double-step stimuli with a small target separation, an ATF as described by Becker and Jürgens is obtained: Dm is about 80 ms while Tw is also about 80 ms. In other words, increasing the target separation results in an increase of Dm by about 60 ms. This indicates that Dm is not fixed within one subject. It is unlikely that the afferent and efferent transmission times of the saccadic system can vary that much. It seems, therefore, improbable that Dm represents the sum of Ta and Te. Dm, nevertheless, reflects the smallest value of D at which the second target step of a double-step stimulus exerts its influence on the amplitude of the first saccade. This moment has to be dependent, at least, on Ta. This notion is supported by the increase of Dm in the ATFs of patient R. This patient had bilateral lesions which probably affected the superior occipital frontal tracts. The lesions might interrupt fibers transmitting visual information to the frontal eye field (which is probably involved in the averaging process, see second half of the discussion), resulting in an increased Ta which in turn yields an increased Dm. Thus, it is likely that Dm equals the sum of Ta and another, unknown, delay-factor.

Becker and Jürgens (1979) proposed that Tw reflects the period during which the position of a target is averaged by the saccadic system. The present investigation provides several arguments in favor of this hypothesis. First, a positive correlation was found between the length of Tw and the saccadic gain: the larger the value for Tw, the more the saccadic gain approaches unity. This finding indicates that saccades are directed more accurately to a target when Tw is larger. This is in agreement with the hypothesis of Becker and Jürgens which states that the saccadic system uses averaging as a means to generate accurate saccades; the averaging of the saccadic amplitude is less dependent on short-lived and random variations of the retinal error signal. However, we found a positive correlation between RT and Tw which indicates that the increase of Tw by the saccadic system occurs at the expense of an increased saccadic reaction time. Second, there were positive correlations between the length of Tw and the parameters expressing the variation of saccadic amplitudes, that is, the larger the value of Tw, the larger the variation of amplitudes. This is not quite in agreement with the above mentioned hypothesis of Becker and Jürgens. Nevertheless, both points suggest that Tw is somehow related to the determination of saccadic amplitudes.

There are two points which are not accounted for by the Becker and Jürgens model. First, Tw equals zero in the ATFs obtained by means of double-step stimuli with a large target separation. In terms of the Becker and Jürgens model, this implies that no averaging occurs prior to the execution of large visually guided saccades. As a result, large saccades should be more inaccurate than small ones. It has been shown that the saccadic gain decreases with large saccades (Carpenter, 1977). Perhaps the saccadic system is organized in such a way that only small saccades are prevented from being inaccurate by the averaging mechanism. This might be related to the fact that most naturally occurring saccades have an amplitude of 15 ° or less (Bahill et al., 1975). Apparently, the more frequently occurring saccades are performed more accurately. Second, our investigation indicated that Dm and Tw are interdependent. A relatively large Tw coincides with a relatively small Dm and vice versa although this is partly due to methodological factors.

We hypothesize that the interdependency of Dm and Tw as well as the fact that Tw can be zero reflect the existence of a mechanism by which the saccadic system controls the length of Tw, Dm being inversely proportional to Tw. For small saccades, which are frequently executed, Tw is set to a certain value. For large saccades Tw is set to zero, because averaging apparently is not necessary.

The way in which Tw is set by the saccadic system may be influenced by lesions affecting the regions involved in the determination of Tw. The findings in the patient group suggest that cortical lesions typically result in an increase of Tw for saccades directed contralaterally to the lesion, while thalamic lesions typically result in an increase of Tw for saccades directed ipsilaterally to the lesion or a decrease of Tw for saccades directed contralaterally to the lesion. This indicates that the cerebral cortex and the thalamus each may exert opposite influences on Tw.

In the Becker and Jürgens model, the saccadic reaction time is the sum of several delay factors reflecting stages of the preparation of a saccade. These factors are Ta, Td, Tw and Te. Td is the time needed for the decision to make a saccade while Tw represents the time needed for the computation of the saccadic amplitude. Ta and Te represent afferent and efferent transmission times. As Becker and Jürgens suggested that Dm = Ta + Te, it was expected that the assessment of Dm, Tw and RT would yield the value for Td: Td = reaction time −Tw −Dm. However, this equation is useless since Dm does not equal Ta + Te. As only RT and Tw could be determined experimentally, the delay factors Ta, Td and Te could not be derived. The concept that averaging is a stage in the preparation of a saccade which takes time is supported by the positive correlation between RT and Tw: a large Tw coincides with a large RT.

Becker and Jürgens (1979) hypothesized that channels exist for the preparation of horizontal leftward and rightward saccades which are largely independent. Although this view is confirmed by the strong asymmetries in saccadic performance which were observed in a number of patients, some objections can be raised. According to the model, unilateral lesions should result in deficits of saccades directed to one side only. However, in the present investigation, many patients with unilateral lesions had bilateral saccadic deficits involving homologue parameters in most cases. There were no indications that these deficits were due to large lesions affecting the normal hemisphere. Thus, our results indicate that, at cortical and thalamic levels, the saccadic system is not strictly divided into separate subsystems for saccades directed to the left and saccades directed to the right. This is supported by the various anatomical connections between visuomotor centres on both sides (Schwartz & Goldman-Rakic, 1984; Leichnetz, 1981). Although the results of most single-unit, stimulation and ablation studies in monkeys suggest that visuomotor centres predominantly control contralaterally directed saccades, there are some indications that the frontal eye field, inferior parietal lobule and thalamus are involved in the control of ipsilaterally directed saccades as well. Stimulation of one frontal eye field sometimes evokes ipsilaterally directed saccades (Bruce et al., 1985), the visual fields of some frontal eye field neurons cover the ipsilateral field (Goldberg & Bushnell, 1981). In the inferior parietal lobule, some neurons have bilateral or ipsilateral visual receptive fields and ablation in humans of the inferior parietal lobule may result in bilateral saccadic abnormalities (Lynch, 1980). Some pulvinar and internal medullary lamina units discharge prior to saccades in all directions (Petersen et al., 1985). Guitton et al. (1985) showed that unilateral ablation of the frontal eye field in humans quite often caused bilateral deficits. Bilaterally increased reaction times were associated with unilateral posterior parietal lesions (Pierrot-Desseilligny et al., 1987).

The role of the superior colliculus, cerebral cortex and thalamus in the decision and averaging processes

The absence of ATF deficits in the patient with bilateral superior colliculus lesions constitutes a finding which is quite remarkable, as, together with the frontal eye field, the superior colliculus is involved in the initiation of saccades and the determination of saccadic amplitudes (Bruce & Goldberg, 1985). Saccades were tested a long time (189 days) after the infarct in our patient. The infarct was, however, still visible on CT-scanning at the time of the eye movement recording. This finding can be explained by assuming that, after the infarct, the function of the superior colliculus was taken over by the frontal eye fields. This assumption is supported by the fact that the most severe saccadic deficits are observed directly after acute functional inactivation of the superior colliculus (Hikosaka & Wurtz, 1986).

On the other hand, lesions affecting the frontal eye field, inferior parietal lobule, pulvinar or lateral posterior nucleus were associated with ATF deficits or deficits of SCAT.

One patient with thalamic lesions had a severely decreased value of LEVL for saccades directed contralaterally to the lesion. As LEVL reflects the saccadic gain, this finding might be due to involvement of the rostral thalamic internal medullary lamina which was affected in this patient but not in the other patients with thalamic lesions (Figure 5). This structure contains cells with saccade related activity (Schlag & Schlag-Rey, 1984) while monkeys with a lesion in this area show a saccadic amplitude deficit (Albano & Wurtz, 1982).

Abnormal values of Dm and/or Tw were especially associated with lesions in the frontal eye field, pulvinar or lateral posterior nucleus. We hypothesize that these structures are involved in the setting of Tw as mentioned above. The frontal eye field might be involved in the averaging process itself. This is supported by several lines of evidence. First, it has been shown that averaged saccades can be elicited by simultaneous electrical stimulation of two sites in the frontal eye fields. This evokes a saccade of which the amplitude is a weighted average of the amplitudes of saccades resulting from stimulating the two sites separately (Robinson & Fuchs, 1969). The same holds for simultaneous stimulation of the superior colliculus or frontal eye field and superior colliculus. Second, we presented evidence for a relation between Tw and saccadic amplitudes. Third, stimulation and single unit experiments indicate that the frontal eye field is involved in the determination of saccadic amplitude and direction (Bruce & Goldberg, 1985; Bruce et al., 1985). Fourth, saccade related unit activity has been found in the pulvinar (Acuna et al., 1983; Petersen et al., 1985).

In conclusion, the results of our study support an important part of the Becker and Jürgens model, namely the significance of Tw. The results suggest that the length of Tw is, at least, determined by the frontal eye field and thalamus. The significance of Dm is not clear. It was not possible to establish which structure is involved in the decision process.

References

Acuna, C., Gonzalez, F., & Dominguez, R., *Sensorimotor unit activity related to intention in the pulvinar of behaving Cebus apella monkeys*, Experimental Brain Research **52(3)** (1983), 411-422.

Albano, J.E.,& Wurtz, R.H., *Deficits in eye position following ablation of monkey superior colliculus, pretectum and posterior-medial thalamus*, Journal of Neurophysiology **48** (1982), 318-337.

Bahill, A.T., Adler, D.,& Stark, L., *Most naturally occurring saccades have an amplitude of 15 degrees or less*, Investigative Ophthalmology **14** (1975), 468-469.

Becker, W., & Jürgens, R., *An analysis of the saccadic system by means of double step stimuli*, Vision Research **19** (1979), 967-983.

Bevington, P.R., "Data reduction and error analysis for the physical sciences," McGraw-Hill, New York, 1969.

Brodal, A., "Neurological anatomy in relation to clinical medicine," Oxford University Press, New York, 1981.

Bruce, C.J., & Goldberg, M.E., *Primate frontal eye fields: I. Single neurons discharging before saccades*, Journal of Neurophysiology **53** (1985), 603-635.

Bruce, C.J., Goldberg, M.E., Bushnell, M.C.,& Stanton, G.B., *Primate frontal eye fields: II. Physiological and anatomical correlates of electrically evoked eye movements*, Journal of Neurophysiology **54** (1985), 714-734.

Burde, R.M., Savino, P.J.,& Trobe, J.D., "Clinical decisions in neuro-opthalmology," The C.V. Mosby Company, St. Louis, 1985.

Campos-Ortega, J.A., Hayhow, W.R., & Clüver, P.F. de V, *A note on the problem of retinal projections to the inferior pulvinar nucleus of primates*, Brain Research **22** (1970), 126-129.

Carpenter, R.H.S., "Movements of the eyes," Pion, London, 1977.

Goldberg, M.E., & Bushnell, M.C., *Behavioral enhancement of visual responses in monkey cerebral cortex. II. Modulation in frontal eye fields specifically related to saccades*, Journal of Neurophysiology **46** (1981), 773-787.

Guitton, D., Buchtel, H.A.,& Douglas, R.M., *Frontal lobe lesions in man cause difficulties in suppressing reflexive glances and in generating goal - directed saccades*, Experimental Brain Research **58** (1985), 455- 472.

Hikosaka, O., & Wurtz, R.H., *Saccadic eye movements following injection of lidocaine into the superior colliculus*, Experimental Brain Research **61** (1986), 531-539.

Leichnetz, G.R., Spencer, R.F., Hardy, S.G.P., & Astruc, J., *An anatomical view of the role of cerebral cortex in eye movement: projections from the prefrontal cortex to the superior colliculus and oculomotor complex in the monkey*, in "A.F. Fuchs, & W. Becker (Eds.), Progress in oculomotor research," Elsevier/North-Holland, New York, 1981, pp. 177-184.

Lynch, J.C., *The functional organization of posterior parietal association cortex*, Behavioral Brain Science **3** (1980), 485-534.

Marquardt, D.W., *An algorithm for least-squares estimation of nonlinear parameters*, Journal of the Society for Industrial and Applied Mathematics **11** (1963), 431-441.

Mazzocchi, F., & Vignolo, L.A., *Computer assisted tomography in neuropsychological research: a simple procedure for lesion mapping*, Cortex **14** (1978), 136-144.

New, P.J., & Scott, W.R.S., "Computerized tomography of the brain and orbit (EMI scanning)," Williams and Wilkins, Baltimore, 1975.

Nieuwenhuys, R., Voogd, J., & Van Huijzen, C., "The human central nervous system. A synopsis and atlas," Springer-Verlag, Berlin, 1978.

Ottes, F.P., Van Gisbergen, J.A.M., & Eggermont, J.J., *Metrics of saccade responses to visual double stimuli: two different modes*, Vision Research **24** (1984), 1169-1179.

Petersen, S.E., Robinson, D.L., & Keys, W., *Pulvinar nuclei of the behaving rhesus monkey: visual responses and their modulation*, Journal of Neurophysiology **54** (1985), 867-886.

Pierrot-Desseilligny, C., Rivaud, S., Penet,C., & Rigolet, M.H., *Latencies of visually guided saccades in unilateral hemispheric cerebral lesions*, Annals of Neurology **21** (1987), 138-148.

Robinson, D.A., & Fuchs, A.F., *Eye movements evoked by stimulation of frontal eye fields*, Journal of Neurophysiology **32** (1969), 637-648.

Schlag, J.,& Schlag-Rey, M., *Visuomotor functions of central thalamus in monkey. II. Unit activity related to visual events, targeting, and fixation*, Journal of Neurophysiology **51** (1984), 1175-1195.

Schwartz, M.L., & Goldman-Rakic, P.S., *Callosal and intrahemispheric connectivity of the prefrontal association cortex in rhesus monkey: relation between intraparietal and principal sulcal cortex*, Journal of Comparative Neurology **226** (1984), 403-420.

Van Buren, J.M., & Borke, R.C., "Variations and connections of the human thalamus. II. Variations of the human diencephalon," Springer-Verlag, Berlin, 1972.

5
Reading Processes

READING AND SPATIAL COGNITION: REFLECTIONS FROM EYE FIXATIONS

MARCEL ADAM JUST AND PATRICIA A. CARPENTER

Carnegie Mellon University, Pittsburgh

Philosophers of science have often pointed out that the development of particular instruments can influence which scientific concepts emerge in a domain. For example, the development of the microscope and later the electron microscope was extremely influential in establishing the concept of the cell as a fundamental unit in biology. The relation between instrumentation and content is often harder to substantiate in psychology and the social sciences than in the natural sciences. The research tools in psychology are seldom as identifiably technological as the microscope. However, the study of eye fixations is one example of a technologically-based approach used in cognitive psychology. Moreover, it proves to be an instance in which the methodology has had a demonstrably important influence on the emerging theoretical concepts. In this paper we will examine that influence in the domains of reading and spatial cognition.

Using eye fixation behavior to learn about properties of thought is not new. Reading researchers recorded eye fixations at the beginning of this century. But despite the historical continuity with pioneering researchers like Dearborn, Huey, and Buswell, there are also discontinuities between earlier approaches and current research. Contemporary research uses the eye fixation method in conjunction with an information processing approach, which analyzes cognition in terms of symbol manipulation. The unique contribution of the eye-fixation method is that it provides a trace of ongoing symbol manipulation, which allows us to infer many of the sequential and temporal properties of specific cognitive processes. The resulting theories also suggest some general principles of the organization of thinking.

This chapter describes some of our research results in the area of reading and spatial cognition that have been enabled by the eye fixation method. To illustrate some of the progress, we will describe some current research projects and compare them to related projects of ten years ago. In particular, we can compare the current state of knowledge to the state of the art circa 1976 as described in our article of that year entitled "Eye fixations and cognitive processes" (Just & Carpenter, 1976).

In addition to research results, the chapter develops two subthemes. One concerns the implications of the eye fixation findings for theories about the *organization of thought*. This methodology has revealed a rich layer of computation underlying even seemingly simple processes, such as mental rotation, or recovering from a misinterpretation of a garden-path sentence. The revelation of intermediate states of computation has reinforced the theoretical analyses, so that they have become much more fine grained.

A second theme is that there are systematic *individual differences* in the way people think; the eye fixation analysis has made the differences and the systematicity apparent. Coarser measures, such as reaction times or error patterns fail to reveal how an individual performs a particular trial. However, the process tracing methods that can be applied to eye fixation patterns reveal the strategies of individual subjects.

Reading

Our understanding of how people read and comprehend language has increased a great deal in the last decade. Much of the new knowledge concerning the oculomotor, perceptual and cognitive processes in reading is due to the analysis of the time course and location of eye fixations.

In the early 1970's, the major eye fixation findings focused on perceptual processes. One of the main issues was the size of the perceptual span. Studies in which the text changed during reading have suggested that readers acquire some visual information about upcoming words, particularly their lengths and perhaps some of their letters (such as the beginning and ending letters) (Rayner, 1975). Taken together, these studies supported the idea of a small semantic span (McConkie, Zola, Blanchard, & Wolverton, 1982). In general, a word that lies to the right of the point of regard is *not* recognized extrafoveally unless it happens to be short, very frequent, and linguistically constrained. This description applies primarily to function words, articles, and prepositions.

Cognitive processes

Since the mid-1970's, research has focused not only on perceptual processes, but also on the cognitive processes in language comprehension. The eye fixation method became a valuable tool for investigating linguistic computations as research interest began to focus on what happened to the information the reader *was fixating*, not just the information he wasn't fixating. We noticed that there was considerable systematicity in the time readers spent on particular words. Readers spent more time on words that required more difficult computations, such as a more complex inference. When we analyzed the time a reader spent on individual words, it became clear that a great deal of processing was done on-line, word by word.

To analyze eye fixations during reading, we had to address the fact that not all words are directly fixated. To determine the distribution of fixated words, we analyzed the eye fixations of college students who were reading scientific reports from a popular magazine (Just & Carpenter, 1980; Carpenter & Just, 1983). Readers fixated over 80 % of the content words (adjectives, adverbs, nouns, and verbs) and over 40 % of the function words (such as conjunctions, articles, and prepositions). Thus, the words that readers tend to not directly fixate are short, frequent, and linguistically constrained.

Immediacy of interpretation. The way that comprehenders deal with the sequential nature of language is to try to interpret each successive word of a text as soon as they encounter it, and integrate the new information with what they already know about the text and its subject matter. We have referred to this processing strategy as the *immediacy of interpretation.* A reader tries to digest each piece of the text as he encounters it (Just & Carpenter, 1980, 1987). The immediacy of interpretation entails many levels of comprehension: encoding the word, accessing its meaning, associating it with its referent, and determining its semantic and syntactic status in the sentence and the discourse. It is important to note that although the attempt at interpretation is immediate, the text can force postponement by withholding essential information. In such cases, the postponement is out of necessity rather than strategic choice. The default strategy is to interpret immediately.

The immediacy of interpretation can be contrasted with a different strategy for dealing with the sequential nature of language, namely a wait-and-see strategy. A reader can always increase the probability of correctly interpreting a given word or phrase if she postpones interpreting it until she sees what follows in the sentence. Wait-and-see strategies have been proposed by several researchers (Kimball, 1973; Marcus, 1980). Comprehenders using the immediacy strategy still use the context that follows a piece of text to help interpret that piece, but they do so by elaborating or amending an already existing interpretation, rather than waiting for the context before making any interpretation.

The clearest evidence for the immediacy strategy is that the time spent looking at a word is strongly influenced by the characteristics of that word (e.g. Just & Carpenter, 1980; Carpenter & Just, 1983). The gaze duration on a word is directly related to the word's length (measured in number of letters), an effect we attribute to the encoding of the visual form of the word. Thus, each word is encoded while it is being fixated. The gaze duration on a word is also related to the word's normative frequency in the language, an effect we attribute to the process of accessing the word's meaning in the mental lexicon (Just & Carpenter, 1987). Readers spend longer on a rare word like *sable* than on a common word like *table*, an effect we attribute to accessing the word's meaning. Thus, the meaning of each word is being accessed while the word is being fixated.

These two effects are illustrated in Figure 1, which shows the average gaze duration on fixated words. These times were generated by college students reading scientific texts, but we have obtained similar results for a variety of different texts and tasks. The downward slopes of the lines in Figure 1 indicate the decrease in gaze duration with the logarithm of the word's frequency. Each of the lines in the figure corresponds to words of a particular length measured in number of characters in the word; the progression of lines (from bottom to top) indicates the increase in gaze duration with word length, independent of frequency.

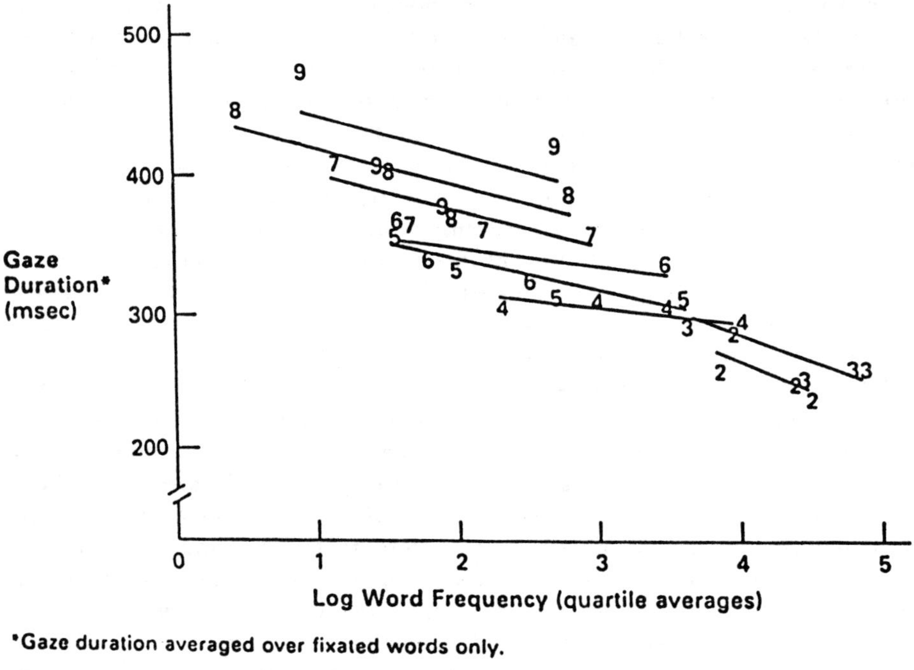

Fig. 1: The average time a reader spends looking at a word (in milliseconds), as a function of the logarithm of the word's frequency. More frequent words (those with a larger log frequency) are looked at for less time than less frequent words. The eight lines represent words of different lengths–words that are two letters long, three letters long, up to nine letters long. Each point represents the mean of a quartile of the words of that length. Source: Carpenter & Just, 1983, Figure 17.2, p. 288. Used with permission of Academic Press.

Unusually long gaze durations can also be produced by words that present a difficulty because of their role in the syntax or semantics of a sentence. For example, a reader will pause longer on a semantically anomalous word compared to an appropriate word of comparable length and frequency. A reader will also pause longer on a word that signals an unusual syntactic construction, or a demanding syntactic computation. These kinds of results indicate that the semantic and syntactic analyses of each word must be occurring while the word is being fixated. Thus, the evidence indicates immediacy at several levels of interpretation, such as the lexical (Just & Carpenter, 1980; Just & Carpenter, 1983), syntactic (McDonald & Carpenter, 1981), and text levels (Dee-Lucas, Just, Carpenter, & Daneman, 1982). If a word introduces an increase in the processing load at any of these levels, there is an increased gaze duration on that word. All these results constitute strong support for the immediacy of interpretation. Thus, the varying processing burden imposed by the successive words of a text is borne as soon as it is encountered.

Why immediacy works. There are two aspects of language use that minimize the costs and maximize the benefits of immediacy. The costs (such as making an incorrect interpretation) are low because it generally *is* possible to compute the correct interpretation of a word when it is first encountered. Wait-and-see proponents focus on contrived sentences presented without context, in which a reader has so little knowledge that he has no choice but to wait-and-see. However, normal context and normal sentences make it possible for the reader to develop strategies that succeed on an overwhelming proportion of the sentences people normally process. Readers use their knowledge of the context and their knowledge of relative frequencies of alternative interpretations in choosing the most likely interpretation. The benefit of immediacy is that it reduces the memory load of retaining information in an unprocessed form while waiting and seeing.

The claim of immediacy was a strong counter-proposal to the prevalent thinking about language processing. Before the eye fixation results became known, the most commonly accepted assumption was that the bulk of processing occurred at the ends of clauses or sentences, a subtle legacy of the linguistic theory of transformational grammar. In transformational grammar, it only made sense to consider syntactic transformations as operating on the syntactic structures of an entire clause or sentence. However, when this assumption was imported into psychology, it implied that readers did not syntactically and semantically process words until the ends of major syntactic boundaries. The dramatic evidence that gaze duration on a word was influenced by its lexical and syntactic properties proved that some processes were executed as the reader encountered each successive word, and not postponed until clause or sentence boundaries.

It is important to emphasize that the temporal unit of analysis in these studies is not the individual fixation duration, but the gaze duration. The gaze is the sum of uninterrupted fixations on a unit, typically the word or phrase. One reason for analyzing the duration of gazes rather than individual fixations is simply that our theory addresses processes that operate on words. A second reason is that this level reveals considerable systematicity. We will return to the issue of the unit of analysis in the third section of the paper which discusses the eye fixation method.

Individual differences

The eye fixation method has been useful not only in understanding the processing of information at various linguistic levels, but also in examining differences among readers, including those in unusual populations, such as speed readers and dyslexics.

Speed reading. We have used eye fixation studies to analyze the reading of very skilled readers; people who graduated from a speed reading course (Just & Carpenter, 1987). The distribution of fixated words and the distribution of gaze durations for speed readers varies systematically from those for normal readers. Speed readers fixate only every third word or so on average, often leaving two or three consecutive words unfixated. Moreover, they show no evidence of extracting semantic information from unfixated words. Consequently, when they are speed reading, their level of comprehension is considerably lower than when they are reading normally, particularly for non-redundant details. Speed readers also spend 33% less time (compared to normal readers) on those words that they do fixate. The analysis of eye fixations has revealed how speed readers scan a text and how they distribute their processing time, telling us where the circumscribed advantages of speed readers lie and where they don't lie.

Working memory capacity. The eye fixation method has also been useful in analyzing the source of comprehension skill differences among normal college readers. One source is the capacity of working memory during language processing. Working memory consists of currently activated propositions, both those that are newly computed and those that are retrieved from long-term memory. The main role of working memory in comprehension is the transient storage of partial computations to support the continuous flow of symbol manipulation. In contrast to traditional theories of short-term memory, working memory is viewed as both a computational and a storage arena (Baddeley & Hitch, 1974). In general, poorer comprehenders have a lower working memory capacity when processing language.

Much of our research on the role of working memory in comprehension makes use of the reading span task developed by Daneman and Carpenter (1980). The task requires subjects to read a set of unrelated sentences and, at the end of the set, recall the final word of each sentence. For example, consider the following set of two sentences:

When at last his eyes opened, there was no gleam of triumph, no shade of **anger**.

The taxi turned up Michigan Avenue where they had a clear view of the **lake**.

After reading these two sentences, the subject tries to recall the words *anger* and *lake*. Each subject was presented with sets containing from two to seven sentences, in order to determine the largest set size from which he could reliably recall all of the sentence-final words. The largest such set size was defined as his reading span. The rationale behind the test was that the comprehension processes used in reading the sentences would consume less of the working memory resources of the better readers. This would leave the better readers with more capacity to store the sentence-final words.

This task has two important virtues. One virtue is that it measures performance when both the processing and storage capabilities of working memory are being used simultaneously. The second virtue is that the reading span assessed by this procedure provides an excellent index of an individual's reading comprehension ability and consequently, is a useful psychometric instrument. By contrast, measures of passive short-term memory span, such as the ability to recall a list of digits or unrelated words, are not significantly correlated with reading comprehension performance.

The initial study demonstrated that skilled readers have greater working-memory capacity in reading than less skilled readers (Daneman & Carpenter, 1980). The greater capacity for computing and storing information may arise from a variety of sources, rather than a single one. For the good reader, many processes may be both faster and more automatic, including encoding, lexical access, semantic and syntactic analysis. Working-memory capacity is a property of the processing system that is the aggregate of several factors that could contribute to the individual differences in reading.

The reading spans of college students, which ranged from 2 to 5.5, were highly correlated with their reading comprehension test scores, with these correlations lying between 0.5 and 0.6 in various experiments. The correlation with reading span was even higher when specific comprehension abilities were considered individually. For example, the ability to answer a factual question about a passage was correlated between 0.7 and 0.9 with reading span in various studies. The correlation between conventional digit-span or word-span tests and reading comprehension was considerably lower, as it usually is.

Reading in the span task. Because the reading span test provides such a good index of reading ability, it is worthwhile to directly examine the reading behavior in the test itself and characterize the differences between subjects who are able to recall many words, typically four or five, and those who recall very few, typically two words. In particular, the eye fixation behavior has the potential of revealing which component processes of comprehension, such as word encoding or lexical access, distinguish among readers of differing spans and, by inference, differing levels of reading skill. The procedure was similar to the usual administration of the span test (see Carpenter & Just, 1988 for a more detailed description of the study). The subjects read a set of sentences aloud and tried to recall the final word of each sentence, while their eye fixations were recorded.

The general description of the eye fixation behavior was that the subjects read each sentence normally until they reached the last word of the sentence, at which time they tried to memorize that word. People with high spans read the sentences faster. The mean gaze duration on each word was 278 ms for the high-span subjects, and 355 ms for the low-span subjects. This result excludes the time on the final words in the sentences, in which the subjects were memorizing as well as reading.

The findings of most interest were the individual differences in the way that word frequency modulated subjects' gaze durations, particularly when the subjects were reading a sentence while maintaining the final words from previously-read sentences. Most of the reading speed advantage of the high-span subjects came from faster lexical access rather than faster word encoding. This conclusion comes from the regression analysis relating gaze duration to word length and word frequency, for all but the final words in the sentences. The regression analysis produces very similar word length parameters for readers of all spans, but produces smaller word frequency parameters for readers with high spans, as shown in Figure 2 for two replications of the experiment.

These results suggest that better readers read faster, partly because they can do lexical access faster, and they use their extra time for task-specific requirements. In this case, the task specific requirement is maintaining the storage of sentence-final words. The analyses reported below localize the effect of the load constituted by the sentence-final words on the reading of subsequent sentences.

While the first sentence of each screen is being read, there are no sentence-final words being stored. Thus, the reading characteristics on the first sentence typify a normal no-load situation, in contrast to the reading of subsequent sentences. The interesting result is that the low-span subjects read very similarly under load and under no load, while the high-span subjects adapt to the load condition. In particular, the high-span subjects have a lower lexical access parameter under the load condition.

The effect of reading under load was selective, not just in which group of readers it affected, but also in the locus of the effect. Only the lexical access parameter, and not the word encoding parameter was affected by load. (Recall that the lexical access parameter relates gaze duration to word frequency, while the word encoding parameter relates gaze duration to word length.) As the lower panels of Figure 2 show, the word encoding parameter remains approximately unchanged for both high and low-span subjects under load or no load. The process of word encoding may be so automatic that it is not affected by the load imposed by storing a final word from a previous sentence. By contrast, the lexical access process does show the selective effect of load on the high-span subjects. We interpret this result to indicate that high-span subjects activate less of the meaning of a word or activate the meaning to a lesser degree under load. This type of modification to "normal" reading is similar to what

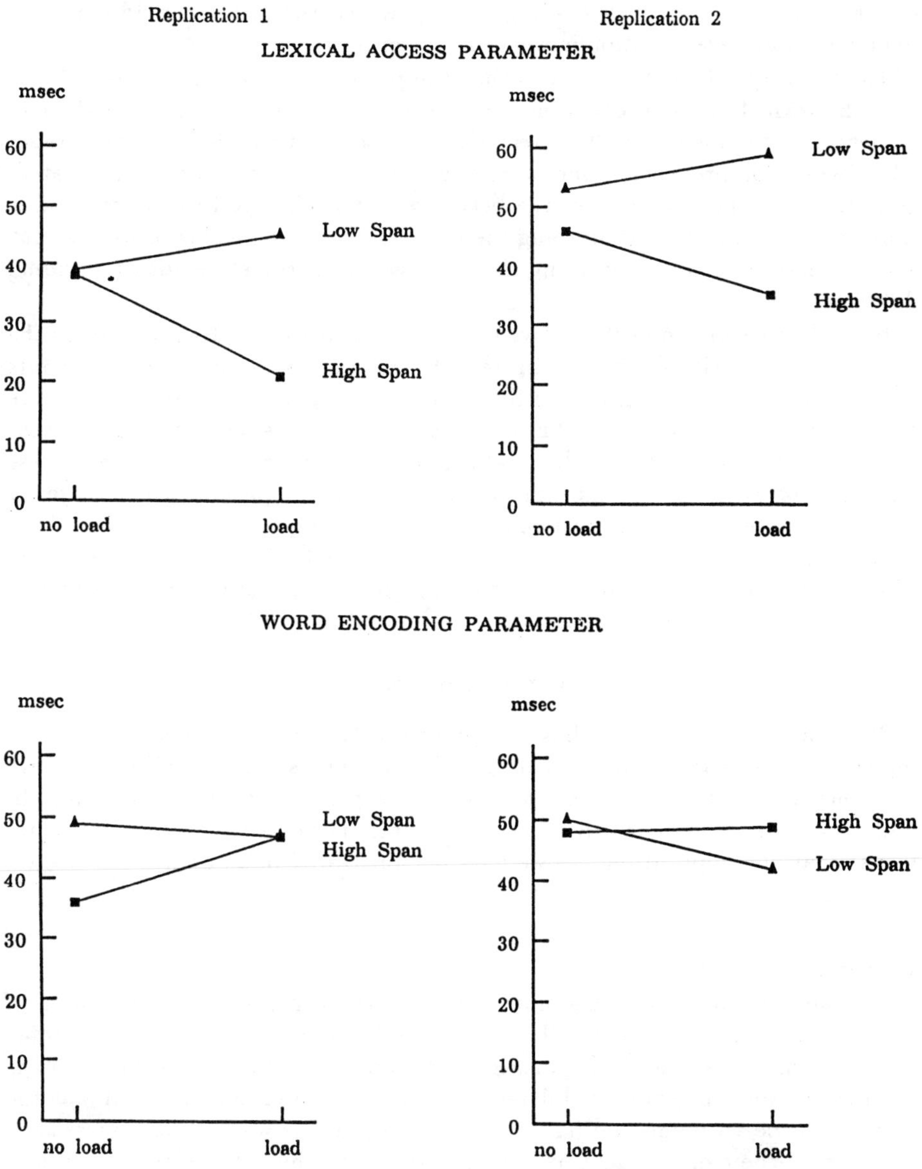

Fig. 2: Readers with high spans show a lower lexical access parameter (the top graphs) when reading with a memory load than do readers with low spans. By contrast, the word encoding parameter (the lower graphs) are similar. Replication 1 represents data from the memory span task in which the words were unrelated; replication 2 represents data from the memory span task in which the words formed a sentence.

we have observed in speed reading, during which the relation between word frequency and gaze duration is weakened even more.

The main result of this study is that the presence of a memory load affects only the lexical access process, not word encoding, and only for the high-span readers, not for low-span. This result reveals some of the detail of the trade-off between comprehension and storage when storage demand is manipulated, and pinpoints the flexibility of the better readers. The eye fixation method is thus not only useful for examining the time course of particular processes, but also for describing and analyzing the processes that correlate with individual differences.

Both the method and substantive results have contributed to a revision in the theoretical analysis of reading. In part, because eye fixation analysis permits an analysis of comprehension on-line, current research and theories are more oriented toward the processes that constitute comprehension as it occurs, rather than focusing exclusively on the final products of comprehension. The process tracing aspect of the eye fixation method is also compatible with computer simulation models, which must provide a step-by-step characterization of the component processes in order to derive final products. In addition, the results of such studies have contributed to a change in the unit of theoretical analysis in text comprehension, from sentences to individual words.

Spatial Cognition

The study of eye fixations has also proven to be extremely effective for tracing the processes in spatial reasoning tasks, as well as reading. Obviously, eye fixations are often closely associated with the process of visual encoding. In addition, under some circumstances, eye fixations can be used to monitor internal spatial computations, as we have demonstrated in an analysis of mental rotation.

Cognitive processes

The analysis began by examining the classic mental rotation paradigm of Shepard and Metzler (1971). They presented subjects with unfamiliar three dimensional figures, as shown in Figure 3, and asked them to decide whether the figures were the same or different. The important empirical result was the response time to judge two figures as being the same was a linear increasing function of their discrepancy in orientation, both when the trajectory was in the picture plane and when it was in depth. The results suggested that subjects were mentally rotating their representation of the object. But little was known about the underlying processes, aside from the correlation between response time and the angular disparity between the two depicted objects. However, it was possible to obtain a very detailed description of the processes by analyzing

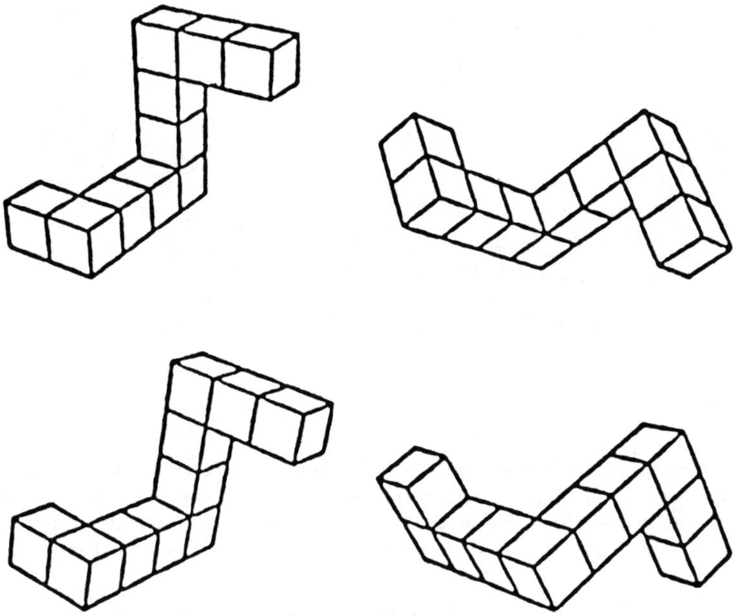

Fig. 3: The upper pair of figures are the Same and can be rotated into congruence. The lower pair of figures are Different; they are mirror image isomorphs.

the nature of eye fixations as people performed the task (Just & Carpenter, 1976).

The analysis of eye fixations made it possible to distinguish several different steps in the solution and to map those steps onto a precise model of the task. One general result from the eye fixation analysis is that rotation is not a holistic process. It is analytic in two ways. First, subjects rotated different parts of the figure at different times. Second, the rotation was not ballistic, but rather, it appeared to be interspersed by comparisons or checks to determine if the two figures were sufficiently close in represented orientation. More specifically, three component processes occurred in judging whether two figures were the same or different:

(1) *Initial search*: searching for two potentially corresponding segments of the two presented figures,

(2) *Rotation*: rotating and comparing the representations of those parts of the figure,

(3) *Confirmation*: confirming that the same transformation would bring the other parts into congruence.

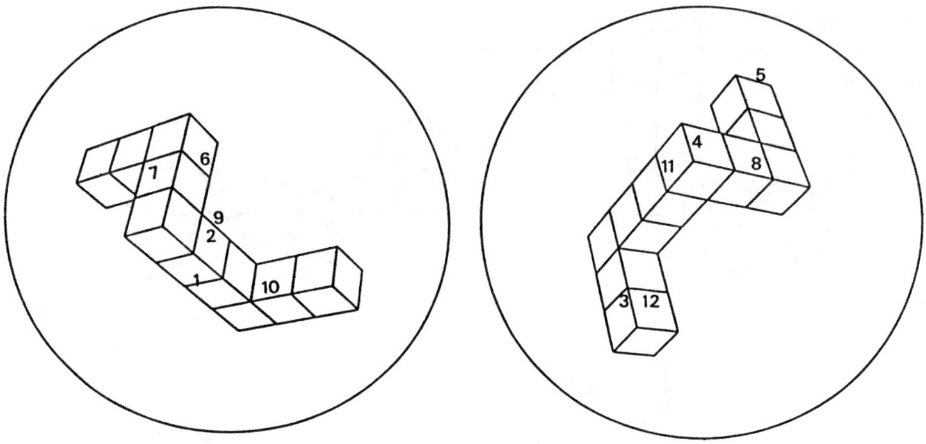

Fig. 4: The figure indicates the sequence of fixations on a correct Same trial in which the disparity was 80 degrees. The subject's total response latency was 3574 ms, of which 9% had no visible eye spot. See Table–Fig. 4 for the locus and duration of the fixation. Source: Just & Carpenter, 1976, Figure 5, p. 449. Used with permission of Academic Press.

Tab. - Fig. 4: Locus and duration of the fixations

Fixation	Figure	Location	Duration (msec)
1.	Left	Central joint	200
2.		Central joint	301
3.	Right	Open arm	167
4.		Central joint	150
5.		Closed arm	167
6.	Left	Closed arm	200
7.		Closed arm	317
8.	Right	Closed arm	501
9.	Left	Central joint	250
10.		Open arm	200
11.	Right	Central joint	484
12.		Open arm	317

Figure 4 shows the eye fixations during a typical correct Same trial and underneath in Table - Fig. 4 is a sequence of gazes which is separated into the three stages. Fixations at the beginning of a trial were associated with the search for corresponding segments of the objects. They .appeared to be initially identified on the basis of some local features, such as the length of the extreme arm or whether the third side of the end was visible. The next part of the protocol is the most distinctive. It is the part associated with the rotation and comparison process. This part was characterized by repeated fixations between corresponding parts of the left and right figures. The number of switches between corresponding segments and the duration of this component increased systematically with increasing disparity in the orientation of the two figures. The last part of the trial typically consisted of fixations on the other extremity, the segment that was not involved in the initial rotation and comparison process. These fixations were associated with a confirmation stage in which the subject determined whether the same trajectory applied to this segment would bring the two representations into alignment.

The analysis revealed how complex objects are decomposed into simpler segments. It revealed the piecewise rotation in which the spatial transformation was applied to one segment at a time. The transformation itself was stepwise, with each step being followed by an eye movement from one figure to the other. The fact that subjects decompose both the figure and the transformation process suggests limitations on working memory storage and computation capacities. Such limitations are a salient aspect of linguistic processing, but they are now also manifested in spatial processing. This general characteristic of thought, the decomposition of structure and process into simple constituents, is made particularly evident by the eye fixation behavior.

Individual differences

A second thrust of the spatial cognition research has been concerned with individual differences in visual problem solving, most recently, with problems adapted from traditional psychometric tests of spatial ability. The goal has been to explore and explain some of the qualitative and quantitative differences in spatial ability as measured by various psychometric tests (Just & Carpenter, 1985; Carpenter & Just, 1985). One of the main findings is that objects are represented within some reference framework – a cognitive coordinate system. The choice of cognitive coordinate system can determine whether or not a given test item will be solved, and influences how long the solution takes. Furthermore, some coordinate systems are used only by those people who are high in spatial ability, as measured by psychometric tests.

The theory we developed was initially intended to explain processing in the Cube Comparisons test, a test of visualization that is a part of the Guilford-Zimmerman test, but the theory has been generalized to apply to many other tests of spatial ability. Figure 5 presents a sample problem. Each problem consists of drawings of two cubes described as children's blocks. The subject is told to assume that each block has a letter or number on each of its six faces with the constraint that the same figure cannot appear more than once on a block. The subjects' task is to determine whether the two drawings could represent the same block (although possibly in different orientations).

The results showed that most subjects used a rotation strategy that involves mentally transforming the representation of an object's orientation. The theory

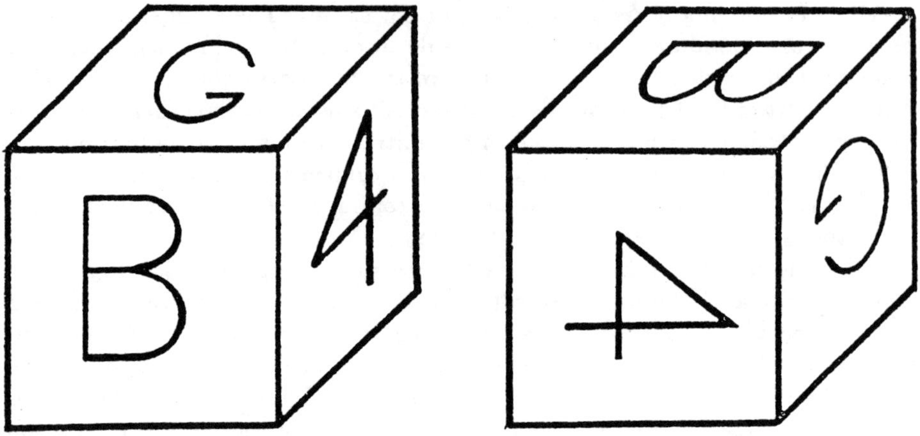

Fig. 5: Example of a 180 degree-3 Matches problem. Source: Just & Carpenter, 1985, Figure 4, p. 154. Copyright 1985 by the American Psychological Association.

of cognitive coordinate systems explains the differences in the ways individuals of low and high spatial ability solve problems from psychometric tests of spatial ability. The theory is instantiated as two computer simulation models that not only solve the problems, but also match the response times for the two groups, as shown in Figure 6.

Three major characteristics differentiated the performance of the two groups, and of the corresponding simulation models. The low spatial subjects rotated a cube only around axes perpendicular to the faces of the cube, whereas the high spatial subjects used shorter trajectories when possible. Also, the low spatial subjects rotated at a slower rate. Finally, the low spatial subjects made more errors in tracking cube faces through "hidden" trajectories. The difference between the trajectories chosen by the low and high spatial subjects in the Cube Comparisons task (both of whom used mental rotation) can be viewed in terms of a difference in cognitive coordinate systems. The subjects who rotated around non-standard axes were able to use that non-standard direction as one of the axes of their cognitive coordinate system. The low spatial subjects almost never used a cognitive coordinate system that did not closely correspond to the cubes' axes or to the main axes of the visual environment.

There were two other possible strategies, in addition to mental rotation, for solving the psychometric problems. The second strategy makes use of codes that are invariant with respect to the object's orientation in space. Subjects using orientation-free codes in the Cube Comparisons task coded the orientation of one letter relative to another on the same cube, without reference to any larger coordinate system external to the cube. Then, the codes for the

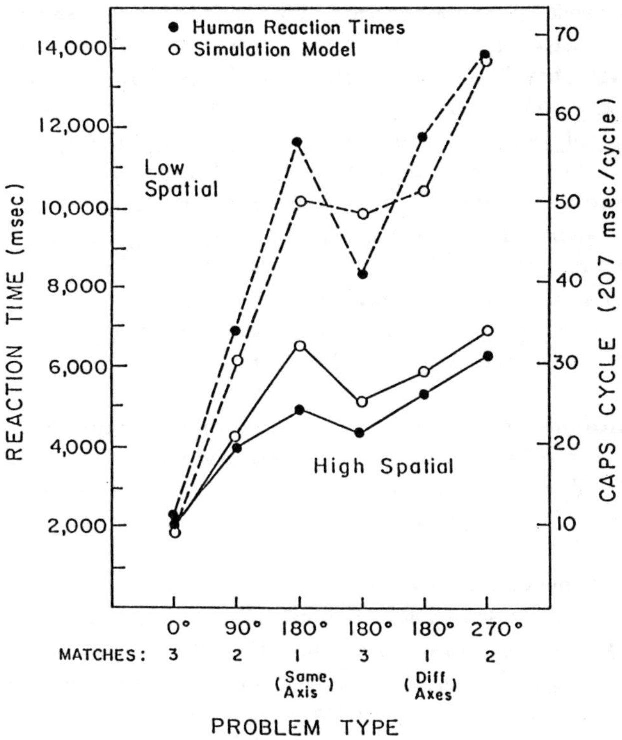

Fig. 6: Human reaction times (left axis) and simulation model cycles (right axis) in the Cube Comparisons task. Source: Just & Carpenter, 1985, Figure 6, p. 158. Copyright 1985 by the American Psychological Association.

left and right cubes can be directly compared without any mental rotation. A third strategy, perspective change, is also possible but infrequently used to solve the problems in the Cube Comparisons test, in the Vandenberg Mental Rotation test, and other similar tasks. In this strategy, the object's orientation in space is kept constant, but there is a change in the representation of the observer's position, and hence his or her view of the object. In this case, the object's position and the observer's position are both coded within a cognitive coordinate system that includes both the observer and the object, and whose origin corresponds to the object's position.

This account of spatial ability can provide an alternative interpretation of some previous psychometric results, as well as clarify a few mysteries within the psychometric literature. The psychometric literature on spatial ability has been preoccupied with a controversy over whether spatial ability consists of a single unitary ability or several distinct component abilities. The controversy exists in part because some of the factors are not stable across populations or across tests, and because different researchers have sometimes used different labels to describe a factor arising from similar tests. The present theory suggests that the varying psychometric descriptions of these factors may refer to three distinct processes engendered by the use of different coordinate systems. The visualization (rotation) factor may result from mental manipulation within an extrinsically defined coordinate system. The object in this case is represented with respect to an axis that is usually provided by the visual environment or the retinal upright. The factor described as spatial orientation seems to be a mixture of two distinct processes, feature-matching and perspective change. The feature-matching strategy may result from an orientation-invariant object-referenced coordinate system, while the perspective change strategy may result from a coordinate system that includes both the object and the observer, with the object at the origin.

The empirical investigations, using eye-fixation techniques in addition to conventional experimental approaches, revealed new strategies that are commonly used in performing a decades-old psychometric test. Moreover, individual differences in spatial ability, which is what these tests were intended to measure, were highly correlated with the selection of strategies. The choice of strategy, in turn, depended on the cognitive coordinate system that the subject adopted. Thus, this research has uncovered an important new determinant of spatial ability, and the characterization of the different types of processing has been formalized as a family of computer simulation models. Moreover, these simulation models have been incorporated into the same theoretical framework as a model of the reading process (Just & Carpenter, 1987). The framework constitutes a first approximation theory of the human processing system, and permits us to integrate the models of processing in individual tasks. The eye fixation studies have revealed important new facts about how people think, and the new insights are being expressed as a coherent theory of human thought.

THE EYE FIXATION METHODOLOGY

The most general assumption in both the research on reading and spatial cognition is that the locus of the eye fixation can indicate which symbol is being processed. In this section, we will describe this and other assumptions of the methodology and compare it to other methodologies for studying cognition.

Converging lines of evidence from very diverse tasks support the assumption that under some conditions, subjects look at the location that corresponds to a concept they are currently processing, in addition to the tasks described in this chapter. In tasks in which the behavioral units are relatively large and easily verbalized (such as cryptarithmetic tasks), the pattern of eye fixations correlates well with subject's verbal reports (Russo & Rosen, 1975; Newell & Simon, 1972; Winikoff, 1967). But even operations that appear to be too rapid for verbal protocols are still revealed by the eye fixations. A good example are the first 5 seconds of the scan paths of chess masters looking at a board position (de Groot & Jongman, 1973; Tichomirov & Posnyanskaya, 1966). These eye fixations reveal a check of the relations among the pieces in play.

In some cases, the link between fixations and processing arises simply because the task involves encoding new information from the display. While the new information is encoded, the person remains at the same location, and only moves to a different functional unit when he needs to acquire different information. However, there are a number of reasons why a subject might continue to fixate an area after the relevant information has been encoded. If the processor is busy operating on the most recently encoded information, there is no reason for it to direct the eye to seek other information. So the eye may remain stationary simply because it is not instructed to move. An alternative view of the persistence of the gaze is that the processor might actively instruct the eye not to move during the processing of the most recently encoded information. The reason for avoiding new fixations might be that a saccade automatically initiates an encoding activity that could interrupt the ongoing processing. This explanation accounts for the relation between eye fixations and cognitive processes in tasks such as reading, that involve cycles of visual encoding followed by higher levels of comprehension processes.

Another possible explanation for the correlation between eye fixations and cognitive processes is that symbols in working memory may be indexed to particular spatial locations. Consequently, eye fixations fulfill a place-keeping role. This seems to be a particularly plausible assumption when a subject is using visual imagery. When the time comes to retrieve or operate on a symbol in the image, the eye may fixate the location from which the symbol was originally encoded. It may be this mechanism that produces fixations on the referent of the symbol being processed.

Process tracing methodologies. The eye fixation method permits an analysis of the thinking that intervenes between the stimulus and the response. Hence, it is possible to characterize this as a *process tracing method.* The eye fixation method can reveal the duration and interdependencies of the intervening component processes, and in some cases, the sources of error. A related feature of this methodology is that the structure of individual trials can be analyzed, in addition to the differences arising between experimental conditions. The occurrence of a component process can be identified and its duration can be measured within a trial, without using any subtractive technique. This property distinguishes the eye fixation method from more traditional research methods, such as reaction time methods, which rely on analyzing the differences between conditions in order to estimate the duration of a particular process.

In some ways, the eye fixation method is similar to the the analysis of concurrent verbal reports, another process tracing technique. Both have the advantage of allowing the investigator to make inferences about the processes that occur within individual trials. Also, both methods can provide information about the content of the thought. For eye fixations, the information about content depends upon an analysis of what is fixated in the visual display; for verbal reports, it depends upon an analysis of what the subject says.

The ways in which the eye fixation method differs from the verbal report method illuminates some of its distinctive characteristics. The verbal report method is, of course, most compatible with tasks that involve easily verbalizable concepts. However, because the process of reporting may be slow and attention-consuming, the reports may alter the time course of the main process of interest. In this respect, the eye fixation method is more versatile and less obtrusive. The eye fixation method is useful for both verbal and more spatially oriented processing; the restriction is that there must be relevant information to be encoded from a visual display. In addition, the method appears to be most useful for computationally intensive tasks that are performed under speeded conditions. Eye movements are relatively fast and automatic, and need not detract from the main task. A second consequence of speed of eye fixations is that the method can be sensitive to processes that are themselves too rapid or automatic to verbalize, reflecting processes that might not reach consciousness. Of course, the eye fixation method and the verbal report method are not mutually exclusive. In a number of problem solving tasks, we have found it useful to ask subjects to report their thoughts while we record their eye fixations or to report verbally immediately *after* they perform a task. Often the two sources of evidence provide converging insights that would be difficult to obtain from either source by itself.

The units of analysis: words and gazes. In a developing science, there is often a problem in finding the appropriate level of aggregation. Ambrose Bierce said that learning history by reading newspapers is like measuring rainfall by counting raindrops. He was commenting on an inappropriate level of aggregation for a given purpose. Newspapers provide current events on a day-by-day basis that simply fails to capture the nature of slower-moving historical patterns. A parallel may be drawn to the issue of the appropriate unit of analysis for cognitive research using eye fixations. Our proposal is that the individual eye fixation is analogous to an individual raindrop. Either individual raindrops or individual eye fixations can have inherent interest for researchers of those phenomena. However, eye fixations are not necessarily the appropriate unit for researchers who are interested in cognition.

The unit of analysis we have typically used is the gaze. The gaze aggregates over consecutive individual fixations on the same functional unit of the stimulus. Our previous and current research has demonstrated that the gaze is generally a more appropriate and fruitful unit for analyzing cognitive processes.

The functional processing unit is the one that most closely corresponds to the mental operations that are performing the symbol manipulations. For example, in the analysis of mental rotation, each gaze consisted of any number of consecutive fixations on the same arm or angle of the Shepard and Metzler figure (Just & Carpenter, 1976). Each gaze was associated with a particular stage of processing. The model had little to say about the distribution of fixations within a gaze. In the research on the Cube Comparisons task, the gaze consists of consecutive fixations on a letter on one face of a cube. Again, the process model accounts for the mental operations relevant to this unit, not individual fixations on a letter.

In reading, the gaze durations on words, rather than the duration of individual fixations, provide the best unit for analyzing cognitive processes. The word is a useful unit because it has sufficient temporal and spatial resolution to reflect many of the processes that occur in language. By contrast, the analysis of too large a segment, such as an entire sentence, or too small a unit, such as individual letters, would not provide as good a match to the visual resolution of the perceptual system or to the tempo of language processes. Gaze durations show sensitivity to linguistic processes, and at the same time show considerable systematicity. Thus, both pragmatic and theoretical reasons point to the gaze as an appropriate unit for cognitive research.

Summary

At this point, we can bring together the three themes that were developed in both reading and spatial cognition. First, eye fixation research has made many substantive contributions to our models of both kinds of thinking, and has also illuminated the commonalities between them. Furthermore, we can now operate on much more refined issues that in many cases have arisen from results that were enabled by the eye fixation method.

Second, the eye fixation method is useful for the study of individual differences in cognition. This method has been useful for analyzing the processes that correlate with reading skill, and for analyzing the processing differences between those of high and low spatial skill. Although it has always been known that there are differences among individuals in cognitive processing, eye fixation studies have made those differences much more concrete and quantifiable.

Finally, the process tracing method itself has contributed to a new conception of human thought that has not been evident from other measures. Thought seems to be characterized by a "divide and conquer" strategy, decomposing complex objects and processes into manageable pieces. William James said that "The mass of our thinking vanishes for ever, beyond hope of recovery, and psychology only gathers up a few of the crumbs that fall from the feast." But 100 years later, James' comment is no longer accurate, thanks largely to the analyses of eye fixations. The intensive tracing of processes as they occur has allowed us to understand not only the general pattern of eating during the feast, but also to follow the consumption of each dish by each individual.

Acknowledgement

This work was supported in part by contract number N00014-85-K-0584 from ONR, grant number MH-29617 from NIMH, and Research Scientist Development Awards MH-00661 and MH-00662 from NIMH.

References

Baddeley, A. D., & Hitch, G., *Working memory*, in "G. H. Bower (Ed.), The psychology of learning and motivation (Vol.8)," Academic Press, New York, 1974.

Carpenter, P. A., & Just, M. A., *What your eyes do while your mind is reading*, in "K. Rayner (Ed.), Eye movements in reading: Perceptual and language processes," Academic Press, New York, 1983, pp. 275-307.

Carpenter, P. A., & Just, M. A., *Spatial ability: An information processing approach to psychometrics*, in "R. Sternberg (Ed.), Advances in the psychology of human intelligence (Vol.3)," Erlbaum, Hillsdale, NJ, 1985, pp. 221-253.

Carpenter, P. A., & Just, M. A., *The role of working memory in language comprehension*, in "D. Klahr & K. Kotovsky (Eds.), Complex information processing: The impact of Herbert A. Simon," Erlbaum, Hillsdale, NJ (to appear).

Daneman, M., & Carpenter, P. A., *Individual differences in working memory and reading*, Journal of Verbal Learning and Verbal Behavior **19** (1980), 450-466.

Dee-Lucas, D., Just, M. A., Carpenter, P. A., & Daneman, M., *What eye fixations tell us about the time course of text integration*, in "R. Groner & P. Fraisse (Eds.), Cognitive processes and eye movements," Deutscher Verlag der Wissenschaften, Amsterdam, 1982, pp. 155-168.

deGroot, A. D., & Jongman, R., "Perception and memory in chess: An experimental analysis of the master's professional eye (RITP Memorandum No. 024)," University of Amsterdam, Holland, 1973.

Gaarder, K. R., "Eye movements, vision and behavior," Hemisphere Publishing Corporation, Washington, DC, 1975.

Just, M. A., & Carpenter, P. A., *The semantics of locative information in pictures and mental images*, British Journal of Psychology **66** (1975), 427-441.

Just, M. A., & Carpenter, P. A., *Eye fixations and cognitive processes*, Cognitive Psychology **8** (1976), 441-480.

Just, M. A., & Carpenter, P. A., *A theory of reading: From eye fixations to comprehension*, Psychological Review **87** (1980), 329-354.

Just, M. A., & Carpenter, P. A., *Reading skills and skilled reading in the comprehension of text*, in "H. Mandl, T. Trabasso, & N. Stein (Eds.), Learning and comprehension of texts," Erlbaum, Hillsdale, NJ, 1983, pp. 307-329.

Just, M. A., & Carpenter, P. A., *Cognitive coordinate systems: Accounts of mental rotation and individual differences in spatial ability*, Psychological Review **92** (1985), 137-172.

Just, M. A., & Carpenter, P. A., "The psychology of reading and language comprehension," Allyn and Bacon, Newton, MA, 1987.

Kimball, J. P., *Seven principles of surface structure parsing in natural language*, Cognition **2** (1973), 15-47.

Marcus, M. P., "A theory of syntactic recognition for natural language," The MIT Press, Cambridge, MA, 1980.

McConkie, G. W., Zola, D., Blanchard, H. E., & Wolverton, G. S., "Perceiving words during reading: Lack of facilitation from prior peripheral exposure (Technical Report

No. 243)," University of Illinois, Center for the Study of Reading, Urbana-Champaign, IL, 1982.

McDonald, J. L., & Carpenter, P. A., *Simultaneous translation: Idiom interpretation and parsing heuristics*, Journal of Verbal Learning and Verbal Behavior **20** (1981), 231-247.

Newell, A., & Simon, H. A., "Human problem solving," Prentice-Hall, Inc, Englewood Cliffs, NJ, 1972.

O'Regan, J. K., *Moment to moment control of eye saccades as a function of textual parameters in reading*, in "P. A. Kolers, M. E. Wrolstad, & H. Bouma (Eds.), Processing of visible language (Vol.1)," Plenum Press, New York, 1979.

Rayner, K., *The perceptual span and peripheral cues in reading*, Cognitive Psychology **7** (1975), 65-81.

Russo, J. E., & Rosen, L., *An eye fixation analysis of multialternative choice*, Memory & Cognition **3** (1975), 267-276.

Shepard, R. N., & Metzler, J., *Mental rotation of three-dimensional objects*, Science **171** (1971), 701-703.

Tichomirov, G. K. & Posnyanskaya, E. D., *An investigation of visual search as a means of analyzing heuristics*, Voprosy Psikhologii **12** (1966), 39-53.

Winikoff, A., "Eye movements as an aid to protocol analysis of problem solving behavior," Unpublished doctoral dissertation, Carnegie-Mellon University, Pittsburgh, Pennsylvania, 1967.

THE EFFECTS OF SPATIALISATION ON THE PROCESSING OF AMBIGUOUS PRONOMINAL REFERENCE

JOEL PYNTE [1], ALAN KENNEDY [2], WAYNE S. MURRAY [2], AND PIERRE COURRIEU [1]

[1]Centre de Recherche en Psychologie Cognitive, Université de Provence
[2]Department of Psychology, University of Dundee

In this paper we consider the processing of ambiguous sentences and the use of these to address issues in eye movement control.

In sentences ⟨a⟩ and ⟨b⟩ the antecedent of the pronoun 'il/elle' is ambiguous until the final disambiguating phrase is encountered (for example, (1) or (2) below). The pronoun could be assigned either to the first or the second noun phrase since both are of the same gender. The ambiguity derives, of course, from the lack of a neutral pronoun in French which could be used to distinguish between animate and inanimate nouns.

⟨a⟩ Cette clause surprend la bourgeoisie car elle est ...

(1) ... imposée sans debat.
(2) ... habituée à la concurence.

⟨b⟩ L'éléctorat refuse ce referendum car il est ...

(1) ... formulé de façon ambigue.
(2) ... embarassé par le question.

In the absence of such formal cues, the reader, encountering an ambiguous pronoun, has to rely on the *meaning* of the sentence if it is to be disambiguated. In the particular case of sentence types ⟨a⟩ and ⟨b⟩, for example, the proposition containing the ambiguous pronoun is introduced by a statement of causality. This means that whatever noun phrase is bound to the pronoun will be considered as the 'cause' of the state of affairs described in the first clause. Thus, the initial assignment of the pronoun could be based on intuitions about the assignment of causality.

In the case of sentences containing a stative verb, such as *surprendre* or *refuser*, 'implicit causality' (Garvey & Caramaza, 1974) is associated with that noun-phrase which plays the semantic role of 'stimulus' (e.g. *referendum*) as opposed to 'experiencer' (e.g. *éléctorat*). Indeed, the stimulus is, by definition 'someone or something *giving rise* to a certain experience,' whereas the experiencer is 'someone *having* a certain experience' (e.g. Brown & Fish, 1983; Chafe, 1970; Comrie, 1981; Fillmore, 1968). Two English examples are given below.

⟨a⟩	Something (Stimulus)	impresses	somebody (Experiencer)
⟨b⟩	Somebody (Experiencer)	admires	something (Stimulus)

Following the previous analysis, the verb 'to impress' conveys the notion that the one who 'is impressed' (i.e. the experiencer), is so by virtue of some property inherent in the stimulus, just as the one who 'admires' is supposed to do so by virtue of some property of what is being admired. Another important factor identified by Brown and Fish (1983) is the relative range of the referents associated with each noun phrase: if something impresses a lot of people, it is probably because of some property likely to impress. Conversely, if a lot of things impress one particular person, this person will be considered as responsible for the ensuing mental state (i.e. will be 'impressionable').

If we now return to the example sentence types ⟨a⟩ and ⟨b⟩, it becomes clear in each case that the disambiguating phrase is consistent with the attribution of causality in continuation (1), but not in continuation (2). We will refer to (1) as a 'Consistent' termination and to (2) as an 'Inconsistent' termination. It is important to note, however, that the inconsistent termination, though a little surprising, remains perfectly acceptable for a French native speaker. We are dealing here with semantic intuitions and not with formal cues (such as masculine *vs* feminine or animate *vs* inanimate). Their violation does not lead to anomaly. In the absence of semantic as well as formal cues (or when semantic cues have failed as in continuation (2) of sentences ⟨a⟩ and ⟨b⟩)the reader may, as a last resort, rely on general heuristics. For example, the reader may bind the pronoun to the first-mentioned noun-phrase in the sentence (see Sidner, 1983, for a discussion) or to the noun-phrase associated with the same grammatical function, the *parallel function* strategy, (Sheldon, 1974).

In summary, in sentence types ⟨a⟩ and ⟨b⟩, assignment of the pronoun may be determined by, at least, the four following rules:

(1) Assign the pronoun to the stimulus
(2) Assign the pronoun to the more-specified referent
(3) Assign the pronoun to the first-mentioned noun
(4) Assign the pronoun to that noun which plays the same grammatical role in the sentence as the pronoun

As stated above, rules (1) and (2) are essentially semantic. To use them, the reader must construct a representation of the sentence's meaning. Rules (3) and (4) are general pronoun assignment heuristics. They are concerned with word-order and word-position; that is, to employ them, it is necessary to know in what order the nouns occur in relation to the verb.

If we consider the disambiguation offered by the alternative 'Consistent' and 'Inconsistent' terminations, it is clear that in the Inconsistent case the semantically-determined referent must be abandoned and a new assignment made. In the case of sentence type (b) the new assignment will be consistent with 'general heuristics' such as rules (3) and (4) which involve positional cues. What the consequences of such reassignment are, in processing terms, remains to be determined.

It has, however, recently been claimed (Kennedy, 1987) that fluent readers locate potential antecedents of pronouns by accessing a spatial code. For example, antecedents may be checked by means or large regressive saccades, which depend for their success on the reader having coded previously-inspected text in terms of relative spatial coordinates. This code is, we presume, derived at the time of initial inspection. The evidence for the Spatial Coding Hypothesis rests on direct observations of eye movements (Kennedy & Murray, 1987; Murray & Kennedy, 1988) and also on inferences drawn from self-paced reading tasks in which spatial coding is manipulated (Kennedy & Murray, 1984). When the reader is deprived of differential spatial information (for example, when the words of a text appear in a single location) a processing deficit is found.

In the first experiment reported here, two conditions in a self-paced reading task were contrasted. First, one in which phrases appeared successively on a display in the same physical location (a Non-Spatialised Mode); and second, one in which phrases also appeared successively, but in their appropriate physical locations (Spatialised Mode). In each condition, subjects had equivalent access to words in the sentence, but only in the second case was it possible to assign them to differential spatial locations at the time of initial reading. Examples of the presentation methods are illustrated below:

	Non-Spatialised Mode		Spatialised Mode		
time 1		Le chat	Le chat		
time 2		mange		mange	
time 3	Le chat mange	la souris	Le chat	mange	la souris

The role of spatial coding in reading can be assessed by comparing reading times when the whole sentence is presented, following either Spatialised or Non-spatialised self-paced presentation. Clearly, if spatialisation allows the reader to establish better cues for the process of later reanalysis (where this is called for) we should anticipate less penalty extracted by the Inconsistent condition in the Spatialised Mode. We are, thus, predicting an interaction between Mode of presentation and Consistency, with a smaller difference between Consistent and Inconsistent terminations in the Spatialised Mode than in the Non-Spatialised Mode.

Experiment I

Method

Subjects. Forty students in the Psychology Department of the Université de Provence participated in the experiment. They were all native French speakers. The subjects were volunteers and not paid for their participation. The subjects were designated as either "poor" or "good" readers, at the beginning of the experiment, on the basis of their reading speed and answers to a questionnaire concerning a short passage. Good and poor readers were equally distributed between the two modes of presentation.

Materials. The experimental materials were 16 pairs of sentences similar in form to ⟨a⟩ and ⟨b⟩ above. The two sentences in each pair differed in termination. This was either 'Consistent' or 'Inconsistent' according to 'semantic' rules (1) and (2). Eight pairs were, like sentence ⟨a⟩, based on a verb of the type 'to impress.' The other eight were, like sentence ⟨b⟩, based on a verb of the type 'to admire.'

Procedure. Sentences were presented on the screen of an Apple IIe computer via a self- paced presentation procedure. Subjects pressed a button to display successively the subject phrase; the verb; the object phrase; a statement of causality containing the ambiguous pronoun; a past participle or adjective which disambiguated the sentence; and the final segment of the sentence. The segments are indicated by slashes in the following example:

Cette clause/surprend/la bourgeoisie/car elle est/imposée/sans debat.

In the Spatialised mode, each segment was presented in its appropriate physical location on the screen, up to the final segment. At that point the whole sentence was displayed. That is, the final segment appeared *only* as part of the whole-sentence display. In Non-Spatialised presentation, all the segments began at the same physical location, on the right of the display. However, the final segment was again only presented as part of a whole-sentence display. This was physically in register with the preceding displays. These two conditions only differ in what happens before the final whole-sentence presentation takes place. What is manipulated is the degree to which subjects can assign appropriate spatial coordinates to the presented words. The experimental materials were mixed with 40 fillers. The subject's task was to decide, by pressing a button, whether the sentences made sense or not. Obviously, this was a yes response for all the experimental materials. The fillers contained a mixture of sentences demanding a yes or no response.

Results and discussion

The dependent variable was a global 'Reading Time' recorded in the whole-sentence reading phase. The results summarised in Figure 1 are based on medians, calculated for each Subject in each experimental condition.

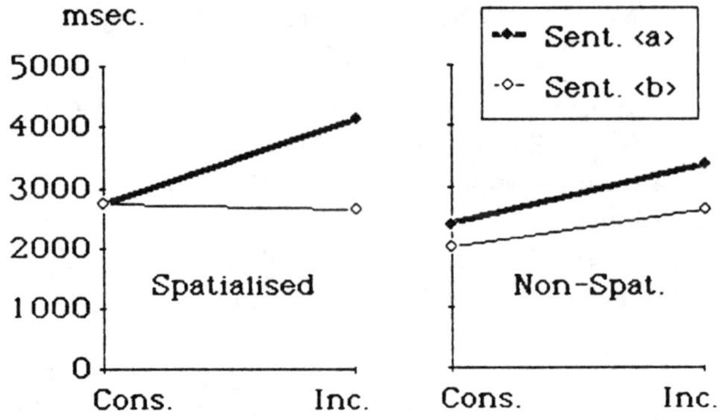

Fig. 1: Total reinspection times (Experiment 1).

An analysis of variance was conducted, with Mode of Presentation, Sentence Type, Consistency and Reading Skill as factors. Our concern was primarily with the Mode by Consistency interaction. Put simply, this prediction was not confirmed, since the outcome was somewhat complicated by differences between the two sentence types. There was an overall interaction between Type of Sentence and Consistency $F(1,32) = 11.38$, $p < 0.01$, as well as a significant interaction between Mode of presentation, Type of Sentence and Consistency, $F(1,32) = 4.38$, $p < 0.05$. Reading skill did not interact with any of the other three factors, and will not be considered further.

Let us first consider the Consistency by Sentence Type interaction. It will be evident that in the case of sentence ⟨a⟩, above, all four rules converge to bind 'elle' to 'cette clause,' which is the stimulus; the noun whose referent is more restricted; the first mentioned noun; and the one with the same syntactic function as the pronoun. Thus, it is not surprising that an Inconsistent termination leads to a relatively long 're-reading time,' since no alternative assignment rules are available for making a new assignment. However, in ⟨b⟩ rules (3) and (4) determine a different assignment from rules (1) and (2). That is, rules (1) and (2) bind 'il' to 'ce referendum,' whereas rules (3) and (4) bind it to 'l'éléctorat.' In the case of inconsistent terminations an alternative assignment was thus available via rules (3) and (4). This leads to a weaker bias and could explain why reinspection time was consistently shorter in this condition.

The nature of the Mode by Consistency by Sentence Type interaction was pursued by analyses for the two modes separately. In the Non-Spatialised condition, there was a significant effect of Sentence Type, $F(1,16) = 18.41$, $p < 0.01$ and of Consistency, $F(1,16) = 8.14$, $p < 0.02$. The interaction did not approach significance. In the Spatialised condition, however, there was a highly significant interaction between Sentence Type and Consistency, $F(1,16) = 10.57$, $p < 0.01$. As indicated in Figure 1, this obviously results from the fact that, in the Spatialised Mode, an effect of Consistency is only found for one type of sentence. Thus, at least for Type ⟨b⟩ structures, our hypothesis is confirmed.

It is necessary, however, to explain why spatialisation apparently does not facilitate reassignment in the case of Type ⟨a⟩ sentences. A possible interpretation could be the fact that no heuristic, at the pycholinguistic level, is available in the case of Type ⟨a⟩ sentences to perform a new assignment. Indeed, the assignment suggested by the disambiguating phrase is inconsistent with all four rules. Put another way, spatialisation may only facilitate pronoun assignment when spatial cues are likely to be used by a processing heuristic employed at a psycholinguistic level. This interpretation does not, however, cope with the fact that for Type ⟨a⟩ sentences, the extra processing time attributable to Inconsistency is *greater* (though not significantly so) in the Spatialised Mode than in the Non-Spatialised Mode. Such a result is, at least, compatible with an alternative hypothesis according to which processing differences between the two Modes originate at the time of *initial inspection*. Possibly all available rules for dealing with the ambiguity, including rules of the form (3) and (4), are applied 'on-line' in order to arrive at an initial assignment. From this perspective, the Consistency effect observed in sentences of Type ⟨a⟩ in the Spatialised Mode would be interpreted as a 'Bias' effect (difficulty in abandoning an original interpretation, rather than in finding another). It is fairly obvious that Type ⟨a⟩ sentences, in which all the rules pull the same way, are more strongly biased than Type ⟨b⟩ sentences, in which different rules pull in opposite directions. What then of the Non-Spatialised condition? The data suggest in this case that the Bias manipulation produces no differential effect at all, as if Subjects were equally (and weakly) biased in both types of sentence. We shall return to this point in the General Discussion section.

It is clear from Experiment I that the availability of differential spatial information influences the processing of this type of ambiguous sentence. Unfortunately, however, the results do not offer unequivocal support for the Spatial Coding Hypothesis. The difficulty is that a measure of global Reading Time gives only a very sketchy idea of the underlying processes which lead to global variations in processing time. At worst, the measure can be actually misleading (Kennedy & Murray, 1987). Experiment II provides the necessary fine-grain analysis by means of concurrent eye movement measurement.

Experiment II

Experiment II allows for the effects of spatialisation to be examined during both initial reading and later reinspection. Although the results from Experiment I suggest that the manipulations of Sentence Type, Consistency and Mode should modify the total *amount* of reinspection, it is possible that the *location* of these fixations may not be affected by the manipulations. That is, subjects may simply look longer in some conditions than in others, but *where* they look may be unaffected. This question can only be addressed by direct eye movement measurement examining the patterns of reinspection (indexing reanalysis) following the two presentation modes.

Method

Forty subjects participated in the Experiment. They were unpaid volunteer Students of Psychology at the Université de Provence. None had participated in Experiment I. Experiment II was identical in all respects to Experiment I, except for changes consequent on the need to measure concurrent eye movements. This necessitated the calibration of the equipment from time to time and minor modifications in the instructions to subjects to remove any possible ambiguity as to whether they were free to reinspect the materials.

Eye movements were recorded using a conventional infra-red limbus-tracking device mounted on spectacle frames. The subject's head movement was restricted by the use of a head support frame and dental composition bite bar, while their horizontal line of regard was sampled every 10 ms from the right eye. Overall accuracy of the system was approximately plus or minus one character position.

Results and discussion

There were no clear differences in initial inspection strategy between the two modes of presentation - apart, of course, from the incidence of larger and more frequent saccades in the Spatialised condition, where the phrases were presented in different spatial locations. Clear differences did, however, emerge in the inspection strategies employed by the two groups of subjects with the presentation of the final, whole-sentence, display.

The range of whole-sentence reinspection times was less than in Experiment I, probably as a result of the changed experimental conditions. The overall pattern of findings was, however, very similar. Taking the two experiments together, there was no tendency for any of the experimental manipulations to interact with Experiment. The distribution of fixations during the whole-sentence display for both Consistent and Inconsistent terminations is shown in Figures 2 and 3. Figure 2 contrasts the two modes of presentation and Figure 3 the two sentence types. Note that only the first five segments are included. The final segment, for which the range of values was much greater, will be considered separately.

The effect of consistency. As shown in Figures 2 and 3, an Inconsistent termination generally resulted in more fixations on each of the segments. An exception was the Object in the case of Non-Spatialised presentation for sentences of Type ⟨b⟩. Analysis over the five segments showed a significant main

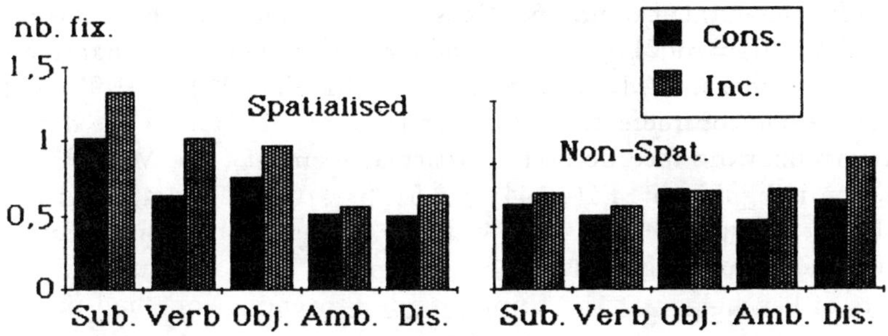

Fig. 2: Patterns of reinspection for the two modes of presentation.

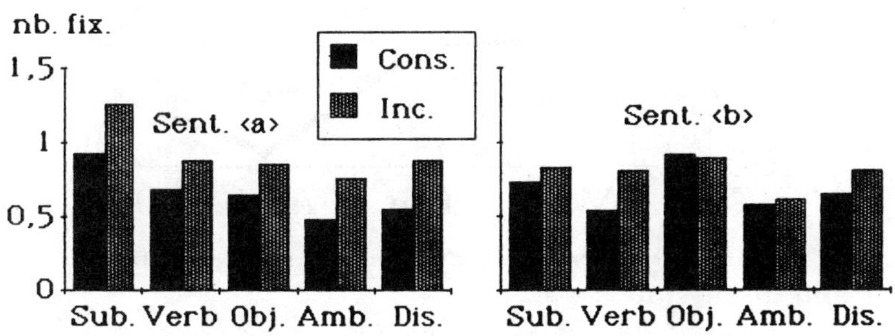

Fig. 3: Patterns of reinspection for the two types of sentences.

effect of Consistency, $F1(1,36) = 9.30$, $p < 0.01$; $F2(1,12) = 7.46$, $p < 0.05$. In addition, the Consistency by Mode by Segment interaction was significant, $F1(4,144) = 3.94$; $p < 0.01$; $F2(4,48) = 3.74$, $p < 0.05$. The largest effect of Consistency was observed on the Verb segment in the case of Spatialised presentation, and there was a significant interaction between Consistency and Mode, $F1(1,36) = 5.67$, $p < 0.05$; $F2(1,12) = 3.88$, $p < 0.10$, on this segment.

The distribution of fixations on the two modes. Following Spatialised presentation, subjects made more fixations on the initial segment, with a significant Mode by Segment interaction, $F1(4,144) = 7.81$, $p < 0.01$; $F2(4,48) = 21.48$, $p < 0.01$. This is consistent with the operation of rules (3) and (4), since the initial segment is also the first noun and the subject of the sentence. Following Non-Spatialised presentation, however, subjects spent more time in the region of the ambiguous pronoun (which is, of course, physically closer).

This pattern of results is very robust. The same results are found if one considers just the position of the very first fixation. A significant effect of Mode is found for the number of first fixations on the initial noun, $F1(1,36) = 7.05$, $p < 0.05$; $F2(1,12) = 39.21$, $p < 0.01$, and for the number of first fixations on the ambiguous segment, $F1(1,36) = 8.74$, $p < 0.01$; $F2(1,12) = 51.97$, $p < 0.01$. Similarly, if one considers Gaze duration (that is, the sum of the durations of the various fixations recorded on a particular segment), the Mode by Segment interaction is significant, $F1(4,144) = 8.51$, $p < 0.01$; $F2(4,48) = 15.48$, $p < 0.01$. Figure 4 illustrates the effect of Mode of presentation on the duration of Gaze for the various segments.

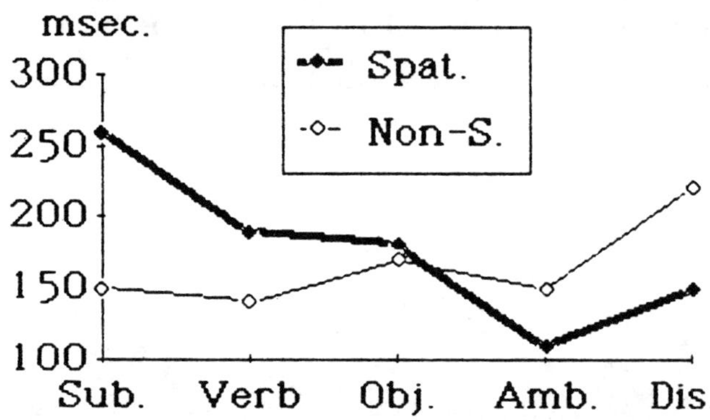

Fig. 4: Reinspection times for the two modes of presentation.

The distribution of fixations for the two sentence types. Figures 3 and 5 reveal a tendency to reinspect the noun which has the semantic role of 'stimulus' - which is, of course, the noun with the greater chance of being the antecedent according to rules (1) and (2). The Segment by Sentence Type interaction evident in Figure 3 is significant, $F1(4,144) = 4.69$, $p < 0.05$; $F2(4,48) = 3.52$, $p < 0.05$. It is also significant when we consider Gaze duration (Figure 5) rather than number of fixations, $F1(4,144) = 5.01$, $p < 0.05$; $F2(4,48) = 3.35$, $p < 0.05$. This appears to be primarily due to the Subject and Object. The interaction of Sentence Type over these two segments also was highly significant, $F1(1,36) = 13.94$, $p < 0.01$; $F2(1,12) = 20.48$, $p < 0.01$.

The final segment. It is when we examine the time spent reinspecting the final segment (Figure 6) that we come closest to recovering the general form of the whole-sentence inspection times. This is partly because the final segment times are so long - with Gaze durations of the order of a second or more. It seems unlikely that this amount of time is simply a reflection of the processing difficulty of the final segment alone. It is much more likely that the results reflect the overall difficulty of the sentences, and the fact that subjects are thinking at this point. The interaction in final segment Gaze duration between Mode, Sentences Type and Consistency is significant by subjects, F1(1,36)

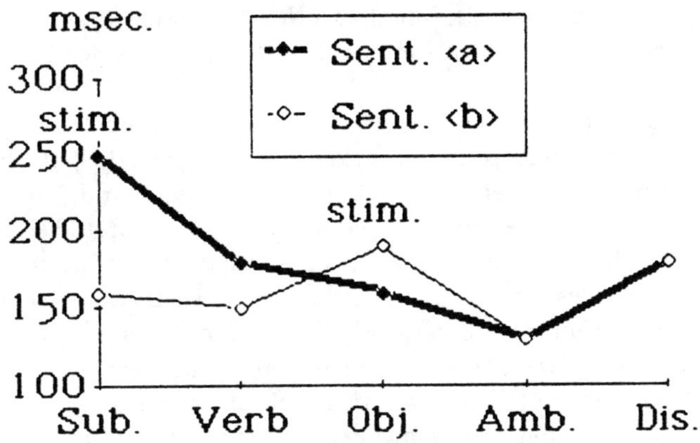

Fig. 5: Reinspection time for the two types of sentences.

= 5.49, $p < 0.05$, but not by items, $F2(1,12) = 1.38$, n.s. When separate analyses are conducted for the two Modes, the interaction in the Spatialised Mode, apparent in Figure 6, approaches significance $F1(1,18) = 4.19$, $p = 0.06$; $F2(1,12) = 3.31$, $p < 0.10$, whereas there is no evidence of any effect of Consistency in the Non-Spatialised condition.

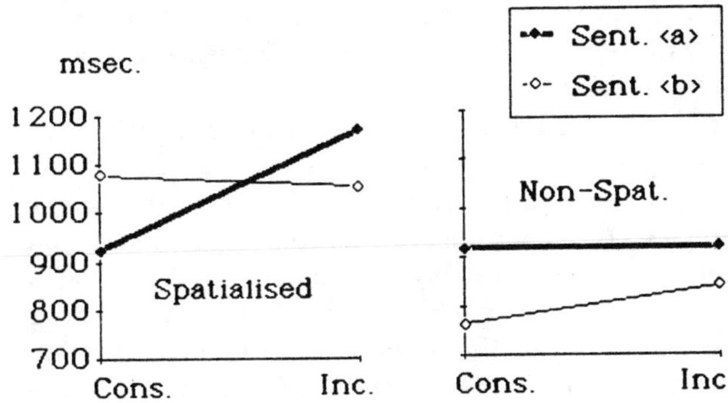

Fig. 6: Reinspection times (end of sentence).

General Discussion

The aim of the two experiments reported here was to compare total re-reading times and patterns of reinspection following Spatialised and Non-Spatialised presentation of ambiguous sentences. Our initial hypothesis was that more reinspection would be necessary in the case of terminations inconsistent with 'semantic' rules (1) and (2), but that a Non-Spatialised presentation would inhibit assignment via the operation of rules (3) and (4), since these are based on positional cues.

Neither of these predictions received unequivocal support from the whole-sentence reading times in Experiment I. While it is true that Spatialised presentation produced a strong interaction between Consistency and Type of sentence (Figure 1), this pattern of results is capable of being interpreted in a number of ways. We believe the most likely explanation is that in this Mode (and only in this Mode) all four rules were applied at the time of segment-by-segment initial reading. Thus, one Sentence Type was effectively more strongly 'biased' than the other. Put another way, Inconsistent terminations were *highly* inconsistent in the case of sentences of Type ⟨a⟩, in which all four rules pull in the same direction, leading to a particular problem for subjects receiving Inconsistent Type ⟨a⟩ sentences in the Spatialised Presentation Mode. In contrast, with Type ⟨b⟩ sentences, in which the two sets of rules pull in opposite directions, Inconsistent terminations were apparently *not* perceived as inconsistent at all.

Subjects in the Non-Spatialised Mode were apparently unable (or, at least, unwilling), during the initial segment-by-segment presentation, to compute relationships demanding positional information. In other words, unlike subjects in the Spatialised Mode, they were simply less able to make use of rules like (3) and (4), and were forced to rely solely on the 'semantic' rules like (1) and (2) in arriving at an initial assignment. In such circumstances, the same effect of Consistency will be found for the two Types of sentences, since rules (1) and (2) apply equally in the two cases.

Clearly, this interpretation is several steps away from the proposition that Spatialisation simply confers a global advantage at the time of reinspection. The results suggest an additional effect of Presentation Mode on *initial* assignment strategies. In Experiment II, an important finding was that a great amount of time was spent 'thinking' (at the end of the sentence) rather than truly 'reinspecting' (the first five segments). Moreover, the results concerning 'thinking' time were close to those obtained with the more global 're-reading' measure from Experiment I: Mode interacted with Consistency and Type of sentence, confirming that an effect of Spatialisation can be found independently of reinspection strategy. We are forced to the conclusion that Non-Spatialised presentation removes from the reader important positional cues and hence disrupts syntactic operations at the time of segment-by-segment reading. This can be readily tested using a measure of syntactic judgement following sentential presentation under the two Modes, and we hope to report on this at a later date.

It is nevertheless true that differences in reinspection strategy *were* found following the two Modes of presentation. All subjects were apparently attracted to the 'stimulus. However, the first noun (the co-referent using rules (3) and

(4)) and the verb were *only* the focus of more reinspections following Spatialised presentation. Again, we are led to the conclusion that all four rules were used in the Spatialised Mode, whereas only rules (1) and (2) were apparently used in the Non-Spatialised Mode. Put another way, the same (unknown) causes which prevent subjects in the Non-Spatialised condition from initially binding the pronoun to the first noun, when the first noun is *not* the stimulus, apparently inhibit their reinspection of it.

Acknowledgement

The research reported here was supported by grants from the United Kingdom Economic and Social Research Council (AK and WSM) and from the British Council (AK).

References

Brown, R., & Fish, D., *The psychological causality implicit in language*, Cognition **14** (1983), 237-273.

Chafe, W.L., "Meaning and the structure of language," The University of Chicago Press, Chicago, 1970.

Comrie, B., "Language universals and linguistic typology," The University of Chicago Press, Chicago, 1981.

Fillmore, C.J., *The case for case*, in "E. Bach & R.G. Harms (Eds.), Universals in linguistic theory," Holt, Rinehart, and Winston, New York, 1968, pp. 1-87.

Garvey, C., & Caramazza, A., *Implicit causality in verbs*, Linguistic Inquiry **5** (1974), 459-464.

Kennedy, A., *Eye movements, reading skill and the spatial code*, in "J. Beech & A. Colley (Eds.), Cognitive approaches to reading," Wiley, Chichester, 1987, pp. 169-186.

Kennedy, A., & Murray, W.S., *Inspection times for words in syntactically ambiguous sentences under three presentation conditions*, Journal of Experimental Psychology: Human Perception and Performance **10** (1984), 833-849.

Kennedy, A., & Murray, W.S., *The components of reading time: Eye movement patterns of good and poor readers*, in "J.K. O'Regan & A. Lévy - Schoen (Eds.), Eye movements: From physiology to cognition," Elsevier North Holland, Amsterdam, 1987, pp. 509-520.

Murray, W.S., & Kennedy, A., *Spatial coding in the processing of anaphor by good and poor readers: Evidence from eye movement analyses*, Quarterly Journal of Experimental Psychology (1988) (to appear).

Sheldon, A., *The role of parallel function in the acquisition of relative clauses in English*, Journal of Verbal Learning and Verbal Behavior **13** (1974), 272-281.

Sidner, C.L, *Focussing in the comprehension of definite anaphora*, in "M. Brady & R. Berwick (Eds.), Computational models of discourse," MIT Press, Cambridge, Mass., 1983, pp. 267-330.

SOME PROPERTIES OF EYE MOVEMENT CONTROL DURING READING

GEORGE W. MCCONKIE, N. RODERICK UNDERWOOD, GARY S. WOLVERTON, AND DAVID ZOLA

Center for the Study of Reading, University of Illinois at Urbana-Champaign

During the past 15 years a number of studies have been carried out to investigate the size of the region from which visual information is acquired and used during eye fixations while reading. For reviews see Rayner and Pollatsek (1987) and McConkie (1983). These studies have used Eye Movement Contingent Display Control research techniques, in which the text display is changed from fixation to fixation in response to the reader's eye movements (McConkie, Zola, Wolverton, & Burns, 1978; Reder, 1973). In most of these studies, the computer is programmed to monitor the eye movement data as a saccade is in progress and as soon as the location of the following fixation can be identified or predicted, to make a change in the displayed text. This change involves replacing letters at selected distances to the left and right of the fixation location with either a masking pattern or with other letters. During the following fixation, then, there is a region of normal text in central vision, typically referred to as a *window*, with the masking pattern or erroneous letters outside the window area. In an experiment, the size and offset of the window is manipulated in order to determine the smallest window that does not interfere with reading. The size and offset of that window is taken to indicate the reader's perceptual span; that is, the region within which useful visual information is obtained during fixations, information of the type distinguishing the patterns inside and outside the window.

It has been pointed out that the perceptual span established from this research may not indicate the region that is attended during individual eye fixations (McConkie, 1983; Rayner & Pollatsek, 1987). The region attended may actually vary from fixation to fixation, with the perceptual span obtained from existing studies giving an indication of the total region within which readers attend during individual fixations. Thus, the region attended during a fixation may lie within, but be smaller than, the perceptual span obtained by existing studies. Consonant with this proposal is current evidence that the text may be attended in word-related units (McConkie, Zola, Blanchard, & Wolverton, 1982; Rayner, Well, & Pollatsek, 1980).

The study described in this paper was designed to investigate whether information from specific visual regions is acquired on only some eye fixations during reading. However, the data analysis resulted in a detailed investigation of the various patterns of response that occur when readers encounter erroneous letters at different locations in their visual field, together with the frequency of occurrence of each pattern. These patterns revealed characteristics of eye movement control during reading, which is the focus of the present report.

Using Eye Movement Contingent Display Control, regions of erroneous letters were inserted into the text at specified regions on selected eye fixations as college students read newspaper articles displayed on a computer screen. In the control condition, the text remained normal during the selected eye fixations. In three experimental conditions, all letters more than a certain distance to either the left or to the right of the currently fixated letter were replaced with other letters during that fixation, and then the text returned to normal during the following saccade. The data analysis was concentrated on identifying the eye movement patterns that resulted and estimating the frequency of each.

Methods

Subjects

Twelve college students participated in this experiment. All were native speakers of English and above average in reading ability and had normal uncorrected vision. Each subject participated for two one-hour sessions.

Apparatus

The text was displayed one line at a time on a computer-controlled cathode-ray tube (CRT) that refreshed the line of text 300 times per second, allowing the entire line to be changed within just over 3 ms. The subject held a button that, after being pushed, called up the next line of text within less than 100 ms. The CRT was 48 cm from the reader's eyes. At that distance, three letters subtended 1 ° of visual angle.

Eye movements were recorded using a modified Biometrics Model SC limbus reflection eye movement monitor (Young & Sheena, 1975) that was interfaced to a computer and was sampled 1000 times per sec. The computer program allows changes to be made in the displayed line of text in response to specified characteristics of the reader's eye behavior (McConkie, Zola, Wolverton, & Burns, 1978).

Materials

Sixteen passages were selected from daily newspaper articles. Each was edited and formated to be 20 lines long with up to 72 characters per line. Five questions were prepared for each passage to use as a retention test. These included a variety of question types, including multiple-choice, true-false, sentence completion, and short answer questions.

Experimental manipulations

The study involved one control and three experimental conditions. Certain eye fixations were selected for potential experimental manipulation. In the control condition, no change was made in the text during such a fixation. In an experimental condition, as soon as the saccade neared completion and the location of the following fixation could be determined, a display change occurred. In the first experimental condition, the *Left-0 condition*, all letters that lay to the left of the directly fixated letter were replaced by other letters. The replacement letters were maximally distinguishable from the original letters within the constraint of maintaining the same general word shape. This was accomplished by dividing all lower-case letters into three sets: ascenders, descenders and those that neither ascend above the others nor descend below the line. The replacement letter in each case was that letter within the same set as the original that was most visually dissimilar from the original, as established by norms collected earlier (Zola, 1982).

In the second experimental condition, the *Right-3 condition*, all letters that lay more than three letter positions to the right of the directly fixated letter were replaced in the same manner. In the third experimental condition, the *Right-5 condition*, all letters more than five letter positions to the right were replaced. An example of the appearance of a line of text during a selected eye fixation in each of the four conditions is presented in Figure 1. During the following saccade, in each case, the original line of text was returned to the screen, so the text was normal during the following fixation. Thus, the erroneous letters were present in the text for a single eye fixation.

Condition	Appearance of the Line of Text
Control	The issuance of the stamp was the result of the
Left – 0	Xfn brromevn ui hfe stamp was the result of the
Right – 3	The issuance of the stmaj xmr hfn snrokh ui hfn
Right – 5	The issuance of the stamj xmr hfn snrokh ui hfn

Fig. 1: Examples of the appearance of part of a line of text during a critical fixation in the four conditions of the experiment. The carat indicates the letter toward which the eyes were directed.

The algorithm which made the changes in the display occasionally failed in two different ways. Sometimes a saccade was so short that the algorithm failed to detect it, and hence failed to remove the errors following the fixation on which they appeared. This only happened with saccades of less than one letter position in length. Second, blinks and other eye-lid movements were sometimes initially interpreted as saccades, causing display changes to be triggered in the absence of saccades. Both types of instances were later identified and the data removed. Thus, the only cases used in the final data analyses were those that were consistent with the above description.

Design

Each subject read all 16 passages. No display changes occurred on the first two or last two lines of the passage. On all other lines, four critical fixations were identified: the fixation following the 2nd, 4th, 6th, and 8th forward saccades. On each line, the four experimental conditions were assigned to these four fixations in a counterbalanced order. Thus, each line on which at least 8 forward saccades were made had three fixations with erroneous letters present and one control condition fixation, with at least one normal fixation separating each of these. In each passage, then, each subject could encounter each condition up to 16 times, for a total of 256 possible instances in each condition over the experiment. Four versions of each passage were prepared, so that on a given line of text the order in which the conditions occurred was counterbalanced across subjects.

Procedure

Subjects read the passages silently as their eyes were being monitored. A bite bar and forehead rest were used to stabilize the head. In order to familiarize the subjects with the task, two warm-up passages were read at the beginning of each experimental session, similar to the experimental passages and with similiar experimental manipulations being made. A retention test was administered immediately following the reading of each passage in the study and the subjects received immediate feedback on their test performance. This procedure placed emphasis on reading the passages for their content. A calibration task was administered immediately before and after reading each passage (McConkie, 1981).

Data reduction

Data associated with a critical fixation were excluded from analysis if any of the following were true: a blink or other eye movement disturbance occurred on the critical fixation or within two saccades following; the saccade prior to the critical fixation was regressive; a small saccade followed the critical fixation during which the modified text was not replaced by the original; or the Index of Accuracy (McConkie, 1981) was greater than 1.5, indicating the possibility of greater than a 1.5 character position error in the identified fixation location. The resulting number of remaining instances in each condition, combined across subjects, ranged from 1072 to 1098.

The following terminology is used to discuss the eye movement data analyzed for this study. A fixation is indicated by *F* and a saccade by *S*. F0 is the critical fixation on which letters were replaced, or the equivalent fixation in the control condition, and F1 is the following fixation. S0 is the saccade preceding the critical fixation, S1 is the saccade following it, and S2 is the saccade following fixation F1. Thus, the eye movement sequence is designated S0-F0-S1-F1-S2. In most cases fixation F2, the next fixation, was the F0 fixation for another condition. Dependent variables studied were the durations of fixations F0 and F1, and the frequency and lengths of progressive and regressive movements on S1 and S2.

Results

Table 1 presents the average fixation durations, frequency of regressions and saccade lengths for F0 and S1, and for F1 and S2 following forward S1 saccades. Where sufficient data were available to obtain stable medians for the individual subject's fixation durations and saccade lengths, the effects of the experimental conditions were tested by ANOVA, with each subject contributing one median to each condition. Otherwise, data were pooled across subjects and a median of the entire distribution is reported without a statistical test. Frequency data (percent of regressions) were converted to proportions and tested. Table 1 indicates significant differences where statistical tests were deemed appropriate.

Tab. 1: Eye movement data averages.

Cond/ N	F0 Duration	Saccade S1 Percent Regress	Saccade S1 Length Forward	Saccade S1 Length Regress	F1** Duration	Saccade S2** Percent Regress	Saccade S2** Length Forward	Saccade S2** Length Regress
Left-0 (1091)	231*	33.6*	7.7	3.0	223*	41.6*	7.3	6.9
Right-3 (1098)	205	13.6*	7.1*	4.0	231*	25.5*	7.3	3.6
Right-5 (1072)	204	14.9	7.6	4.3	222*	21.6*	7.2	4.5
Control (1085)	210	16.8	7.7	3.7	210	17.6	7.6	4.0
Stat Test	$F(3,33)$ $=9.32$ $p<.001$	Individual z tests	$F(3,33)$ $=7.57$ $p<.001$		$F(3,33)$ $=5.20$ $p<.01$	Individual z tests		

* Significantly different from Control Condition value ($p<.05$).

** Only data following forward S1 saccades are included in these statistics.

All three experimental conditions produced data that were significantly different from the control condition, but the specific patterns of these differences varied from condition to condition. Thus, as expected, the regions of letter replacement were within the general perceptual span for these readers and the erroneous letters produced effects on at least some eye fixations. However, only the Left-0 condition caused an increase in the duration of F0 fixations, those on which the errors were present. All three conditions showed greater time spent on the next F1 fixation. Additional regressions were induced by the Left-0 condition on saccade S1, and by all conditions on saccade S2. The number of regressions was decreased by the Right-3 condition on saccade S1. S1 forward saccades were shortened by condition Right-3, and it appears that saccade S2 regressions were lengthened in condition Left-0, although there was insufficient data to test this properly. The basis of these differences is discussed below.

The frequency of effects problem

Interpretation of these effects is complicated by the frequency of effects problem (McConkie, Zola, & Wolverton, 1985). That is, if the average fixation duration in an experimental condition is 30 ms greater than that for the control condition, this could be because the experimental manipulation increases all fixations by 30 ms or because the manipulation affects 25% of the instances by adding 120 ms to their duration. Either interpretation (and many others) is consistent with the finding of a 30 ms difference, but the psychological significance of the result may differ greatly depending on which interpretation is correct.

Two methods were used with the present data to deal with the frequency of effects problem. First, where appropriate, the frequency and size of effects were estimated using the Frequency of Effects Analysis (McConkie, Zola, & Wolverton, 1985). This method was applied to changes in fixation duration and saccade length. Second, in frequency data the change in frequency was estimated by subtracting the frequency of the control condition from that of the experimental condition. This approach was used with the frequency of making regressive saccades.

Frequency of Effects Analysis. The Frequency of Effects Analysis involves comparing the frequency distribution of a variable (say, fixation duration) from an experimental condition with that from the control condition. It is assumed that, were it not for the experimental manipulation, the two distributions would be very similar. The difference in shape between the distributions, resulting in a statistically significant difference between their means, is assumed to be due to an experimentally-induced change of amount e in the values of a proportion P of the cases in the experiment condition. Thus, P is the proportion of cases affected by the manipulation, or frequency of effect, and e is the size of the effect when it occurs. The goal of the analysis is to estimate these two parameters.

These estimates are obtained by an iterative procedure for identifying the values of the parameters which, when applied to the distribution from the control condition, transform it to a distribution most similiar to that obtained in the experimental condition.

The Frequency of Effects Analysis is appropriate to apply in cases where a frequency distribution from the experimental condition differs significantly from that of the control condition, and the following two assumptions are reasonable:

(1) *Stability assumption.* The frequency and size of the effect are constant across the frequency distribution categories. (Of course, other models can be developed in which these parameters do change across categories).
(2) *Data selection assumption.* There are no influences operating that select data entering into the experimental condition frequency distribution in a way that is different from that in the control condition frequency distribution.

Table 2 presents the frequency and size of effect estimates for appropriate variables and conditions. In the Left-0 condition the F0 fixations, those during which the erroneous letters were present, showed an average increase of 21 ms. However, the Frequency of Effects Analysis estimated that this resulted from 21% of the cases being influenced by the experimental manipulation, with an increase of 151 ms in the duration of those affected fixations. Similarly, in the Right-3 condition, the F1 fixations showed an average increase of 21 ms. Here, the Frequency of Effects Analysis estimated that this resulted from 36% of the cases being affected, with an average effect in these cases being an increase of 54 ms. Finally, in the Right-3 condition, forward saccade length increased an average of .6 letter positions. The Frequency of Effects Analysis estimated that this effect occurred on 100% of the cases.

Tab. 2: Results of the frequency of effects analyses.

Condition	Data	Mean Diff	Parameter estimates	
Left-0	F0 Duration	+21 ms	.21	151 ms
Right-3	S1 Forward length	-0.6 cp*	1.00	-0.7 cp
Right-3	F1 Duration	+21 ms	.36	54 ms

*cp=No. of character positions

In each of the cases to which the Frequency of Effects Analysis was applied, a wide range of values for P and e were tested, and a single minimum was observed in the sum of squares surface, without other local minima. Figure 2 presents plots of the sum of squared differences between the predicted and obtained distributions for a range of values on one parameter while holding the other parameter constant at its optimal value. These curves show that in each case there is a clear minimum, though the width of the region varies.

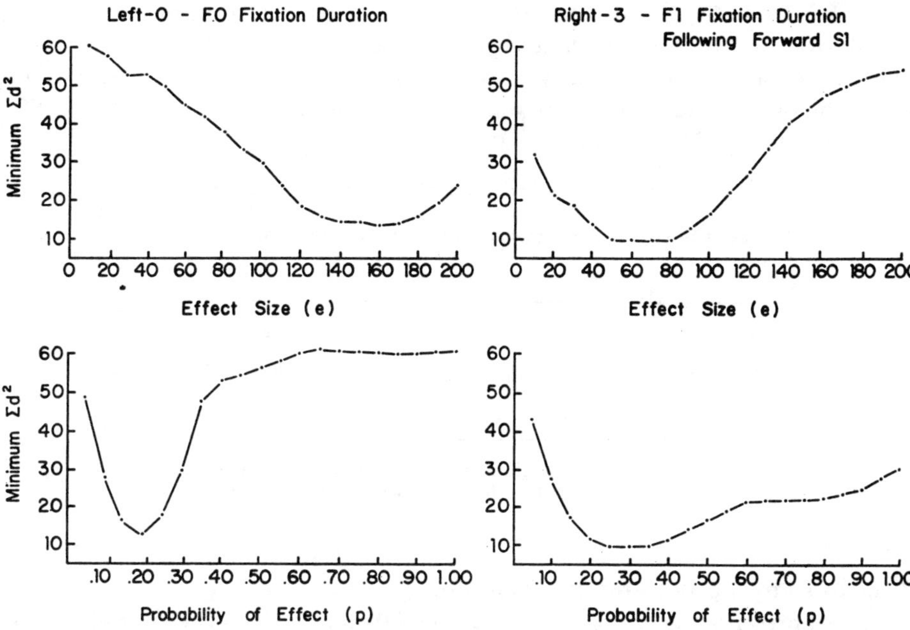

Fig. 2: Goodness of fit plots for parameter combinations from the Frequency of Effects Analysis. Each plot shows, for different values of one parameter, the minimum sum of squared deviations between the experimental condition and modified control condition frequency distributions that could be obtained by varying the other parameter. The plots demonstrate that reasonable estimates of the parameters of the model are possible.

An alternative model was also used to assess the frequency of effects, one assuming that the effect sizes produced were normally distributed and including a third parameter for the standard deviation of this distribution. Adding this third parameter made very little difference in the estimates obtained for P and e, and hence the results are not reported here.

Frequency of Regressive Influence. For each of the experimental conditions, the difference was obtained between the proportion of regressive saccades in the experimental and control conditions. This proportion was then divided by the proportion of forward saccades in the control condition to yield a new proportion that was entitled the Frequency of Regressive Influence score. A positive score indicates more regressions in the experimental condition, and a negative score indicates fewer regressions. The score estimates the proportion of forward saccades from the control condition that were turned into regressive saccades in the experimental condition if the score is positive and gives a proportion increase in the frequency of forward saccades when the score is negative. Table 3 presents the Frequency of Regressive Influence scores for saccades S1 and S2 for the three experimental conditions. The frequency of regressions was increased greatly in condition Left-0 on both saccades S1 and S2. In the other conditions, there was an increase in regressive saccades on S2, but a decrease on S1.

Tab. 3: Estimates of the frequency of regressive influence.

Condition	Frequency of Induced Regressions on:	
	Saccade S1	Saccade S2
Left-0	.20*	.29*
Right-3	-.03	.09*
Right-5	-.02	.05*

* Number of regressions was significantly different from the number in the control condition, $p<.05$.

Relation among dependent variables

Table 4 presents the durations of fixations F0 and F1 when they were followed by forward saccades versus regressive saccades. These data make it clear that the increase in F0 fixation durations observed in the Left-0 condition is strictly the result of increased time on fixations preceding a regressive movement. Fixations preceding a forward movement showed no effect of the errors at all. Note the agreement between the Frequency of Regressive Influence score, suggesting that regressions were induced in 20% of the cases, and the Frequency of Effects Analysis results, indicating that 21% of the cases showed an increased fixation duration.

Table 4 further indicates that the average fixation duration for F0 fixations preceding regressions is only 84 ms greater than that for the control condition, yet the Frequency of Effects Analysis suggested an increase of 151 ms for affected fixations. This apparent discrepancy is resolved by assuming that only the induced regressions showed an increased fixation duration and that the naturally-occurring regressions showed no effect. If 17% of the regressions were naturally occurring and showed an average fixation duration of 189 ms as in the control condition and 21% fixations were followed by induced regressions with an average duration of 189+151=340 ms as suggested by the Frequency of Effects Analysis, the average fixation duration for the entire set of fixations preceding regressions in the Left-0 condition would be expected to be 272 ms, very close to the 273 ms average reported in Table 4.

F1 fixation durations preceding S2 regressions show no increase in any condition, but all conditions show increased fixation durations preceding S2 forward

Tab. 4: Average fixation durations of data partitioned by the direction of the following saccade.

Fixation	Condition	Direction of Prior Saccade	
		Forward	Regressive
F0	Control	204	189
	Left-0	208	273
	Right-3	203	176
	Right-5	200	175
F1	Control	203	194
	Left-0	235	192
	Right-3	234	192
	Right-5	225	205

saccades. Thus, the cases of increased fixation duration identified by the Frequency of Effects Analysis are strictly among fixations preceded by a forward saccade. Taking the Left-0 condition data, we again find that the average fixation duration preceding F2 forward saccades is increased by only 32 ms in comparison with the control condition, substantially less that the 112 ms effect estimated by the Frequency of Effects Analysis. As with F0 fixations, this discrepancy is reconciled by assuming that the effects were only observed on part of the fixations preceding forward saccades, not on all of them.

Patterns of eye movement response to encountering errors

From the complex set of results revealed in the above analyses, it is possible to identify specific patterns of eye movements during reading in each condition, and to estimate the frequency with which each pattern occurred. Patterns for the Left-0 and Right-3 conditions are presented in Figures 3 and 4. The Right-5 condition is very similiar to that of the Right-3 condition, but with fewer significant effects, and therefore, not included here. Taking Figure 3 as an example, the four components of the eye movement sequence are presented along the top of the figure: F0 duration, S1 direction and length, F1 duration and S2 direction and length. Underneath each of these components is a list of the differences observed between the data in this condition and that of the control condition. For the Left-0 condition, for example, there was a 21 ms increase in F0 fixation duration, 100% increase in the number of regressive S1 saccades, a shortening of these saccades by 0.7 character positions, a 13 ms increase in the duration of F1 fixations, a 135% increase in S2 regressions, and a 2.9 character position increase in the length of S2 regressive saccades.

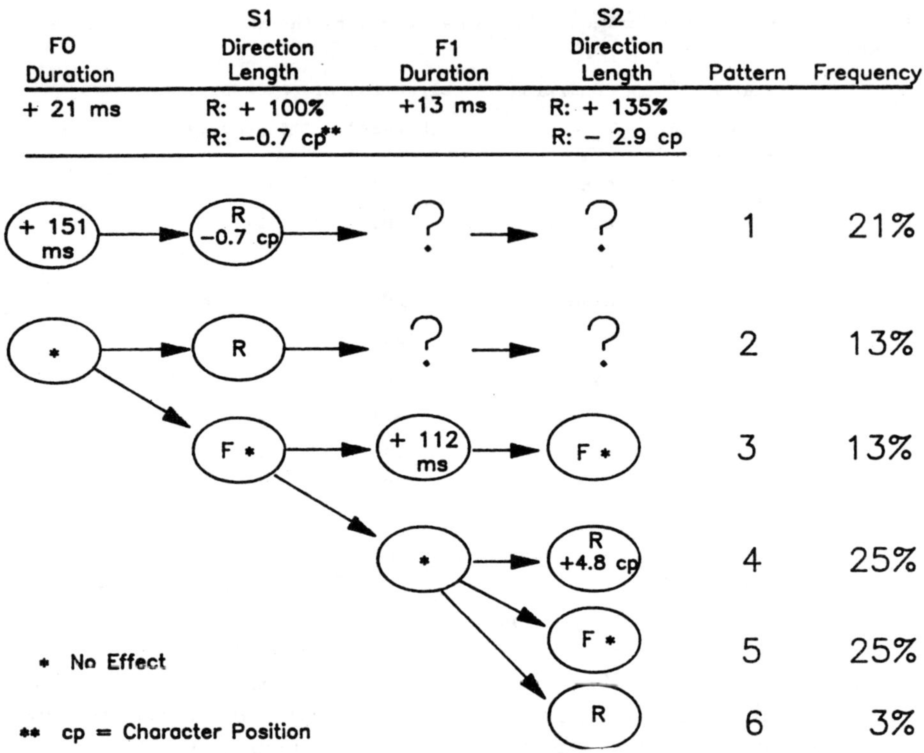

Fig. 3: Eye movement patterns in the Left-0 condition.

Figure 3 next presents a series of observed eye movement patterns in the form of branching trees. Each pattern is identified by a number on the right side of the figure in order to facilitate reference to the figure. Also, the frequency of each pattern is indicated, as calculated from the data reported above.

In describing the patterns, under F0 and F1 duration wherever the data are significantly different from those of the control condition the difference is listed; where there is no difference from the control, an asterisk is entered into the figure. Under S1 and S2 saccades, the letter *F* or *R* is entered to indicate whether the saccades in that pattern were forward or regressive. In addition, if the average length of the saccades differed from similar saccades in the control condition, a positive or negative number is listed to indicate the size and direction of this difference, measured in character position units. If no significant difference exists, an asterisk is entered to note this fact. Finally, there

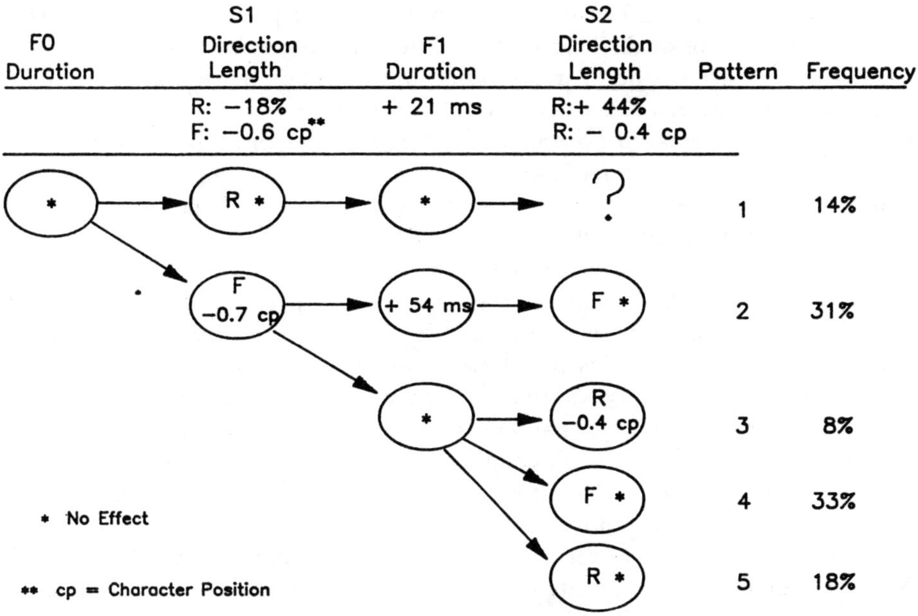

Fig. 4: Eye movement patterns in the Right-3 condition.

are patterns in which it was impossible to determine whether the experimental condition differed from the control. In these cases, a question mark is entered into the table.

Left-0 condition. Six eye movement patterns are detectable in the Left-0 condition, three of which show effects of the experimental manipulation. Pattern 1, occurring 21% of the time, is the only pattern showing an effect on fixation F0. In these cases the F0 fixation was increased by 151 ms and was followed by a shorter than normal regressive saccade. The regression took the eyes back into the region where letters had been replaced on fixation F0, but, of course, the errors were not then present on the next fixation, F1. Pattern 2, occurring 13% of the time, was also characterized by a regressive S1 saccade but in these cases both F0 and S1 showed no effects of the experimental manipulation. Further analysis of F1 and S2 could not be carried out since it was impossible to identify whether an individual case with a regressive S1 saccade was part of Pattern 1 or Pattern 2.

All other patterns showed F0 fixations of normal duration followed by forward saccades of normal length. Cases in Pattern 3 are characterized by long F1 fixation durations, increased by 112 ms, and then a normal S2 forward saccade. Cases in Pattern 4, on the other hand, showed F1 fixation durations of normal length, followed by particularly long regressions on saccade S2. S2 regressions in condition Left-0 averaged 6.9 character positions. However, this is an underestimate of the length of the Pattern 4 regressions, since they constituted only part of the S2 regressions in the data. If we assume that S2 regressions in Patterns 1, 2 and 5 were of normal length, then Pattern 4 regressions must have averaged over 8.8 character positions in length, 4.8 character positions longer than normal, taking the eyes back into the region where letters had been replaced, even though those errors were no longer physically present during the preceding fixation, F1.

If Pattern 4 S2 regressive saccades were indeed taking the eyes back to the region where errors had occurred, then we would expect a correlation to exist between the lengths of S1 forward saccades and S2 regressive saccades in the Left-0 condition. While this correlation was only .11, an examination of the scatter plot showed a very unusual pattern with two distinct legs. For S2 regressive saccades less than 4 character positions in length, S1 forward saccades ranged from 1 to 16 letter positions in a leg showing a slope of zero. However, for S2 regressions over 4 character positions there was a second leg, showing a strong linear relationship to S1 saccade length. The correlation between the lengths of S2 regressions over 4 character positions and S1 saccades was .49. No other condition in the study showed a similar scatter plot, and similar correlations for other conditions ranged from .06 to .11, whether calculated on the full data or on a restricted range of S2 regression length. Apparently, only within the Pattern 4 cases was there a relationship between the lengths of these saccades, as the eyes were being taken back into the region where errors had existed on a prior fixation.

In the remaining patterns, 5 and 6, no evidence of any effects from the presence of errors was observed. This constitutes 28% of the cases in the present data. There could be additional cases in Pattern 2 in which the errors produced no effect, but this could not be further established.

One further analysis was carried out on Left-0 condition data to determine whether effects were present on still later fixations. This was complicated by the fact that if F0 was followed by two forward saccades, in most cases the next fixation, F2, would be the F0 fixation for another condition. However, data were selected in which either S1 or S2 were regressive, thus postponing the implementation of the next experimental manipulation. In these cases, the average F2 fixation duration was 206 ms, as compared to 205 ms for similarly-selected fixations in the control condition, thus providing no evidence for a lingering influence.

In summary, six eye movement patterns were identified, three of which showed specific effects of the presence of erroneous letters on fixation F0. Two patterns, totaling 28% of all cases, showed no identifiable effects, and three patterns totally 59% of the cases did show effects. One pattern was indeterminate in this regard. Only 21% of the cases show an effect on the fixation on which the errors were present, or on the immediately following saccade. Most effects occurred only later. The effects observed tended to be specific to certain fixations or saccades. For example, no pattern showed both an increased duration on F1 and an increased likelihood of regressing on S2.

Right-3 condition. Figure 4 presents the eye movement patterns identified in data from the Right-3 condition. None of the five identified patterns shows an effect on fixation F0. In Pattern 1 where S1 is regressive, the data do not differ from similarly-selected data in the control condition, though the sample size is too small to give an adequate comparison for saccade S2 data. Also, the number of occurrences of this pattern is smaller than in the control condition, since errors in the right visual field reduced the frequency of S1 regressions. All other patterns are characterized by a forward saccade on S1, and all show a shortening of that saccade. In Pattern 2, the F1 fixations were increased by 54 ms, followed by a forward saccade of normal length.

In Pattern 3, the F1 fixations were normal but shorter-than-normal regressions were then induced on saccade S2. While all S2 regressions average 0.4 character positions shorter than corresponding regressions in the control condition, Pattern 3 regressions constitute only part of these and hence must be shorter still. These shortened regressions took the eyes to a text region where erroneous letters had been present on fixation F0, though they were no longer present during the F1 fixation preceding the regression. The average S1 saccade length of 7.7 would have taken the eyes to the fifth letter position within the region of replaced letters. Thus, a regression of less than 3.6 character positions on saccade S2 would keep the eyes within this region.

Patterns 4 and 5 constituting 33% and 18% of the data respectively show no further influence of the errors beyond the initial shortening of saccade S1. Thus, there is no evidence of additional processing time being required by the presence of the errors, except to the extent that a shortened saccade might result in the occurrence of an additional fixation.

An additional analysis was conducted to determine whether, in the Right-3 and Right-5 conditions, the F0 fixation duration might show effects if erroneous letters had appeared within the word being fixated. Cases were selected in which, had they been in the Right-3 condition, the first word containing errors would have ended within 5 character positions to the right of the directly fixated letter. These cases in the Right-3 condition contained errors in the word directly fixated, or, in the case of very short words, in the word that began immediately to the right of the letter position fixated. In the Right-5 condition, these cases never contained errors in the directly fixated word, but only in the following word. The median fixation durations for these cases were as follows: Control condition, 204 ms (N=217); Right-3 condition, 205 ms (N=215); and Right-5 condition, 209 ms (N=175). Thus there was no evidence for effects on fixation F0 when errors were in the directly-fixated word.

In summary, five separate patterns were identified in the Right-3 condition data. None of the patterns showed any effect on the duration of fixation F0. The presence of errors reduced the frequency of S1 regressions by 18% but the remaining cases containing such regressions showed no effect of the errors. In all other cases the S1 forward saccade was shortened. Beyond this, no further effects were observed in two patterns, totaling 51% of the cases. In the patterns showing effects, these appeared either as an increased F1 fixation duration followed by a normal forward saccade, or as a short regression on S2 following a fixation of normal length. No pattern showed increased F1 fixation durations followed by short induced S2 regressions. Data from the Right-5 condition showed similar patterns but with fewer significant effects.

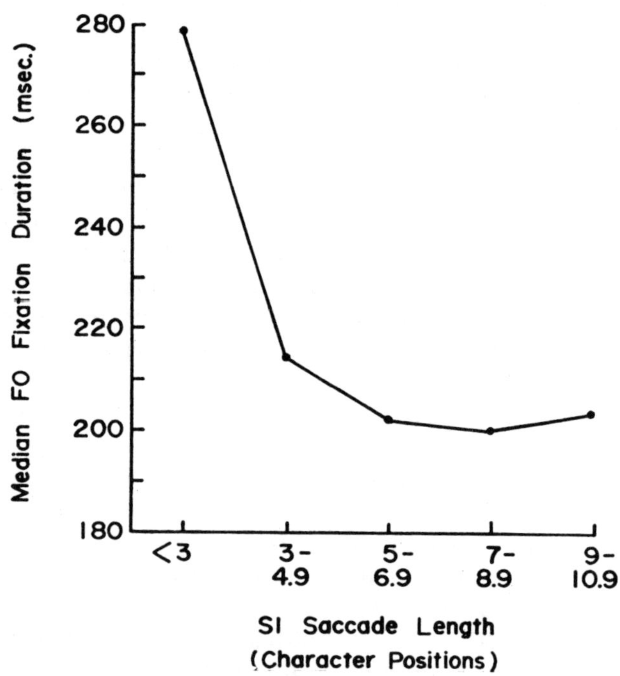

Fig. 5: Duration of fixation F0 as a function of the length of the following saccade S1. Data are taken from the control condition.

Relation of fixation durations and saccade lengths

A final analysis examined the relationship between the durations of fixations and the lengths of forward saccades that immediately follow them. In the control condition these correlations were low, ranging from -.27 to .24 for individual subjects, and averaging .04 across subjects, agreeing with results from

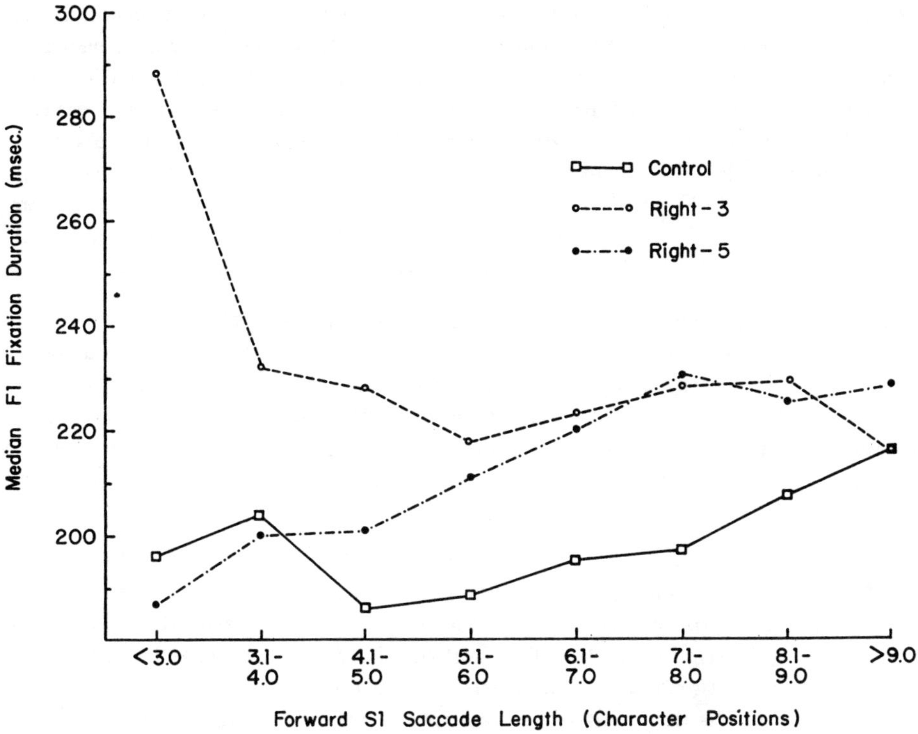

Fig. 6: Duration of fixation F1 as a function of the lengths of the preceding saccade S1 in the Control, Right-3 and Right-5 conditions.

previous studies (Lévy-Schoen & O'Regan, 1979; Rayner & McConkie, 1976). However, further examination indicates that very short forward saccades, those less than three character positions in length, tend to be preceded by particularly long fixations, as shown in Figure 5. This suggests that short saccades are produced on some basis that is qualitatively different than for average and longer saccades (McConkie, 1983).

No such relationship exists between the S1 forward saccade length and the following F1 fixation duration, as shown by the relatively flat control condition curve in Figure 6. However, the Right-3 and Right-5 conditions do show relationships. In the Right-3 condition, saccades less than three character positions in length (those going short of the location of the replaced letters) are followed by exceptionally long fixations. Saccades of other lengths, except for the longest, are followed by fixations that are somewhat longer than those of the control condition. The Right-5 condition, on the other hand, shows an interesting cross-over pattern. For saccades up to 5 character positions in length (those going short of the region of replaced letters) the following fixation durations are very similar to those of the control condition. However, for longer saccades that are taking the eyes into the replacement region, the fixation duration data are similar to those of the Right-3 condition. Thus, there is a rather striking difference between having erroneous letters beginning 3 vs. 5 letter positions to the right of the fixated letter.

Discussion

Encountering errors in the text at different locations in the visual field leads to characteristically different eye movement patterns, but there is also considerable variability in response to errors at the same location. The response to these errors is not just an undifferentiated disruption of the ongoing eye movement activity, but rather is local and specific. This specificity of response enables us to suggest a number of conclusions about the control of eye movements during reading.

(1) The effect of encountering an error during a fixation is sometimes immediate and sometimes delayed, even under similar stimulus conditions. One pattern in the Left-0 condition showed an increased fixation duration on the fixation on which the error was encountered. In another pattern, the first evidence of disruption was on saccade S2, two saccades after encountering the problem.

(2) Encountering a problem in processing during a fixation does not necessarily increase the duration of that eye fixation. In the data presented, only one pattern out of seven in which effects of the errors were observed showed an increase in the duration of that fixation. No pattern containing an increased F0 fixation duration was found in either the Right-3 or Right-5 condition, yet other measures indicated that the errors were being perceived.

(3) There were enough cases in which no effects of the errors were observed to raise the possibility that certain regions within the general perceptual span area are not attended on some fixations. This is harmonious with the above suggestion that somewhat different visual regions may be attended on different eye fixations during reading.

(4) The eyes tend to be drawn to a region of difficulty. In this study, the occurrence of errors sometimes lengthened saccades and sometimes shortened them, and sometimes increased the frequency of regressions and sometimes reduced that frequency. However, in each case, the change produced was that which drew more fixations to the textual region within which letters were replaced.

(5) The target of a saccade can be established on the basis of information obtained prior to the fixation immediately preceding the saccade. Error-induced regressions on saccade S2 tended to take the eyes back to a region containing errors two fixations earlier, even though they were no longer present when the saccade was launched. On other occasions, saccades were directed to the region containing errors encountered on the immediately preceding fixation.

(6) Redirecting the immediately following saccade against the direction of normal progressive movement during reading is a very time-consuming process. When regressions were induced on saccade S1, the F0 fixations were increased by 151 ms. However, no similar penalty occurred on F0 in the Right-3 condition when regressions were cancelled and replaced by forward movements (Pattern 2). Thus, the increased time in the first case came, not just from redirecting eye movements, but from changing the movements of the eyes to send them against the normal direction of movement.

(7) Redirecting the eyes to go against the direction of normal movement on a later saccade exacts no penalty on the preceding fixation duration. In all three experimental conditions, the pattern containing induced regressions on saccade S2 shows no increase in the duration of either fixation F0 or F1. This may mean that the time required to set up a regressive saccade in this case is taken in parallel with other processing activities. Since the average duration of fixations preceding regressions during reading differs very little from those preceding forward saccades, it follows that most regressions are not induced by processing of the text seen during the immediately preceding fixation. This "lagged regression hypothesis" requires specific investigation.

(8) Word-level processing difficulties can be dealt with either by lengthening a fixation or by regressing back to the locus of the problem. We do not know the conditions that determine which option is chosen, since both were exhibited in all experimental conditions of this study. But in the present data, only one pattern showed both an increased fixation duration and a regression in the initial responses to the problem encountered. In all other cases in which an effect was present, it was either one or the other. Furthermore, in the pattern in which both responses were observed (Left-0 condition, pattern 1), the increased fixation duration may have resulted from the time required to change the direction of the following saccade rather than from additional processing time needed on that eye fixation.

(9) Short saccades made during reading, those under about 3 character positions in length, appear to reflect a different processing state than longer saccades do. In the control condition data, short saccades are preceded

by particularly long fixations, and thus may reflect processing difficulties of some type. Further evidence for this is found in the Right-3 condition where short forward F1 saccades are followed by particularly long fixations, even though this is not so in other conditions.

(10) Saccade length and direction appear to be related to the text region attended during the prior eye fixation. In the Right-5 condition, the F1 fixation duration is affected by errors only in cases where the S1 saccade takes the eyes into the region that contained erroneous letters on the previous fixation.

The results of this study indicate that errors of interpretation can be made by ignoring the frequency of effects problem in interpreting differences in averages between experimental and control conditions. Finding a significant difference indicates that some difference probably exists and justifies further exploration of the data to understand the basis for the difference. Assuming that the obtained difference is the actual size of the effect produced by the experimental manipulation can lead to erroneous conclusions.

There is one final implication of the above findings. The monitoring of eye movements is often done, not for the purpose of studying eye movements themselves, but to determine whether some experimental manipulation produces a change in the processing taking place. The main concern is to determine whether the eye behavior is affected in any way by the experimental conditions, without regard to the precise nature of the changes produced. In such a situation, the most sensitive indicator may be a global dependent variable such as reading rate, gaze duration. or time to reach a particular point in the text. Such global variables will reflect the occurrence of all of the various deviations observed in the current study. The cost of this approach, of course, is the loss of precision in understanding the nature of the eye movement response and any relations that this response might have to the processing changes that were caused by the experimental manipulation.

Acknowlegment

The research reported in this paper was supported by NIMH grant MH32884 to the first author and by NIE contract NIE-C-400-76-0116 to the Center for the Study of Reading. The authors express appreciation to Margaret Olson for assistance in collecting and analyzing the data.

N.R. Underwood's present address is Claremont Teachers' College, Claremont, Western Australia, 6010.

References

Lévy-Schoen, A., & O'Regan, K., *The control of eye movements in reading*, in "P.A. Kolers, M.E. Wrolstad, & H. Bouma (Eds.), Processing of visible language," Plenum Press, New York, 1979, pp. 7-36.

McConkie, G.W., *Evaluating and reporting data quality in eye movement research*, Behavior Research Methods and Instrumentation **13** (1981), 97-106.

McConkie, G.W., *Eye movements and perception during reading*, in "K. Rayner (Ed.), Eye movements in reading: Perceptual and language processes," Academic Press, New York, 1983, pp. 65-96.

McConkie, G.W., Zola, D., Blanchard, H.E., & Wolverton, G., *Perceiving words during reading: Lack of facilitation from prior peripheral exposure*, Perception & Psychophysics **32** (1982), 271-281.

McConkie, G.W., Zola, D., Wolverton, G.S., & Burns, D.D., *Eye movement contingent display control in studying reading*, Behavior Research Methods and Instrumentation **10** (1978), 154-166.

McConkie, G.W., Zola, D., & Wolverton, G.S., *Estimating frequency and size of effects due to experimental manipulations in eye movement research*, in "R. Groner, G.W. McConkie, & C. Menz (Eds.), Eye movements and human information processing," North Holland Press, Amsterdam, 1985, pp. 137-147.

Rayner, K., & McConkie, G.W., *What guides a reader's eye movements?*, Vision Research **16** (1976), 829-837.

Rayner, K., & Pollatsek, A., *Eye movements in reading: A tutorial review*, in "M. Coltheart (Ed.), Attention and Performance XII: The psychology of reading," Erlbaum, Hillsdale, NJ, 1987, pp. 327-362.

Rayner, K., Well, A.D.,& Pollatsek, A., *Asymmetry of the effective visual field in reading*, Perception and Psychophysics **27** (1980), 537-544.

Reder, S.M., *On-line monitoring of eye position signals in contingent and noncontingent paradigms*, Behavior Research Methods & Instrumentation **5** (1973), 218-228.

Young, L.R., & Sheena, D., *Survey of eye movement recording techniques*, Behavior Research Methods & Instrumentation **7** (1975), 397-429.

Zola, D., "The perception of words in reading: An exploratory treatise," Unpublished doctoral dissertation, Cornell University, 1982.

CALLOSAL TRANSMISSION IN READING

MARC BRYSBAERT AND GÉRY D'YDEWALLE

Laboratory of Experimental Psychology, University of Leuven

Callosal Transmission in Reading

Eye movements during reading are characterized by a succession of saccades and fixations. Saccades bring new information into the center of the visual field; fixations serve to take up the information. Erdmann and Dodge (1898) already noted that fixation falls almost exclusively on words rather than on the gaps between them "and probably almost always roughly on the middle of the word." The latter finding has recently received considerable attention (Dunn-Rankin, 1978; O'Regan, Lévy-Schoen, Pynte, & Brugaillère, 1984; Rayner, 1978). It is now well established that there is a "convenient viewing position" in the center of a word or slightly left of center (O'Regan & Lévy-Schoen, 1987). The reasons for this are thought to be threefold: sensory constraints (acuity and lateral masking), oculomotor constraints, and processing constraints (lexical and linguistic). A comprehensive review of this subject is given by O'Regan and Lévy-Schoen (1987).

However, the tendency to fixate words centrally poses a problem that has hitherto received little or no attention. The visual system is organized in such a way that everything left of fixation is sent to the right cerebral hemisphere, and everything right of fixation to the left cerebral hemisphere (Bradshaw & Nettleton, 1983). This implies that central fixation of a word splits the word in two halves, the first of which is projected into the right cerebral hemisphere, the second into the left cerebral hemisphere (see Figure 1). As the left cerebral hemisphere has a greater capacity for verbal information processing (Bradshaw & Nettleton, 1983), the first, usually most informative part is also sent to the "wrong" cerebral hemisphere. Does this influence word processing?

First, we will consider whether the division between the two visual hemifields is as sharp as has been suggested. Second, we will examine the potential contribution of callosal connections between the two hemispheres. Third, we will discuss relevant findings in the literature on eye movements. Finally, in sections four and five, we will present some new experiments.

The Nasotemporal Division of the Retina

In mammals, cells of the temporal retina project ipsilaterally and those of the nasal retina contralaterally into the optic tract. This leads to the familiar picture in classic neurology textbooks that shows the nasal (or right) hemiretina

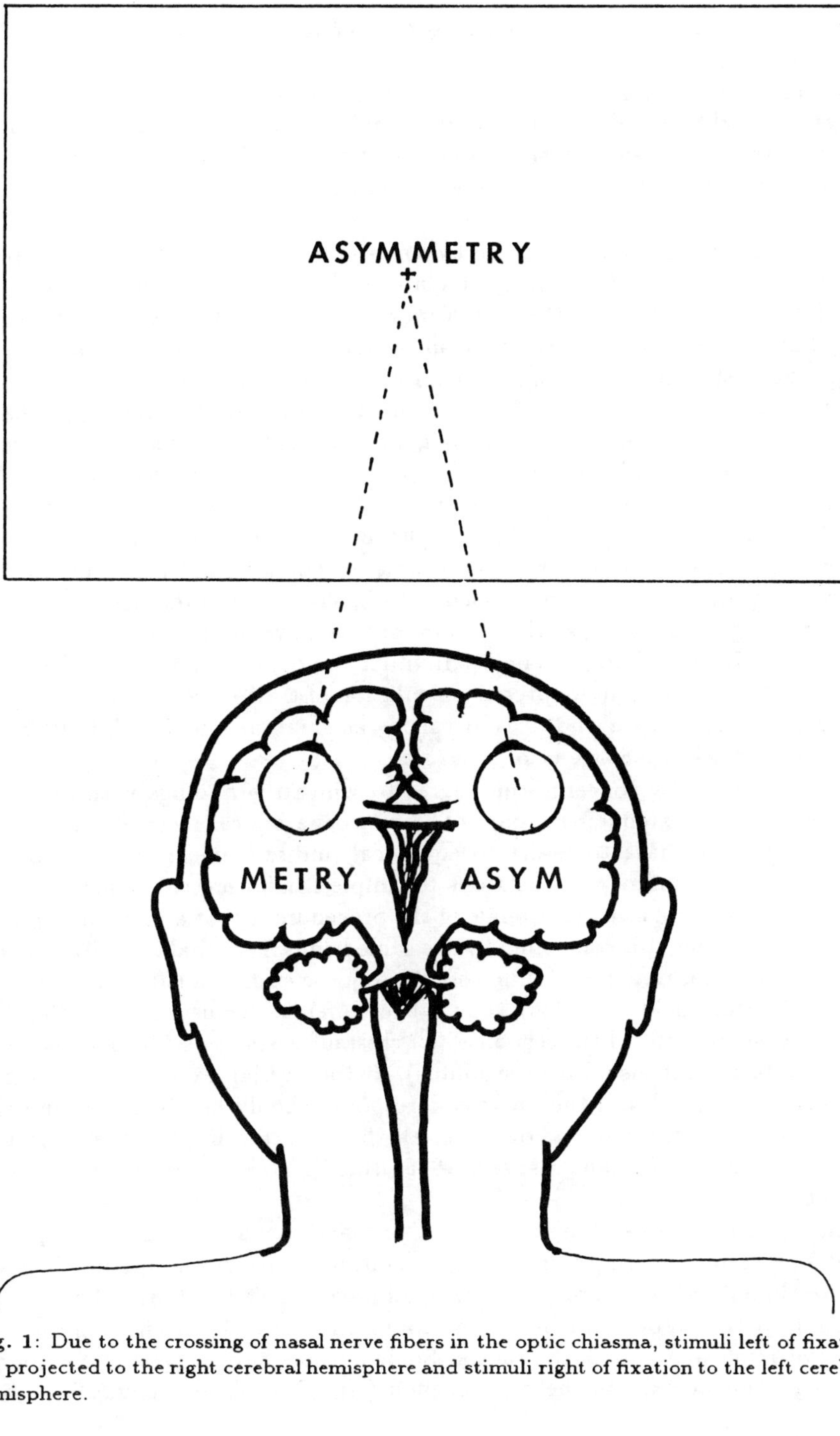

Fig. 1: Due to the crossing of nasal nerve fibers in the optic chiasma, stimuli left of fixation are projected to the right cerebral hemisphere and stimuli right of fixation to the left cerebral hemisphere.

of the left eye corresponding with the temporal (or right) hemiretina of the right eye on the right side of the brain and a similar arrangement on the left. The vertical meridian passing through the fovea defines the border between the two cell populations and is usually represented diagrammatically as a sharp vertical line.

By sectioning one optic tract or by unilateral injection of horseradish peroxidase into the dorsal lateral geniculate nucleus, it is possible to obtain a description of the areas of the retina in which the ganglion cells are affected and that therefore, project to the ipsilateral or the contralateral sides of the brain. Such studies in the cat (Stone, 1966; Terao, Inatomi, & Maeda, 1982) and monkey (Stone, Leicester, & Sherman, 1973; Bunt & Minckler, 1977) have shown that the dividing line separating ganglion cells having crossed axons from those having uncrossed axons is not sharp. Instead, the "line" is represented by a band of about 1 ° within which crossed and uncrossed cells are intermingled. The band, thus, projects bilaterally to the left and right hemisphere.

Two difficulties, however, prevent simple extrapolation of these findings to the reading problem we are concerned with in this paper. First, the fovea does not contain ganglion cells, so the amount of foveal overlap can only be inferred. Bunt and Minckler (1977) believed it might amount to about 3 ° (i.e. the complete fovea), but a more precise calculation of their data indicates that the width probably is at most 1.5° and can be as small as 0.5° (Wyatt, 1978), a position also held by Stone et al. (1973).

Another difficulty concerns the degree to which the findings with cats and monkeys can be extended to man. The neuroanatomical methods cannot be used, so that we have to resort to equivocal, indirect evidence. One line of research involves unimanual reactions to simple stimuli presented slightly next to the fixation points. The rationale of the procedure is that a manual response will be faster when it is controlled by the same hemisphere that initially receives the stimulus information (an "uncrossed" response such as a left-hand response to a left visual field stimulus) than when different hemispheres receive the information and control the response (a "crossed" response such as a left-hand response to a right visual field stimulus). If the overlap exists, the difference between the crossed and the uncrossed response should be absent around the visual midline, but, to our knowledge, all the studies using this method have failed to find the overlap (Harvey, 1978; Haun, 1978; Lines, 1984; Lines & Milner, 1983).

Another line of research involves foveal or macular sparing and gives opposite results. Patients suffering from hemianopia usually preserve a functional region on the "blind" side (for a brief review, see Perenin & Vadot, 1981). This region amounts to 1 ° above and below the fovea and varies between 1 and 4 ° in the foveal/macular part of the retina. Some authors have suggested a bilateral representation to explain the phenomenon (e.g. Bunt & Minckler, 1977), but this is far from being generally accepted (see e.g. Harrington, 1981; Perenin & Vadot, 1981). There may also be a dual blood supply to the region of the occipital pole of the cortex that helps defend striate cortex cells representing the central retina against ischemia, or there may be an enlarged representation of the central visual field at postretinal levels of the retina-geniculate-striate cortex pathway that increases the probability of central field survival for a random lesion.

One last complicating factor is that a growing body of evidence suggests that symptoms of hemispatial neglect not only are based on anatomical grounds but also are largely influenced by attentional factors (Jeannerod, 1987). Kinsbourne and Warrington (1962), for instance, showed that the tendency of right-lesion patients to infer a word from its terminal letters occurred not only when the beginning of the word was situated in the affected right hemifield but also when all the letters were presented well within the intact left field.

Considering all the evidence, it becomes clear that the bilateral representation of the fovea in man is, at best, a working hypothesis that still needs to be proved (we will return to it further on). Even if the overlap exists, it does not completely solve the problem of callosal transmission. The overlap extends only 0.5° to the left of fixation, which means that only one or two letters left of fixation can be processed by the left hemisphere, while the convenient viewing position usually is found between the third and fifth letter.

Interhemispheric Connections

If bilateral projection of the fovea cannot remedy the splitting of words into a left and a right part during reading, it might be that the interhemispheric connections are tight enough to solve the problem without additional costs. For instance, the callosal fibers could be thought of as merely a special case of the normal intrahemispheric corticocortical connections. It has long been known that there are more callosal connections between the areas around the vertical midline than in the areas normally tested in laterality research (Berlucchi, 1972). This hypothesis, however, would be in conflict with much of the work on cerebral asymmetry (for reviews, see Bradshaw & Nettleton, 1983; Hellige, 1983). The right visual field superiority for words is quite well established and all studies involving callosal transmission time have found some delay.

One problem with the extrapolation of laterality findings to reading is the difficulty of disentangling interhemispheric transmission from other mediating factors. For instance, it is impossible to use the difference in recognition time between words in the left and the right visual hemifield as an estimate of callosal transmission time because presenting words left or right of fixation not only sends them to different hemispheres but also places the most informative first part nearer or farther away from fixation. Similarly, it has been shown that estimates of transmission time for many complex situations are too variable to be meaningful as the sole indicators of transmission time (Swanson, Ledlow, & Kinsbourne, 1978). Other variables, such as processing demands, attentional factors, and the like come into play. For one thing, it has repeatedly been shown that crossing the hands or turning the head to the left or the right suffices to alter the results considerably, giving rise to a distinction between hemiretina and hemispace (for a short review, see Heilman, Bowers, Valenstein, & Watson, 1987).

There is only one paradigm that yields a consistent estimate of interhemispheric transmission time: the measurement of simple unimanual reactions to lateralized light flashes as described in the preceding section. These studies consistently show transmission times between 2 and 6 ms (Bashore, 1981; John, Shields, Krahn, & Timney, 1987) that do not change markedly as stimulus eccentricity increases.

It is, however, open to question whether we can extend the findings with light flashes to reading situations. Haun (1978), for instance, already found a difference of 10 ms in vocal reaction times to unilaterally presented letters. Evidence is also growing that information transfer through the corpus callosum occurs at different processing stages (Marzi, 1986), possibly at different rates. Rugg, Lines, and Milner (1984) recorded visual evoked potentials to lateralized flashes. At central sites, the N160 latency component of the evoked potentials was 4 ms shorter contralaterally to the light flash, in conformity with the findings of simple reactions, but at the occipital sites the difference was much larger and amounted to about 14 ms.

Finally, a study relevant here concerns laterality and visual masking (Moscovitch, 1983). Patterned masks can interfere with target perception at central levels by interrupting the processor that integrates sensory information about the target into relational visual features. Thus, it is possible to measure the time it takes for target information to arrive and be processed at the stage beyond which the mask is presumed to operate. By choosing targets known to produce reliable hemispheric asymmetries in traditional laterality studies, it is reasonable to assume that a target presented in the dominant visual field will evade the mask sooner than a target presented in the inferior field by an interval equal to the amount of time it takes to cross the corpus callosum. Moscovitch (1983) used three-letter CVC words presented 0.7° from fixation and obtained a systematic right field advantage of 4 ms, thereby indicating that the interhemispheric transmission time found for simple reactions to light flashes might also be applicable to short words.

It may be concluded that the transfer of part of a word through the corpus callosum takes time. Estimates differ from 2 ms to more than 10 ms for rather simple stimuli. It is not known how long it takes to transfer more complex material; whether transmission occurs in parallel or serially. The possibility of signal degradation during callosal transmission has not been considered, although some authors (e.g. Kimura, 1973) have invoked it to explain hemispheric differences.

RELEVANT FINDINGS IN THE EYE MOVEMENT LITERATURE

Dispersing a word over both hemispheres during reading is likely to involve costs in efficiency. So it might be expected that the best strategy would be to have most of the word sent directly to the specialized hemisphere. As most people have left-hemisphere dominance for verbal processing, direct sending of a word to the dominant hemisphere is achieved by fixating the beginning of the word. This makes the entire word fall in the right visual field. Two findings in the eye movement literature are applicable in this regard. First, the "perceptual span" extends more to the right than to the left (Rayner & Pollatsek, 1987). Second, a closer examination of the convenient viewing position reveals not only an optimum position slightly left of center but also faster processing with fixations in the left half of a word than with fixations in the right half.

The perceptual span is the functional field of view during reading and extends from the beginning of the currently fixated word but not more than 3-4 letters to the left of fixation to about 15 letter positions to the right of fixation (Rayner & Pollatsek, 1987). At first sight, this might be taken as evidence for the influence of laterality on the gaze direction. But then, the same asymmetry should be found for readers of right-to-left orthography, such as Hebrew, which is not the case. An asymmetry to the right has been reported for this orthography (Pollatsek, Bolozky, Well, & Rayner, 1981). Thus, asymmetry of the perceptual span cannot be taken as evidence of hemispheric specialization. This does not imply that influences of hemispheric specialization on word processing have to be excluded completely because it is well documented that different types of information are extracted from different parts of the perceptual span (McConkie & Rayner, 1976; Rayner & Fisher, 1987). Lexical processing probably only occurs in a region of about four letters on each side of fixation. Thus, a shift of asymmetry in the perceptual span for Hebrew indicates only that the processes occurring in the "preview region" (Rayner & Fisher, 1987) are not confined to the left hemisphere. Also, the finding that the mean saccade length for Hebrew is shorter than for English (Pollatsek et al., 1981) is compatible with the suggestion that laterality makes the extraction of lexical information left of fixation more difficult.

The convenient viewing position in words refers to faster processing when the eyes fixate near the middle of the word and has been explained by sensory, oculomotor, and lexical constraints (O'Regan & Lévy-Schoen, 1987). Sensory constraints mostly involve a drop in visual acuity outside the fixation location

(Bouma, 1978) and explain why gaze durations are longer if fixations are imposed at the very beginning or end of a word. Oculomotor constraints refer to the tendency to make more fixations when the eye starts further from the convenient viewing position. They also explain why gaze durations take more time if fixations are directed to the beginning or end of a word. Neither sensory nor oculomotor constraints explain why processing time is shorter with initial fixations in the first half of a word than with fixations in the last half. To do this, a third constraint has been proposed, the lexical constraint. Since the identity of a word can be more often easily guessed from knowledge of its first letters than from knowledge of its last letters in languages such as English and French, it is hypothesized that the first syllables of words might often be a more convenient viewing position. Although manipulation of the most informative part of words does have some effect, the effect is not as strong as might be expected (Holmes & O'Regan, 1987; O'Regan et al., 1984). The left part of a word maintains its superiority over the right to a large extent. We believe that this superiority is due to the need for callosal transmission when a word is fixated to the right. Supporting evidence for this position will be given below.

One last finding about eye movements should be mentioned, although it is not directly related to reading. In oculomotor adaptation studies, it has frequently been found (Deubel, Wolf, & Hauske, 1986; Henson, 1978, 1979; Robinson, 1973) that the essential trigger for rapid oculomotor adaptation is to avoid overshooting the target. According to Henson (1978, 1979), the functional meaning of this resistance against overshooting is to retain the cortical image of the target within the same hemisphere that initiated the primary saccade. This strategy permits re-identification and relocation of the target by the same cortical hemisphere and avoids additional processing delays by information transfer through the corpus callosum (see also Deubel et al., 1986). Whether this thesis can be extended to eye movements during reading will be examined in the following sections.

Gaze Directions for Right- and Left-Hemisphere Stimuli

The above review suggests that if efforts are made to eliminate sensory and lexical constraints, a significant difference should be found between the gaze direction for stimuli processed primarily in the left hemisphere and those processed primarily in the right hemisphere. If a stimulus is more easily processed in the left hemisphere, then the right visual hemifield will have a superiority because of its direct connections to the left hemisphere, and the best strategy for the eye would be to look as far left as possible at the stimulus. Conversely, the same argument predicts a rightward gaze direction for right-hemisphere stimuli.

Tab. 1: Major parameters and results of the experiments about gaze directions for left and right hemisphere stimuli (Brysbaert & d'Ydewalle, 1987 a,b).

	subjects	stimuli	hemisphere aimed at	S-width	presentation time	task of subject	depending variable	results * left eye	results * right eye
exp.1	6 righthanded males	vertically pres. words (capitals) (10 slides)	left	1.3°	not measured	reading aloud	mean gaze direction per slide	+ .69	-1.12
		vertical row of triangles, rectangles and circles (10 slides)	right	1.3°	not measured	looking at the figure row	mean gaze direction per slide	+ .95	- .98
exp.2	19 righthanded males	vertically pres. words (capitals) (20 slides)	left	2.3°	2.1 sec/slide	reading aloud	mean gaze direction	- .54	- .32
		vertical row of irregular polygons (13 slides)	right	2.3°	4.1 sec/slide	looking at the figure row	mean gaze direction	- .33	- .33
exp.3	12 righthanded males	4 horizontal words of 4 letters (10 slides)	left	5.5°	2.2 sec/slide	reading aloud	mean gaze direction per slide	+ .05	- .34
		4 horizontal rows of 4 triangles, rectangles or circles (10 slides)	right	5.5°	2.2 sec/slide	looking at the figure rows	mean gaze direction per slide	+ .48	- .27
exp.4	8 righthanded males and 8 righthanded females	pieces of a rapid serial visual presentation text	left	4.2°	140 msec/slide	reading and reproducing at the end	mean gaze direction per slide	+ .20	
		triangles and rectangles	right	4.2°	140 msec/slide	reacting when triangle	mean gaze direction per slide	+1.00	

* results in degrees relative to the center of the stimuli

A series of four experiments tested this hypothesis (Brysbaert & d'Ydewalle, 1987a, b). Sensory constraints (for the most part, a drop of acuity outside the center of the visual field) were eliminated by the use of large stimuli with high contrast. Lexical constraints were controlled by choosing stimuli with an equal information distribution between the halves. The left-hemisphere stimuli were either vertically presented words written in capitals, horizontally presented words of four letters, or texts divided so as not to favor the first part of the fragments. Capitals are difficult to identify from their first part, because 12 of the 26 letters (A, B, D, etc.) start with the same vertical line and four of the 26 with the same curvature (C, G, O, Q). Similarly, words of four letters have good information distribution because, at least in the language used, Dutch, almost every letter can be changed to get another meaningful word. The right-hemisphere stimuli were visuospatial stimuli (Bradshaw & Nettleton, 1983), symmetric around the vertical midline (e.g. rectangles, triangles, circles, and irregular polygons). The eye movements were recorded by means of a Debic 80 eye tracker based on the corneal reflection-pupil center measurement. Subjects looked monocularly. Table 1 gives a summary of the major parameters and the results of the four experiments.

Three things are to be noted in particular. First, the difference between the gaze direction for left- and right-hemisphere stimuli is always statistically significant in the expected direction ($p < .05$), but not substantial enough to confirm the hypothesis absolutely. Second, the effect is larger for the left eye and almost absent for the right eye, which always leads to a significant eye-by-material interaction ($p < .01$). Finally, the left eye generally looks more to the right than does the right eye.

Several explanations of the effects are possible. However, none of them allows a definitive decision about whether or not cerebral asymmetry influences the gaze direction for left- and right-hemisphere stimuli. Therefore, we will first present corroborating findings from another paradigm and then return to the discussion.

The Convenient Viewing Position for Subjects with Left-Hemisphere and Right-Hemisphere Dominance

The paradigm of spontaneous shifts of gaze direction as a function of stimulus information presented gave very little evidence. Although clearer results might be obtained by refining the dependent variable (gaze direction), we are pessimistic about the final effect. One of the major problems with the paradigm is that we have to rely on *spontaneous* shifts of gaze direction, which seem to be extremely difficult to elicit in an experimental setting. Limiting presentation time to 140 ms (Experiment 4), for instance, did not result in larger differences between the gaze direction for left- and right-hemisphere stimuli, as expected, but in a negative correlation between gaze direction and quality of text reproduction (Brysbaert & d'Ydewalle, 1987a, b). Our subjects seemed to be more willing to accept poor results than to adapt their gaze direction.

O'Regan et al. (1984, Experiment 1) offered a different paradigm to examine the influence of various constraints on word processing. Subjects were asked to fixate a gap between two vertically aligned fixation lines and to read aloud every word presented. The words were presented horizontally in such a way that a different letter location lay between the two lines. The naming latency was recorded and proved to be shortest when the letter left to the middle of the word was presented between the fixation lines. Similar results were obtained with other dependent variables, such as gaze duration and number of fixations and have since been attributed to sensory, oculomotor, and lexical constraints (O'Regan & Lévy-Schoen, 1987). Therefore, naming latency can be used as a reliable estimate of word processing time. Comparing the performance of subjects with a left-hemisphere dominance for verbal stimuli to the performance of subjects with a right-hemisphere dominance for verbal stimuli thus should give an estimate of laterality influence on the convenient viewing position.

The study reported below closely follows the procedure given in O'Regan et al. (1984, Experiment 1). Changes were made largely because of the difficulty of finding subjects with right-hemisphere dominance, as only about 3% of right-handers and 25% of left-handers are thought to be right dominant (Bryden, 1982).

A population of about 300 undergraduate and graduate students were screened. First, they were selected with respect to sex (males are considered to be more lateralized; McGlone, 1980), and with respect to hand, foot, ear, and eye preference (left-side preference for all variables enhances the chances of right-hemisphere dominance; Strauss, 1986). All males with a strong leftward preference were then asked to participate in a tachistoscopic visual hemifield presentation experiment in which four- and five-letter words were used as stimuli. Only two subjects met our criteria for right-hemisphere dominance to a sufficient degree: being male, having a left-hand, left-foot, left-ear, and left-eye preference, and showing no right visual hemifield superiority in the tachistoscopic experiment. We had hoped to find some subjects with a clear left-hemifield superiority which would have been a much stronger indication of right-hemisphere dominance, but we did not succeed, probably because horizontally presented words additionally favor the right visual hemifield due to reading habits (Lambert & Beaumont, 1983).

The two right-dominant subjects and three subjects who met the criteria for left dominance (male, right-hand, foot, ear, and eye preference, and right visual hemifield superiority in the test) were tested with all the conditions. For each subject, 12 to 18 hours of tests were administered over a two-week period.

The subjects obtained corrective glasses from an ophthalmologist if their acuity was less than 10/10. They then went through several practice trials before starting the experiment, which consisted of 30 presentations of a series of 90 three-letter, 96 four-letter, 100 five-letter, 96 seven-letter, and 100 nine-letter words. Thirty presentations were necessary because (a) the subjects were tested binocularly, monocularly with the left eye and monocularly with the right eye, (b) the five-letter words and the nine-letter words had to be presented five times in order to have every letter of the five letter words and every odd letter of the nine-letter words fixated, and (c) we wanted to present every condition, at least, twice. Just as for the five-letter words, every letter of the three- and the four-letter words had to be fixated. Every odd letter of the seven-letter words also had to be fixated.

The three- and four-letter words consisted of three variants: (a) high frequency words, (b) low frequency words that only differed from high frequency words by their first letter, and (c) low frequency words that differed from high frequency words by their last letter. The effects of this manipulation will be discussed elsewhere. All the five-, seven- and nine-letter words were high frequency words.

Subjects were sitting 40 cm in front of a microcomputer screen that presented the stimuli in a random sequence. One character space was 3.1 mm wide so that each letter subtended 0.4°. The subjects were trained to fixate the gap between two vertically aligned lines placed just above and below the horizontal position where the test word was to appear. Lower case words were then presented in such a way that a different (random) letter position lay between the fixation lines. The subjects were instructed to name the word as rapidly and as accurately as possible. The latency time was recorded. Each trial began automatically, half a second after the subject had finished naming the word that was displayed in the previous trial. The fixation lines remained visible. To ascertain that the subjects really fixated the gap, every second to tenth trial, a digit was presented in the gap for 40 ms. The subjects had to read the digit. If they made a mistake, they were warned by a sound. An error rate of more than 10% for the approximately 85 digit presentations automatically led to a new presentation of the entire series. After two or three hours training, this rarely occurred. The presentation of 482 words and about 85 digits took approximately 15 minutes.

The major expectation was to find a different pattern of naming latency as a function of the letter initially fixated for subjects with left-hemisphere dominance and subjects with right-hemisphere dominance. We also wanted to find out whether a nasotemporal overlap would appear in the data and why there always was a difference between the left and the right eye in the experiments reported above. The nasotemporal overlap would appear if no callosal delay is found at the beginning of a word for subjects with left dominance and if no callosal delay is found at the end for subjects with right dominance.

Because the three subjects with left-hemisphere dominance gave very similar results apart from individual speed differences, their data were averaged together (see Figure 2).

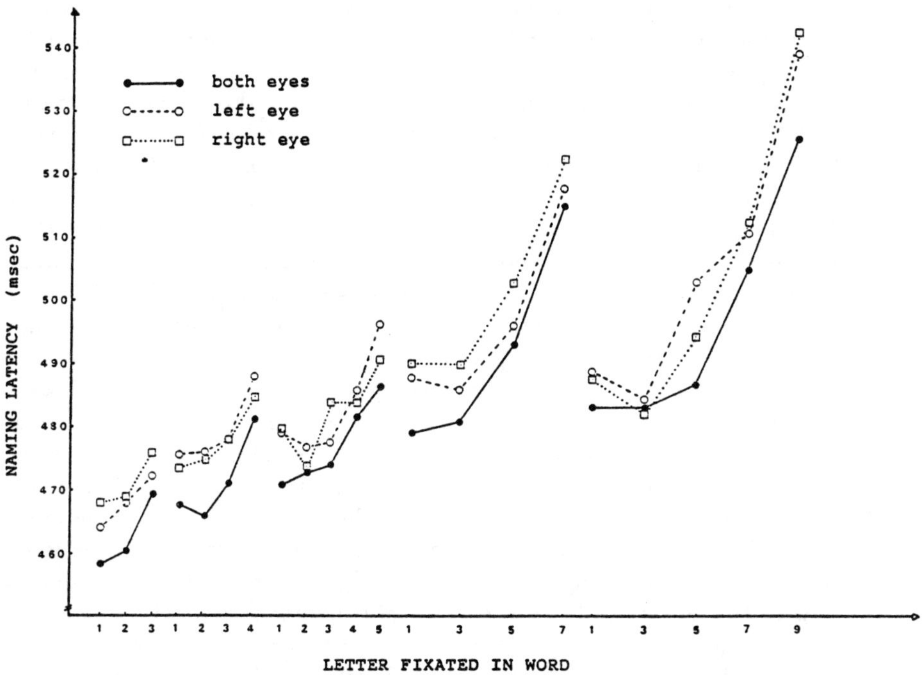

Fig. 2: Naming latency for left hemisphere dominant subjects as a function of eye, word length, and letter initially fixated. Every estimate is an average of at least 200 observations.

Several differences are to be noted between our data and those reported by O'Regan et al. (1984, Experiment 1). First, our subjects are, on the average, 200 to 300 ms faster than those of O'Regan et al. (1984). This is probably due to our subjects being more intensively trained. At least, it gives us certainty that our subjects performed optimally and that the latency differences found as a function of the fixated-letter position at the moment the word appeared are really due to processing constraints. A second difference between our data and those reported by O'Regan et al. (1984) concerns the increase of reaction time for every letter of deviation from the "ideal" initial fixation position. O'Regan and Lévy-Schoen (1987) mention a penalty time of about 20 ms; our data reveal a penalty time of about 6 ms per letter deviation for the words with three, four, and five letters, and about 13 ms for the words with seven and nine letters. More importantly, however, is the finding that a clear superiority of the left-hand side of a word is found for short words, where sensory and lexical constraints are less important. The reaction times for every subject and almost every condition (binocular, left eye, right eye) are shortest when the subject fixates the first letter position in the word that appears. The results of the words with seven and nine letters more closely resemble those of O'Regan and Lévy-Schoen, probably because they are more influenced by sensory and lexical constraints. Still, we find a greater left-hand side superiority than usually reported. Several reasons for this suggest themselves. Perhaps, it is found because we used subjects with strong cerebral dominance. In that case, the superiority will be likely to diminish with females (McGlone, 1980) or left-handers (see below). It might also be that the left-side superiority was strengthened by the training and the long duration of the experiment or that differences between the Dutch and French languages favor word beginnings more in Dutch than in French. Finally, it is possible that sensory constraints are stronger in eye movement studies where the eye-tracking system sometimes does not allow the subject to wear glasses.

At first sight, the data do not support the existence of a nasotemporal overlap. This would have been so, if there had been no differences of latency between the conditions in which the first letter position was fixated at the moment the word appeared and the conditions in which the second letter position was fixated. Certainly for the binocular conditions this is not so. However, because the effects in Figure 2 are likely to be the result of several constraints, a more powerful test will be to compare the latency difference of the left-dominant subjects with the latency difference of the right-dominant subjects.

There is a reliable main effect of 2 to 10 ms for binocular vision (present for every subject and every condition), but no consistent difference between the left and the right eye.

The two subjects with right-hemisphere dominance differed more from one another than the left-dominant subjects, in that one resembled the left-dominant subjects more than the other. Nevertheless, because there are no a priori grounds to exclude the first subject, the data of both subjects are presented together in Figure 3.

Five differences with respect to Figure 2 are to be noted. First, the convenient viewing position lies more to the right. Second, the reaction times for rightward fixations are shorter. Third, the reaction times for leftward fixations are longer. Fourth, both subjects show a consistent non-dominant right eye superiority across all conditions. Fifth, both subjects are reliably faster than the left-dominant subjects.

The shifting of the convenient viewing position to the right and the change of penalty times for deviations to the left and to the right of the convenient viewing position are consistent with the expectations. The finding that the pattern of naming latencies in Figure 2 is not reversed in Figure 3, however, indicates that cerebral dominance is but one influencing factor in addition to

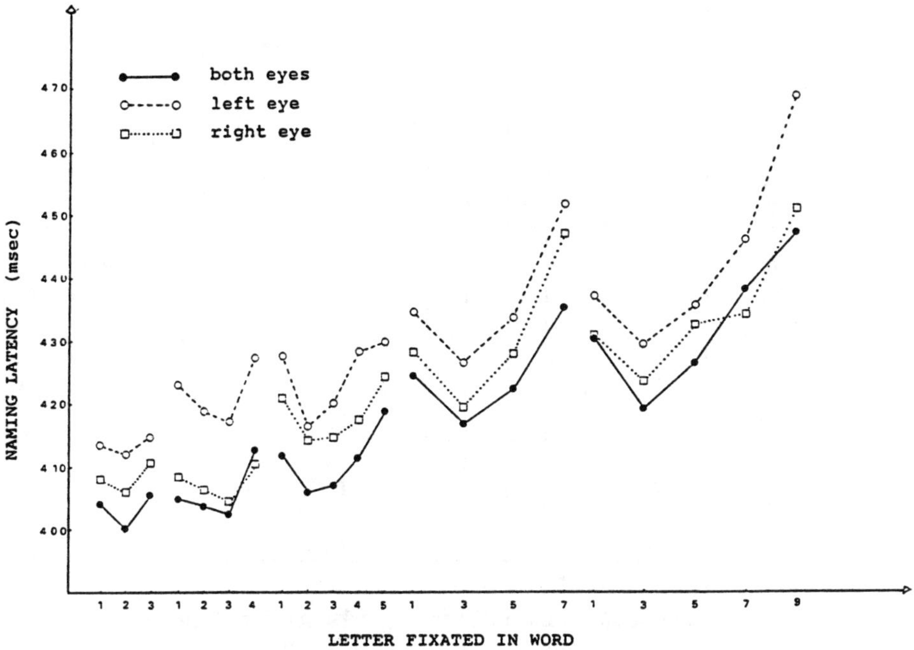

Fig. 3: Naming latency for right hemisphere dominant subjects as a function of eye, word length, and letter initially fixated. Every estimate is an average of at least 200 observations.

those already cited by O'Regan and Lévy-Schoen (1987). By comparing the results in Figures 2 and 3 with their average, it is possible to get an unbiased estimate of the time costs associated with cerebral asymmetry. Figure 4 shows the distribution of the time costs per letter deviation from the beginning of a word for the left-dominant subjects. The data for the right-dominant subjects are the same, apart from a sign change in the abscissa.

The time estimates in Figure 4 are well in agreement with other independent measures of callosal transmission time (Bashore, 1980; John et al., 1987) and seem to indicate that every letter sent to the "wrong" hemisphere is transferred separately and involves a supplemental cost. This cost is likely to lie around 1 or 2 ms, which, depending on word length and fixation location, is about a half to a fifth of the sum of the other influences.

Evidence either in favor of or against the nasotemporal overlap can be derived from the pattern of penalty times. If the callosal overlap exists, no callosal delay will be found between every first and second letter for the left-dominant subjects. Similarly, no callosal delay will be found between the last and second last letters for the right-dominant subjects. This implies that the estimates in Figure 4 should be about 1 ms (i.e. about half the callosal transmission time)

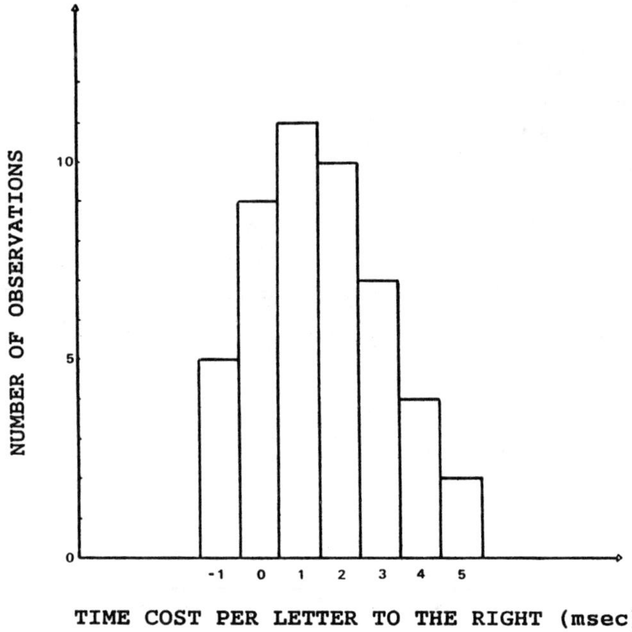

Fig. 4: Frequency distribution of differences in naming latency between fixations on letter 'n' and letter 'n+1': Data for the left hemisphere dominant subjects. Increases were calculated for the conditions with binocular, monocular left and monocular right vision separately.

shorter between the two most leftward and rightward letters than between the middle letters. Apart from the four-letter words, all data argue against the existence of a nasotemporal overlap: the estimates of callosal transmission tend to be slightly smaller in the middle range than at the extremes and are not smaller for three-letter words than for nine-letter words or for any condition.

The superiority of the right eye will be discussed in the next section.

Cerebral Asymmetry and Word Processing: General Discussion

Because there is little evidence for bilateral projection of a small, one degree, band in the middle of the visual field and because callosal transmission is always found to involve time costs, it was hypothesized that the callosal delay would influence reading. The influence could manifest itself in two ways: either by directing fixation to the beginning of a word and thereby allowing a projection of the complete word into the dominant left hemisphere or by enhancing processing time with the time needed to transfer part of the stimulus from the right to the left cerebral hemisphere.

In Brysbaert and d'Ydewalle (1987a, b), we tried to find evidence for an influence of cerebral asymmetry on gaze direction. Gaze directions for stimuli known to be better processed in the left hemisphere were compared with gaze directions for stimuli known to be processed preferentially in the right hemisphere. Although there was a small tendency for looking at the left-hand side of the left-hemisphere stimuli and at the right-hand side of the right-hemisphere stimuli, the evidence was not strong. In view of the findings about processing constraints, the simplest explanation for the lack of a clear effect probably is that the influence of cerebral asymmetry does exist but is too small to dominate other influences (sensory and lexical constraints, habits) and thus to effect spontaneous gaze directions significantly.

Unexpected differences between the gaze direction of the left and right eye were found: the left eye almost always looked more to the right than the right eye and the difference between the gaze direction for left-hemisphere and right-hemisphere stimuli was more clearly present in the left eye. This effect might be a consequence of inequality between the nasal and the temporal retina, though it is not clear how this inequality has to be conceived of. Some authors (e.g. Crovitz & Lipscomb, 1963; Kruper, Patton, & Koskoff, 1971; Maddess, 1975) have reported a superiority of the nasal retina, some (McKeever & Huling, 1970; Neill, Sampson, & Gribben, 1971) found a superiority of the temporal retina, while others (e.g. Parker, Satz, & Horne, 1976) failed to find any difference or were confronted with large interindividual differences (Leat & Woodhouse, 1984).

In Brysbaert and d'Ydewalle (1987a, b), we explained the difference between the gaze directions for the left and the right eye with a double assumption. First, we assumed that the nasotemporal overlap found in monkeys also existed in man. Second, we postulated a superiority of the temporal retina. The double assumption implied that more information is sent to the ipsilateral than to the contralateral cerebral hemisphere in the nasotemporal overlap, which is why the right eye has to look more to the left to get the information directly into the left-hemisphere. The assumption also explains the lack of difference between the gaze directions in the right eye because a superiority of the temporal retina would imply a "dilemma" between sharp visual acuity in the center of the visual field and the better transmission to the wrong hemisphere. The dilemma has less effect for the left eye because the visuospatial stimuli do not require much sharp vision.

However, it is equally possible to explain the difference between the left and the right eye by invoking a superiority of the nasal retina. Such a superiority implies that the left eye has the "choice" for left-hemisphere stimuli between sending information directly to the left hemisphere through the minor ipsilateral connections or indirectly through the superior contralateral connections. The right eye, however, only has the choice between direct sending through the superior contralateral connections or indirect sending through the inferior ipsilateral connections. Because the penalty for indirect sending is greater for the right eye than for the left eye, the right eye will be forced to look more to the left of left-hemisphere stimuli. The same argument predicts a greater force for the left eye to look to the right-hand side of right-hemisphere stimuli than for the right eye, which explains the more rightward gaze direction of the left eye. Differences between penalty times for left- and right-hemisphere stimuli might further explain why the gaze directions of the left eye differed more than those of the right eye.

The experiments about the influence of cerebral asymmetry in gaze directions provided more new questions than definite answers. Therefore, the constraints of callosal transmission on lexical processing were investigated more closely by comparing the naming latency for isolated words in subjects with left-hemisphere dominance and in subjects with right-hemisphere dominance. If callosal transmission does, indeed, influence lexical processing, naming latency should be hampered more for initial fixations at the end of a word when the subject is left dominant than when he is right dominant. The expectation was confirmed: every letter of deviation from the beginning of the word involved a penalty time of about 1 or 2 ms for the left-dominant subjects and an advantage of 1 to 2 ms for the right dominant subjects.

The "cost" per letter sent to the wrong hemisphere agrees well with other measures of callosal transmission time (Bashore, 1981) and seems to suggest that every letter has to be transmitted sequentially. Depending on the letter the subjects were asked to fixate and the word length, the callosal delay was about a half to a fifth of the sum of the other influences suggested by O'Regan and Lévy-Schoen (1987). A penalty time of only 2 ms per letter also explains why the effect of cerebral asymmetry on gaze directions is not very conspicuous. No evidence was found for the nasotemporal overlap.

Differences of naming latency between the left and the right eye are less clear. There are large interindividual differences. Three subjects (among them the two subjects with right cerebral dominance) showed an ipsilateral eye dominance maybe suggesting a superiority of the temporal retina and connections; one subject showed a faint contralateral eye dominance, and the last subject displayed no preference. It is not clear whether these differences are due to interindividual differences (Leat & Woodhouse, 1984) or what their relation is to the findings on gaze directions.

Conclusions

The present experiments provide an answer to the question of whether the division of the visual field into a left and right half constrains reading. It has been shown that the need for callosal transmission when part of the stimulus is sent to the wrong hemisphere tends to direct the gaze in such a way that the greater part of the word can be sent directly to the hemisphere specialized to process it. However, because callosal transmission is not the only constraint, the gaze is rarely directed so that the entire stimulus is sent directly to the specialized hemisphere. A penalty time of about 1 to 2 ms per letter has to be "paid" for this deviation.

The experiments did not support the suggestion of a nasotemporal overlap in the middle of the visual field. The results thus agree with those of studies using unimanual reactions to lateralized light spots (Harvey, 1978; Haun, 1978; Lines, 1984; Lines & Milner, 1983) and are further evidence for either the existence of a difference between man and lower animals with respect to the overlap, or the idea that the nasotemporal overlap has no other function than assisting stereopsis (Bishop, 1975).

Finally, the results suggest a difference between the eyes, possibly due to differences between the nasal and the temporal retina. Evidence is not conclusive, but it does support dominance of the eye ipsilateral to the dominant hemisphere, possibly attenuated by interindividual differences (Leat & Woodhouse, 1984).

Acknowledgement

The authors wish to thank Noël Bovens, Stef Decoene, Patrick Driessen, Patrick Matthys, and Jan Willems for their help at different stages of the experiment.

References

Bashore, T.R., *Vocal and manual reaction time estimates of interhemispheric transmission time*, Psychological Bulletin **89** (1981), 352-368.

Berlucchi, G., *Anatomical and physiological aspects of visual functions of corpus callosum*, Brain Research **37** (1972), 371-392.

Bishop, P.O., *Binocular vision*, in "K.A. Moses (Ed.), Adler's physiology of the eye," Mosby, St. Louis, 1975, pp. 558-614.

Bouma, H., *Visual search and reading: Eye movements and the functional visual field, a tutorial review*, in "J. Requin (Ed.), Attention and Performance VII," Erlbaum, Hillsdale, N.J., 1978, pp. 115-147.

Bradshaw, J.L., & Nettleton, N.C., "Human cerebral asymmetry," Prentice Hall, Englewood Cliffs, N.J., 1983.

Bryden, M.P., "Laterality: Functional asymmetry in the intact brain," Academic Press, New York, 1982.

Brysbaert, M., & d'Ydewalle, G., *Cerebral asymmetry and the gaze directions for verbal and visuospatial stimuli*, Psychological Reports (University of Leuven: Department of Psychology) **65** (1987a).

Brysbaert, M., & d'Ydewalle, G., *Gaze directions and cerebral asymmetry*, in "G. Lüer & U. Lass (Eds.), Fourth European Conference on Eye Movements, Vol. 1: Proceedings," Hogrefe, Göttingen, 1987b, pp. 43-45.

Bunt, A.H., & Minckler, D.S., *Foveal sparing: New anatomical evidence for bilateral representation of the central retina*, Archives of Ophthalmology **95** (1977), 1445-1447.

Crovitz, H.F., & Lipscomb, D.B., *Dominance of the temporal visual fields at a short duration of stimulation*, American Journal of Psychology **76** (1963), 631-637.

Deubel, H., Wolf, W., & Hauske, G., *Adaptive gain control of saccadic eye movements*, Human Neurobiology **5** (1986), 245-253.

Dunn-Rankin, P., *The visual characteristics of words*, Scientific American **238** (1978), 122-130.

Erdmann, B., & Dodge, R., "Psychologische Untersuchungen über das Lesen," Niemeyer, Halle, 1898.

Harrington, D.O., "The visual fields: A textbook and atlas of clinical perimetry," Mosby, St. Louis, Missouri, 1981.

Harvey, L.O., *Single representation of the visual midline in humans*, Neuropsychologia **16** (1978), 601-610.

Haun, F., *Functional dissociation of the hemispheres using foveal visual input*, Neuropsychologia **16** (1978), 725-734.

Heilman, K.M., Bowers, D., Valenstein, E., & Watson, R.T., *Hemispace and hemispatial neglect*, in "M. Jeannerod (Ed.), Neurophysiological and neuropsychological aspects of spatial neglect," North-Holland, Amsterdam, 1987, pp. 115-150.

Hellige, J.B. (Ed.), "Cerebral hemisphere asymmetry: Method, theory and application," Praeger, New York, 1983.

Henson, D.B., *Corrective saccades: Effects of altering visual feedback*, Vision Research **18** (1978), 63-67.

Henson, D.B., *Investigation into corrective saccadic eye movements for refixation amplitudes of 10 degrees and below*, Vision Research **19** (1979), 57-61.

Holmes, V.M., & O'Regan, J.K., *Decomposing French words*, in "J.K. O'Regan & A. Lévy - Schoen (Eds.), Eye movements: From physiology to cognition," North-Holland, Amsterdam, 1987, pp. 459- 466.

Jeannerod, M. (Ed.), "Neurophysiological and neuropsychological aspects of spatial neglect," North-Holland, Amsterdam, 1987.

John, R.St., Shields, C., Krahn, P., & Timney, B., *The reliability of estimates of interhemispheric transmission times derived from unimanual and verbal response latencies*, Human Neurobiology **6** (1987), 195-202.

Kimura, D., *The asymmetry of the human brain*, Scientific American **228** (1973), 70-78.

Kinsbourne, M., & Warrington, E.K., *A variety of reading disability associated with right hemisphere lesions*, Journal of Neurology, Neurosurgery & Psychiatry **25** (1962), 339-344.

Kruper, D.C., Patton, R.A., & Koskoff, Y.D., *Hand and eye preference in unilaterally brain ablated monkeys*, Physiology and Behaviour **7** (1971), 181-185.

Lambert, A.J., & Beaumont, J.G., *Imageability does not interact with visual field in lateral word recognition with oral report*, Brain and Language **20** (1983), 115-142.

Leat, S.J., & Woodhouse, J.M., *Rivalry with continuous and flashed stimuli as a measure of ocular dominance across the visual field*, Perception **13** (1984), 351-367.

Lines, C.R., *Nasotemporal overlap investigated in a case of agenesis of the corpus callosum*, Neuropsychologia **22** (1984), 85 - 90.

Lines, C.R., & Milner, A.D., *Nasotemporal overlap in the human retina investigated by means of simple reaction time to lateralized light flash*, Experimental Brain Research **50** (1983), 166-172.

Maddess, R.J., *Reaction time to hemiretinal stimulation*, Neuropsychologia **13** (1975), 213-218.

Marzi, C.A., *Transfer of visual information after unilateral input to the brain*, Brain and Cognition **5** (1986), 153-163.

McConkie, G.W., & Rayner, K., *Asymmetry of the perceptual span in reading*, Bulletin of the Psychonomic Society **8** (1976), 365-368.

McGlone, *Sex differences in human brain asymmetry: A critical review*, The Behavioral and Brain Sciences **3** (1980), 215-263.

McKeever, W.F., & Huling, M.D., *Left-cerebral hemisphere superiority in tachistoscopic word - recognition performances*, Perceptual and Motor Skills **30** (1970), 763-766.

Moscovitch, M., *Laterality and visual masking: Interhemispheric communication and the locus of perceptual asymmetries for words*, Canadian Journal of Psychology **37** (1983), 85-106.

Neill, D.O., Sampson, H., & Gribben, J.A., *Hemiretinal effects in tachistoscopic letter recognition*, Journal of Experimental Psychology **91** (1971), 129-135.

O'Regan, J.K, & Lévy-Schoen, A., *Eye-movement strategy and tactics in word recognition and reading*, in "M. Coltheart (Ed.), Attention and Performance XII: The psychology of reading," Erlbaum, London, 1987, pp. 363-383.

O'Regan, J.K., Lévy-Schoen, A., Pynte, J., & Brugaillère, B., *Convenient fixation location within isolated words of different length and structure*, Journal of Experimental Psychology: Human Perception and Performance **10** (1984), 250-257.

Parker, R., Satz, P., & Horne, E.P., *Visual pathways, acuity dominance, and visual halffield asymmetry*, The Journal of General Psychology **95** (1976), 233-240.

Perenin, M.T., & Vadot, E., *Macular sparing investigated by means of Haidinger brushes*, British Journal of Ophthalmology **65** (1981), 429-435.

Pollatsek, A., Bolozky, S, Well, A.D., & Rayner, K., *Asymmetries in the perceptual span for Israeli readers*, Brain and Language **14** (1981), 174-180.

Rayner, K., *Eye movements in reading and information processing*, Psychological Bulletin **85** (1978), 618-660.

Rayner, K., & Fisher, D.L., *Letter processing during eye fixations in visual search*, Perception and Psychophysics **42** (1987), 87-100.

Rayner, K., & Pollatsek, A., *Eye movements in reading: A tutorial review*, in "M. Coltheart (Ed.), Attention and Performance XII: The psychology of reading," Erlbaum, London, 1987, pp. 327-362.

Robinson, D.A., *Models of the saccadic eye movement control system*, Kybernetik **14** (1973), 71-83.

Rugg, M.D., Lines, C.R., & Milner, A.D., *Visual evoked potentials to lateralized visual stimuli and the measurement of interhemispheric transmission time*, Neuropsychologia **22** (1984), 215-225.

Stone, J., *The naso-temporal division of the cat's retina*, Journal of Comparative Neurology **136** (1966), 585-600.

Stone, J., Leicester, L., & Sherman, S.M., *The naso-temporal division of the monkey's retina*, Journal of Comparative Neurology **150** (1973), 333-348.

Strauss, E., *Hand, foot, eye and ear preference and perfomance on a dichotic listening test*, Cortex **22** (1986), 475-482.

Swanson, J., Ledlow, A., & Kinsbourne, M., *Lateral asymmetries revealed by simple reaction time*, in "M. Kinsbourne (Ed.), Asymmetrical function of the brain," Cambridge University Press, Cambridge, 1978.

Terao, N., Inatomi, A., & Maeda, T., *Anatomical evidence for the overlapped distribution of ipsilaterally and contralaterally projecting ganglion cells to the lateral geniculate nucleus in the cat retina: A morphologic study with fluorescent tracers*, Investigative Ophthalmology and Visual Science **23** (1982), 796-798.

Wyatt, H.J., *Nasotemporal overlap and visual field sparing*, Investigative Ophthalmology and Visual Science **17** (1978), 1128-1130.

BREAKING DOWN SACCADE LATENCY INTO CENTRAL AND PERIPHERAL PROCESSING TIMES IN A VISUAL DUAL-TASK

ARTHUR M. JACOBS AND ARIANE LÉVY-SCHOEN

Groupe Regard, Laboratoire de Psychologie Expérimentale,
Université René Descartes, Paris

INTRODUCTION

According to a hypothetical model of the control of exploratory saccades presented by the first author at the last ECEM-meeting, the when- and where-decisions of saccade control are determined by the processing of information in peripheral vision (Jacobs, 1987a). As expected, these processings determine saccade size and latency in simple visual search tasks in which subjects scan a more or less homogeneous background in search of a known target (Jacobs, 1986, 1987b; Jacobs & O'Regan, 1987; Rayner & Fisher, 1987). In addition, data from a recent study show that both latency and accuracy of saccades can be directly determined from the ability to locate the target in peripheral vision (Jacobs, 1987c). It is evident, however, that in more complex visual search or reading situations, eye movement parameters depend on both the processing of information in central vision and the (pre)-processing of peripheral information (see Jacobs & Lévy-Schoen, 1987, for a recent review). However, the above statement raises a number of questions.

To illustrate the problem, imagine the following situation. During a single eye fixation in search or reading the brain must carry out two different processes. These are combined in order to produce efficient oculomotor behavior. One we shall label a high-level or cognitive process with regard to the stimulus in central vision and one we shall call a low-level or perceptual process with regard to the stimuli in peripheral vision. Specifically in reading, the information in central vision (e.g. the fixated word) is processed up to a relatively high level (letter recognition, word encoding, case role assignment, etc.), while the information in parafoveal and peripheral vision is (pre)-processed on a lower level (word segmentation, length, shape and possibly, partial letter discrimination; see Coltheart, 1987; Jacobs & Lévy-Schoen, 1987, for recent reviews). Evidence for qualitatively different processes with regard to the information in central and peripheral vision has also been obtained in a simple visual search task. Rayner and Fisher (1987) argued that processing up to the level of decision (about the presence of a target) only occurs within a central region 3-6 letters large, whereas processing of location and partial letter information occurs beyond that region.

There are, at least, three questions of interest in such a situation that have not received sufficient investigation. First, to what extent does fixation duration or saccade latency reflect the duration of each of these processes (central and peripheral)? Second, what is the temporal ordering of these processes? Do they overlap, occur totally in parallel or strictly in series? Third, if they are sequential, which has often been hypothesized in the literature, then what exact order do they follow: a periphery-to-center order (Mackworth, 1965), a left-to-right order (Gough, 1972) or a center-to-periphery order (Rayner et al., 1981; Schiepers, 1980)? These questions not only are important for understanding eye movement control and for elaborating our model of exploratory saccades, but also have general implications for the study of visual perception. To investigate them systematically two things are required: models that predict the dependence of saccade latency on the duration of information processing in central and peripheral vision, and methods that test the predictions. As a first step, the present study introduces a method that separates saccade latency into its parts resulting from processing of information in central and peripheral vision. This can be realized better in a very simplified situation than in a normal visual search or reading situation. The study was the first of a research program that, by use of simplified models and methods, aims at understanding the laws that govern saccade latency in situations in which a perceptual and a cognitive task have to be executed at the same time in different parts of the visual field. The basic experimental idea here was to give simultaneously a perceptual task in peripheral vision (labeled P) and a cognitive task in central vision (labeled C) in order to see how saccade latency varied with the level of complexity of both tasks. We began the study by measuring performance in each of the two tasks (C and P) separately in order to obtain baseline measures and then went on to combine them in a dual-task.

METHOD

Subjects and apparatus

Four subjects (mean age of 27) participated voluntarily in these experiments. They were well familiar with our eye movement recording method, but not pre-trained for the tasks. All subjects had normal vision, three of them were naive about the aims of the study. Subjects sat in an adjustable chair, their head stabilized by a chin/forehead rest. Their eye movements were monitored by a photoelectric, infra-red, iris/sclera reflection technique (O'Regan et al., 1983). The position the eye was fixating was sampled by the computer at a 100 Hz rate. Stimuli were presented on a VELEC VS video monitor using a fast P4 phosphor. Stimulus luminance was about $70\,cd/m^2$, display background luminance was about $0.7\,cd/m^2$. Ambient lighting was photopic. All experiments started with an initial calibration phase.

Task, stimuli and procedure

There were 3 possible experimental situations in which subjects had to make a single saccade to the left or to the right of the fixation point. Figure 1 (a and b) illustrates two of the situations.

(1) Memory search task, SINGLE, CENTRAL (Figure 1a): At time t1 a central fixation mark was presented on a computer screen. The subject's eye position that was monitored was used by the computer to control stimulus presentation. Only when the computer identified correct fixation at the mark, was this replaced by a central digit together with two asterisks ($\star$) in the periphery. The two asterisks served as the saccade landmark. Their purpose was to ascertain whether saccades have constant amplitudes across trials which could be compared with those obtained in the peripheral task described below. The digit specified whether a saccade to the left or to the right had to be made. This had to be done as quickly as possible, allowing for an error rate of 20% or less.

There were 3 levels of difficulty. In the easy condition (C1), only two digits were used. These digits were chosen at random from the set 0-9 at the beginning of the experimental block. One digit was associated with a saccadic response to the left, the other with a response to the right Thus, memory set size was 1x2. In the example given in Figure 1a, appearance of the digit "7" might have required a saccade to the left, whereas appearance of another digit on a differential trial would have required a saccade to the right. In the medium difficult condition, (C2), memory set size was increased to 2x2. Thus at each trial one out of 4 possible digits could appear. In the difficult condition, (C3), memory set size was increased to 3x2.

This Sternberg-type (1966, 1969) of memory search or character classification task was called cognitive in comparison with the "perceptual" task described below. Within the framework of the present experimental logic these labels make sense However, in general, we do not consider them as sharply distinguished, mutually exclusive categories. The structure underlying this memory search task can be best described by Sternberg's model using 4 stages arranged in series, having independent capacity and duration: encoding, serial comparison (stimulus to members of memory set), binary decision and response organization. Traditionally, only the comparison stage is considered to be affected by memory set size. For small memory set sizes as used here ($n < 6$), the search in the comparison stage is understood as being serial and exhaustive.

(2) Letter discrimination task, SINGLE, PERIPHERAL (Figure 1b): A simple letter discrimination task in the periphery similar to Nazir, Heller, and Jacobs (1987) was performed. First appeared a central fixation point. As soon as the computer has tested, by help of our real-time eye movement monitoring system, that the subject's gaze was on this point, the stimulus was presented. It consisted of two letters, one appearing to the left and one appearing to the

right of the central fixation mark. The eccentricity of each letter with regard to the fixation point was 9 letter spaces (about 4.5 degrees) in experiment 1b and 3 letter spaces (about 1.5 degrees) in experiment 3b. Given the typography of the computer screen (16 x 16 pixels) and the viewing distance of 50 cm, the two letters were sufficiently visible at this eccentricity to obtain at least 80% correct responses for all difficulty levels. Subjects had to localize the target letter which was known in advance and constant within one block of trials and make a saccade to it. In the easy condition (P1), the target ("Z") was not visually similar to the distractor ("o"). In the medium difficult condition (P2), they were similar: "a" and "o." In the difficult condition (P3), they were very similar: "c" and "o." Compared to the central task this task could be called perceptual.

The peripheral task is like a visual search task with only two elements (target and distractor). The peripheral task is presumed to be composed of the same 4 elementary processing stages assumed to occur between the stimulus and the response, as the single central task above (e.g. Harris et al., 1977; Harvey & Gervais, 1981; Sterling & Salthouse, 1981). However, since we denote the central task as "cognitive" and the peripheral as "perceptual," we hypothesize that the difference lies in the comparison stage. In the peripheral task this stage compares the internal representation of the target to the two representations corresponding to the letters in peripheral vision. Contrary to the central memory search task, this requires no activation of a previously learned memory set which contains 2, 4 or 6 elements. In addition, we found and know of no convincing evidence showing that the comparison stage in such a two-letter discrimination task is serial and exhaustive, as it is in the central memory search task. Because of these differences, we expected task execution time (saccade latency) to be faster in the peripheral task than in the central task for all levels of task difficulty.

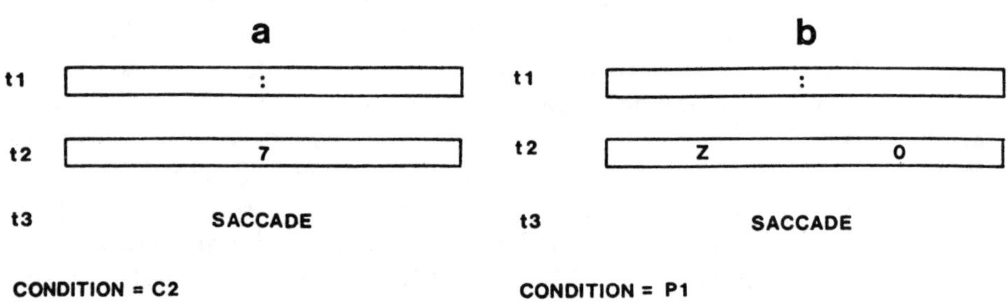

Fig. 1: Two examples of the stimulus situation in the SINGLE tasks. a) Central, memory search task, condition (C2). b) Peripheral, letter discrimination task, condition (P1). In both tasks a central fixation mark was presented at time t1. Then, once the computer had verified that the subjects eye was on the mark, stimuli were presented at time t2, until a saccadic reaction to the left or right occured at time t3.

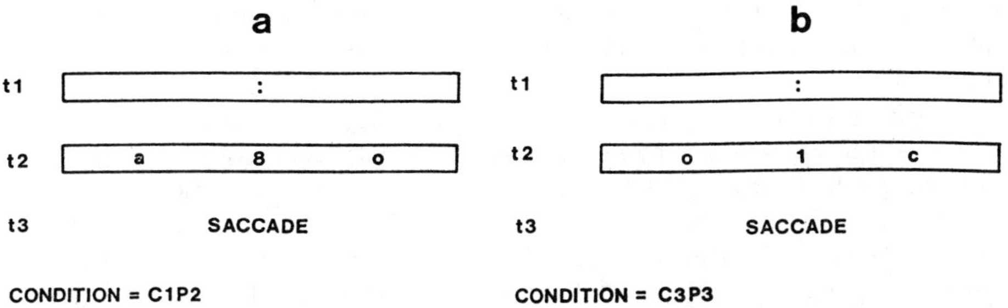

Fig. 2: Two examples of the stimulus situation in the DUAL-tasks, combining the central memory search task with the peripheral letter discrimination task. a) Condition (C1P2). b) Condition (C3P3). (Explanation in the text.) In the Dual-task, after correct fixation of the central mark, both the central digit- stimulus and the peripheral letter stimuli were presented simultaneously, until a saccade occured.

(3) DUAL-task, CENTRAL + PERIPHERAL (Figure 2a and b): The dual-task situation is illustrated in Figure 2. Here both a central digit and two letters in the periphery appeared simultaneously at each trial. Since the two SINGLE task situations had 3 different levels of difficulty, we used 9 (3x3) levels which were denoted C1P1 to C3P3. For example, in condition C1P2 (Figure 2a) the central task was easy, that is, memory set size was 1x2, while the peripheral task was of medium difficulty, that is the letters "a" and "o" were used. The instruction was always to make a saccade to one letter, if a digit belonging to the corresponding previously learned memory set appeared at the central location, and to make a saccade to the other letter, if a digit of the other memory set appeared. Thus, the central stimulus (always a digit) was associated with one of the two peripheral stimuli (always letters) and the subject had to process both the central and two peripheral stimuli in order to make a correct response. In the most difficult dual-task condition C3P3 (see Figure 2b), memory size set was 3x2 and the peripheral letters were hard to discriminate: "c" and "o." Thus, whenever one out of the 3 digits associated with the letter "c" appeared, subjects had to make a saccade to the "c." Otherwise, they had to make a saccade to the "o." The associations between digit sets and letters, as well as the memory sets were chosen randomly at the beginning of each block. Subjects had time to learn accurately which digits were associated with which letters.

Presentation side of the peripheral letters and presentation of the central digit were randomized across trials. In all experiments there were 100 trials per condition plus 30 warming-up trials at the beginning of each experimental block. After an initial calibration phase, the subject started each trial by fixating a central mark. As soon as the computer identified a correct fixation position the stimuli were presented until a saccadic reaction occurred. The dependent variable was saccade latency, measured as the time elapsing between stimulus onset and saccade onset. Subjects followed an accuracy instruction requiring at least 80% correct responses. To encourage accuracy, subjects were informed that in the case of more than 20% errors the entire block would be repeated.

In principle, the hypothetical structure underlying this novel type of dual-task could be represented by serial, stage models (Sanders, 1980; Smith, 1968; Sternberg, 1969; Taylor, 1976), by parallel/continuous stage models (Eriksen & Schultz, 1979; McLeod, 1977; McClelland, 1979), by concurrent or mixed models (Davis, 1957; Harris et al., 1977; Miller, 1982; Schweickert, 1978), or by timesharing models (Tolkmitt, 1973; Sperling & Melchner, 1978). The following is a discussion of various possible models and their predictions on saccade latency.

PREDICTIONS

To derive saccadic latency predictions in the dual-task, four simple models were chosen. These hypothetical models are deterministic, that is, they neglect trial-to-trial variability of the total task execution time as well as the hypothetical intercompletion times of the underlying processes. Table 1 summarizes the 4 models of saccade latency composition in the dual-task conditions and the corresponding predictions. Figure 3 gives a graphic illustration of each model.

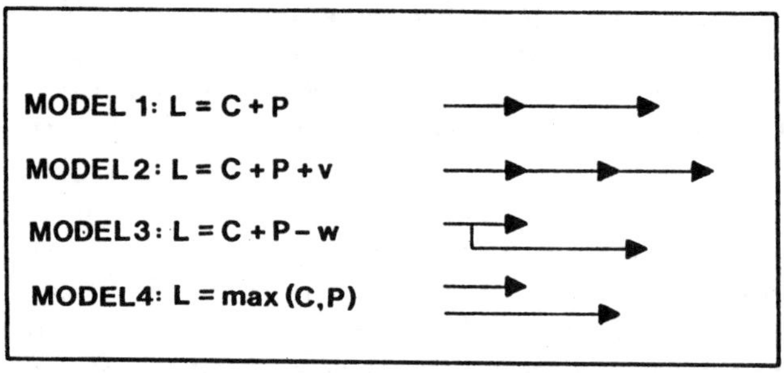

Fig. 3: Graphic illustration of each of the 4 tentative models of saccadic latency. An arrow represents a process corresponding to the central and peripheral tasks, C and P. In model 2, the 3rd arrow represents an inserted, additional process. Each process might be composed of several subprocesses or stages of the type proposed by Sternberg and others.

The straightforward model 1 assumes that saccade latency (L) in the dual-task corresponds to the sum of the times required to do the central (C) and peripheral (P) tasks: L = C+P. The prediction then is a simple addition of supplementary times. For instance, in condition C2P1, that is, the medium difficult central task and the easy peripheral task, it would be: L(C2P1) = C1P1 + (C2-C1). Accordingly, in condition C3P2, latency should be the sum of the latency observed in the baseline condition C1P1 and the differences in latency for conditions C3-C1 and P2-P1. Note that to test the models one cannot compare the data from the two single-task experiments (1a and b) to those of the dual-task experiment (2) simply by adding up the absolute latency values of *two* saccadic responses observed in experiments 1a and b (e.g. L(C2P1) = L(C2) + L(P1)). This would include the deadtime of the oculomotor system (approximately 75 ms; see Becker & Jürgens, 1979) twice in the sum of the single-task latencies and only once in the corresponding dual-task condition. We avoided this problem by comparing the differences. Model 1 was labeled the ADDITIVE model, although other possible assumptions traditionally associated with this type of model (such as seriality and stage or stochastic independence) are implied (Luce, 1986; Taylor, 1976; Townsend & Ashby, 1983).

Tab. 1: Some examples of the predictions of each of the 4 models of saccadic latency for different experimental conditions (explanations in the text).

Model	Condition		Prediction		
(1) L = C + P	C2P1	=	C1P1 + (C2-C1)		
	C3P1	=	C1P1 + (C3-C1)		
	C1P2	=	C1P1 + (P2-P1)		
	C1P3	=	C1P1 + (P3-P1)		
	C2P2	=	C1P1 + (C2-C1)	+	(P2-P1)
	C2P3	=	C1P1 + (C2-C1)	+	(P3-P1)
	etc.				
(2) L = C + P + v	C2P1	=	C1P1 + (C2-C1)	+	"v"
	etc.				
(3) L = C + P - w	C2P1	=	C1P1 + (C2-C1)	-	"w"
	etc.				
(4) L = max(C,P)	C2P1	=	max(C2,P1)		
	etc.				

Model 2 is also an additive, serial type. However, it assumes that a variable time (v) must be added to the sum of the two processing times : L = C + P + v. The variable time reflects the possible extra processing demand (load) resulting from the combined tasks and should vary with task difficulty. This model was labeled the EXTRA-LOAD model. As indicated in Figure 3 and in agreement with Donders' classical idea (1868, 1969), one possibility in the dual-task situation might be the insertion of a new process into the total processing structure, whose function could be to decide a response on the basis of the combined output from the two other processes. The additional, variable time "v" then should reflect the duration of this hypothetical process which should increase when task difficulty increases. Table 1 gives an example of the prediction for condition C2P1.

Model 3 assumes that some processing can be done in parallel and that a variable time (w) must be subtracted from the sum of both processing times. (w) represents the overlap of processing time: $L = C + P - w$. Model 3 was labeled the **PARTIAL OVERLAP** model. One possibility, indicated in Figure 3, is the assumption that the second process starts at a critical moment during the completion of the first process. Such a critical moment might be the completion of a subprocess or stage within the preceding process.

Finally, model 4, labeled the **PARALLEL** model, assumes complete parallel processing with latency corresponding to the maximum of both processing times: $L = \max(C,P)$. Prediction examples derived from models 3 and 4 are also given in Table 1.

Given the structure of the present dual-task, it seems plausible that the central and peripheral tasks share some of the processing elements. Thus, some of the underlying subprocesses (e.g. the encoding stage) might occur in parallel. On the other hand, because of the novelty and complexity of the dual-task, and, given the supposedly strict serial nature of the central memory search task, complete parallel processing is hard to predict, at least, for subjects who are not extensively trained. We therefore favored the partial overlap model (3) for predicting saccadic latency.

EXPERIMENTS

1. Experiments 1a+b: SINGLE-tasks, large eccentricity

A first series of experiments evaluated processing times for central and peripheral tasks in a single task situation to obtain baseline data for the following dual-task experiments. In experiment 1a the central memory search task was used (see Figure 1a). In a second experiment the peripheral letter discrimination task illustrated in Figure 1b was used. The peripheral stimuli were presented at a constant eccentricity of 9 letter spaces from the central stimulus. The combined results of experiments 1a and b are summarized in Table 2. It gives saccadic latency (in ms) for each of the 6 single-task conditions (means over 4 subjects with about 400 observations per mean).

The data in Table 2 show clearly that saccadic reaction time increases with the level of difficulty of the central (C) and the peripheral (P) single task (ANOVA for the central task: $F(2,6) = 38.2$, $p < .001$; and for the peripheral task: $F(2,6) = 6.5$, $p < .05$). The regression line correlating saccadic latency to difficulty of the central task (i.e. memory set size) was characterized as follows: $Y = 54.9*X + 234$. The slope of this function is a measure of the time taken

Tab. 2: Summary of the results of SINGLE-task experiments 1a and 1b Data represent averages over 4 subjects with about 400 measures per mean. The linear equations of the regression functions relating saccade latency (Y) to task difficulty (X) are also given for each single task. In the central task, X represents memory set size. In the peripheral task, X represents target/non-target similarity.

Condition	Latency (ms)	
C1	290.0	Experiment 1a: Central task
C2	339.8	
C3	400.7	Y = 54.9X + 234
P1	186.5	Experiment 1b: Peripheral task
P2	217.6	
P3	264.6	Y = 39X + 144.8

to compare the internal representation of the stimulus to each member of the memory set, activated in short-term memory (Sternberg, 1969). In this case, the memory scanning rate was approximately 55 ms/item. The time to encode the digit and the time to decide and execute the appropriate response are subtracted out of the slope and are contained in the zero-intercept. According to the above equation, these 3 remaining stages together took about 235 ms in the single central task.

For the peripheral task, the slope of the line relating saccadic latency to discrimination difficulty was about 40 ms. Its zero-intercept was at 145 ms. We can conclude from the last finding that encoding, decision and response organization only took about 145 ms, whereas the comparison of target letter and distractor took about 40 ms more for each (arbitrary) step chosen in the various levels of difficulty. Thus, the peripheral letter discrimination task can be executed between 100 to 200 ms faster than the memory search task in central vision. This corresponds to our expectations based on the different structures of the two SINGLE tasks (see bottom of paragraph (2)). If one compares the zero-intercepts for both tasks, the peripheral task took about 100 ms less than the central task. It would be interesting to determine in future research which of the subprocesses, supposed to be contained in the zero-intercept (encoding, target/non-target decision and response organization), is about 100 ms faster in the peripheral letter discrimination task than in the central memory search task, or whether different stage structures must be assumed for both tasks.

2. Experiment 2: DUAL-task, large eccentricity

In a first dual-task experiment, saccadic latency was measured for 9 dual-task conditions, denoted C1P1 to C3P3. The same design and subjects as in experiments 1a+b were used. The mean latencies (100 trials per condition and subject) were analysed using a 2-factor, repeated measures ANOVA: factor C (central task difficulty): $F(2.6) = 166.37$, $p < .001$; factor P (peripheral task difficulty): $F(2.6) = 6.5$, $p < .05$. The interaction was not significant: $F(2.12) = .442$, n.s. The results are summarized in Table 3 below.

Tab. 3: Summary of the results of DUAL-task experiment 2. Data represent average latencies (in ms) for 4 subjects with about 400 measures per mean. m represents the grand means. The linear equations relating the data to the experimental conditions are also given.

	P1	P2	P3	m	linear equations PERIPHERAL	linear equations CENTRAL
C1	344.6	387.1	441.7	391.2	C1: Y = 48.5X + 294	P1: Y = 78.8X + 270
C2	436.4	490.5	564.6	497.2	C2: Y = 64.1X + 369	P2: Y = 71.6X + 326
C3	502.3	530.4	618.7	550.5	C3: Y = 58.2X + 434	P3: Y = 88.5X + 365
m	427.8	469.3	541.7	497.3		

Discussion of results from experiments 1 and 2

We will now analyse the data of experiments 1 and 2 with regard to the 4 models describing the possible composition of saccadic latency in our dual-task. Table 4 summarizes this analysis. The left part of the table (condition) gives predictions of saccadic latency for each of 8 dual-task conditions with condition C1P1 serving as the baseline. For simplicity, the equation chosen (e.g. C1P2 = C1P1+(P2−P1)) corresponds to model 1 (ADDITIVE), from which the equations for models 2 and 3 can easily be derived (see Table 1). In the middle part of the table (results), the observed latency values were inserted into the equations in the leftmost column. "v" gives the time that must be added to the two other times to give a correct result. It thus represents the prediction error for model 1 (and also gives an estimation of the parameter "v"

Tab. 4: Comparison of the results of DUAL-task experiment 2 with the predictions of model 1. For instance, for condition C2P2 the prediction of model 1 would be: L = 344.6 + 31.1 + 48.9 = 424.6 ms. The observed latency, however, was 490.5 ms, yielding an error of 66 ms (further explanation in the text).

Condition	Results (mean latency, ms)	"v"	Model
baseline: C1P1	344.6		
C1P2=C1P1+(P2-P1)	387.1 = 344.6 + 31.1 +	(11)	2
C1P3=C1P1+(P3-P1)	441.7 = 344.6 + 78.1 +	(19)	2
C2P1=C1P1+(C2-C1)	436.4 = 344.6 + 48.9 +	(43)	2
C3P1=C1P1+(C3-C1)	502.3 = 344.6 + 109.8 +	(48)	2
C2P2=C1P1+(P2-P1)+(C2-C1)	490.5 = 344.6 + 31.1 + 48.9 +	(66)	2
C2P3=C1P1+(P3-P1)+(C2-C1)	564.6 = 344.6 + 78.1 + 48.9 +	(93)	2
C3P2=C1P1+(P2-P1)+(C3-C1)	530.4 = 344.6 + 31.1 + 109.8 +	(45)	2
C3P3=C1P1+(P3-P1)+(C3-C1)	618.7 = 344.6 + 78.1 + 109.8 +	(86)	2

of model 2). The mean error for model 1 (across the 8 conditions) was 51.3 ms with a standard deviation of 29 ms. As concerns model 3 the parameter "w" was only predicted to be negative and to vary with task difficulty. Therefore, we cannot determine prediction errors as for model 1. However, it becomes immediately clear from the data in Table 4 that neither model 1 nor model 3 do predict the data, since in all conditions the obtained total latency is more (and not equal to or less) than the sum of the two component times. As concerns model 4, the prediction errors were computed as in the following example: the latency for, say, condition C2P2, obtained in the dual-task, was 490.5 (see Table 3). However, the maximum latency of conditions C2 and P2 obtained in the single tasks was 339.8 (see Table 2). The resulting error was 150.7 ms. The mean error for model 4 (across the 8 conditions) was 164.3 ms with a standard deviation of 51 ms. Thus, model 4 can also be rejected.

The rightmost column of Table 4 gives the model that fits the data: model 2. This EXTRA-LOAD model assumed that some extra time ("v") has to be added to the sum of the processing times for the central and peripheral single tasks when both are combined in the dual-task. The additional time, presumably reflecting the duration of an inserted extra process, should increase with task difficulty. The values given in column 4 of Table 4 show that "v" indeed increases from about 10 to 20 ms in the easiest conditions (C1P2, C1P3) to about 70 to 90 ms in the most difficult conditions (C2P3, C3P3).

Note that none of the 4 tentative, deterministic models has enough structure to predict absolute latency values. This might be achieved by using more refined models and methods in a follow-up study, for example Schweickert's (1978, 1983) critical path analysis. Nonetheless, as a first approximation, the present models allow to discriminate between the main hypotheses under consideration.

The data shown in Table 2 indicate that the memory scanning rate in the single, CENTRAL task was about 55 ms/item. This is a little more than the classical 38 ms/item observed by Sternberg (1966) using manual reaction times. However, it fits well with the 50 ms/item obtained by Gould (1973) using eye fixation durations. To verify whether an extra-load model best predicts the data, it is helpful to compare this rate to the one observed in the dual-task in order to determine if it is slowed down by the second task (peripheral) being executed together with the (central) memory search task. The result from experiment 2 showing the absence of an interaction between central and peripheral tasks would predict no effect. In the dual task we found slopes between 70 and 80 ms/item depending on the condition, but not being significantly different from each other (see Table 3). Thus, there seems to be a 15 to 25 ms difference with respect to the slopes obtained in the single-task. However, a comparison of the combined data from experiments 1a and 2 indicates that there was no significant interaction between the central and peripheral tasks (ANOVA: $F(6.18) = .665$, n.s.), indicating that the difference observed in the slope values is not significant. This finding shows that the dual-task memory scanning rate and thus the comparison stage of the central task does not interfere with the peripheral task. If we have a look at the PERIPHERAL task, the slope in the single task experiments was about 40 ms (see Table 2), whereas, in the dual-task experiment, the mean slope was about 57 ms (see Table 3). Again, no differences between the combined data from experiments 1b and 2 were found (ANOVA: $F(6.18) = 1.5$, n.s.), leading to the interpretation of an absence of task interference.

Interestingly, this result can be interpreted as showing that memory set size (central task) and discrimination difficulty (peripheral task) do not affect the same stage in the dual-task, i.e. the comparison stage. This is consistent with findings presented below indicating that discrimination difficulty affects the encoding stage. In summary, the present analyses show that the two tasks certainly cannot be executed totally in parallel and that they do not interfere with each other. The results favor the view that the two main processes underlying the dual-task are independent and arranged in series. Note that this does not necessarily imply that all subprocesses are also sequential (see final discussion). Finally, with regard to the structure underlying the single tasks, a new process seems to be inserted in the dual-task whose duration varies with task difficulty. Its function probably is to select a correct response on the basis of the combined output from the two main processes C and P.

3. Experiments 3a+b: SINGLE tasks, small eccentricity

Among the possible explanations for the results obtained in the preceding experiments, the idea that the relatively wide spatial separation of the two tasks might have prevented a more efficient, overlapping or parallel processing is plausible as well as easy to test. Since Poffenbergers's (1912) observation, many experimental studies have shown that peripheral stimuli are processed with a significant, eccentricity-dependent delay relative to central stimuli (e.g. Eriksen & Schultz, 1977; Sterling & Salthouse, 1981). Findings from Holmes et al. (1977) are also in agreement with this view, by suggesting that adult subjects use a "central stimulus first" processing strategy. Compatible quantitative estimates of the delay in processing time for peripheral stimuli exist. Based on data from a word recognition study in peripheral vision, Schiepers (1980) proposed a 90 ms/° delay. In a recent study using simple letter-string stimuli in a localization task, Jacobs (1987c) found a 60 to 100 ms/° delay depending on discrimination difficulty. There seems to be agreement that this delay means that it takes longer for peripheral information to become available to some comparison or decision stage, but that retinal eccentricity does not impair the speed of comparing/deciding between possible stimulus representations (Harris et al., 1979; Sterling & Salthouse, 1981). In short, retinal eccentricity should affect the duration of the encoding stage.

According to these considerations, use of a smaller eccentricity for the peripheral stimuli in the present dual-task might allow faster processing and possibly give rise to overlapping or parallel processing. This idea was tested in the next experiments which used an eccentricity of 3 letter spaces instead of 9, as in the preceding experiments. Thus, peripheral stimuli were still clearly separated from the central stimulus (avoiding lateral masking) without being so far in the periphery that a significant delay in processing should result. If stimulus eccentricity affects the encoding stage, as suggested above, one would expect saccade latency in experiment 3b to be shorter than in experiment 1b. Furthermore, if target/non-target similarity also affects the encoding stage as suggested by the results of experiment 2, then, we would expect smaller effects of target/non-target similarity in experiment 3b than in experiment 1b (or no effect at all).

The following experiments exactly replicated experiments 1a and 1b except for the smaller eccentricity of peripheral stimuli. Note that a replication of experiment 1a (central task) was useful, since a smaller eccentricity was used with smaller saccadic amplitudes that might have influenced their latency. The results of both experiments (3a and b) are summarized in Table 5.

Tab. 5: Summary of the results of SINGLE-task experiments 3a and 3b. Data represent averages over 4 subjects with about 400 measures per mean. The linear equations of the functions relating saccade latency to task difficulty are also given for each single task.

Condition	Latency (ms)	
C1	314.9	Experiment 3a: Central task
C2	322.6	
C3	391.4	Y = 38.3X + 266
P1	187.4	Experiment 3b: Peripheral task
P2	202	
P3	192.4	Y = 2.5X + 188.9

Firstly, Table 5 shows that the data of the single central task of experiments 1a and 3a are consistent. Both show a linear effect of memory set size on saccade latency. The latency effect found in the three conditions of the central task was significant (ANOVA: $F(2,6) = 56.7$, $p < .005$). However, the peripheral task had no significant effect on latency when a small eccentricity was used ($F(2,6) = 3.6$, n.s.). This confirms the above hypothesis that discrimination difficulty (target/non-target similarity) interacts with retinal eccentricity, because both factors affect the encoding stage.

4. Experiment 4: DUAL task, small eccentricity

Experiment 4 replicated the dual-task experiment 2, except for the use of a smaller eccentricity for peripheral stimuli. Results indicated that the central task had a significant effect on saccade latency (ANOVA: $F(2,6) = 16.2$, $p < .025$). No significant effect was found for the peripheral task (ANOVA: $F(2,6) = 4.6$, n.s.). The interaction between both tasks was not significant (ANOVA: $F(4,12) = .58$, n.s.). The data are summarized in Table 6.

Tab. 6: Summary of the results of experiment 4 (DUAL-task). Data represent average latencies (in ms) for 4 subjects with about 400 measures per mean. m represents the grand means. The linear equations relating the data to the experimental conditions are also given.

	P1	P2	P3	m	linear equations PERIPHERAL	linear equations CENTRAL
C1	344.6	397.1	390.7	377.2	C1: Y = 23X + 331	P1: Y = 66X + 283
C2	424.3	449.1	484.7	452.7	C2: Y = 30.2X + 392	P2: Y = 42X + 358
C3	476.6	480.8	537	498.2	C3: Y = 30.2X + 437	P3: Y = 73.2 + 324
m	415.2	442.3	470.8	442.7		

Tab. 7: Comparison of the results of DUAL-task experiment 4 with the predictions of model 1 (cf. Table 4; explanations in the text).

Condition	Results (mean latency, ms)	"v"	Model
baseline: C1P1	344.6		
C1P2=C1P1+(P2-P1)	397.1 = 344.6 + 14.6 +	(38)	2
C1P3=C1P1+(P3-P1)	390.7 = 344.6 + 5.0 +	(41)	2
C2P1=C1P1+(C2-C1)	424.3 = 344.6 + 7.7 +	(72)	2
C3P1=C1P1+(C3-C1)	476.6 = 344.6 + 76.5 +	(55)	2
C2P2=C1P1+(P2-P1)+(C2-C1)	449.1 = 344.6 + 14.6 + 7.7 +	(82)	2
C2P3=C1P1+(P3-P1)+(C2-C1)	484.7 = 344.6 + 5.0 + 7.7 +	(127)	2
C3P2=C1P1+(P2-P1)+(C3-C1)	480.8 = 344.6 + 14.6 + 76.5 +	(45)	2
C3P3=C1P1+(P3-P1)+(C3-C1)	537 = 344.6 + 5.0 + 76.5 +	(111)	2

Note that by an interesting coincidence the latency in the baseline condition (C1P1) was identical in experiments 2 and 4 (see Table 4).

The absence of a significant interaction between the two tasks indicates that, as in experiment 2, they do not interfere and are executed by independent processes. The absence of an effect of the peripheral task agrees with the results of experiment 3b in contrast to those of experiments 1b and 2. It is consistent with the idea of an interaction between target/non-target similarity and retinal eccentricity at the encoding stage.

As in experiments 1 and 2, we used the data of experiment 3 and 4 to test the 4 models of saccadic latency in a dual-task. Table 7 summarizes this analysis. It can be seen from Table 7 that the results of experiment 4 are best accounted for by the extra-load model 2, since in all conditions an additional time "v," which varies with task difficulty, must be added to the equation of model 1. The mean error for model 1 was 71 ms with a standard deviation of 33 ms. The mean error for model 2 must, at least, be as big as for model 1, because of the negative parameter "w." The mean error for model 4 was 108.5 ms with a standard deviation of 32 ms.

These findings agree with the analysis done in Table 4, but go against our hypothesis. It then appears that even if the peripheral stimuli are only 3 letters away from the central stimulus, partial overlap between the two components of the dual-task is not possible.

Discussion

The main question underlying the present study was how saccadic latency is influenced by the durations of different information processings operating in central and peripheral vision. Closely related to this question was the problem of knowing whether a cognitive task in central vision could be executed in parallel with a perceptual task in peripheral vision. Two main results were obtained with regard to these questions. First, in the dual-task experiments, the central and peripheral tasks did not interfere and a parsimonious interpretation of the data is that both tasks are executed by independent processes arranged in series. This did not depend on the eccentricity of the peripheral stimuli since the same pattern of results emerged in experiments 2 and 4 using large and small eccentricities, respectively. Second, a comparison of results from the single and dual-tasks to 4 tentative models of saccadic latency showed that the so-called EXTRA-LOAD model (model 2) best described the data. This model assumed that in the dual-task, the combination of both tasks requires an extra-process which integrates the output of the memory search task with the output of the letter discrimination task into a single response decision. The data of the 4 experiments thus suggest that in the visual dual-task introduced here, saccade latency is composed of three additive, independent components: the time taken to process the central stimulus, the time taken to process the peripheral stimuli, and the time taken to combine the outputs of both processes into a correct response command.

Note that these interpretations concern a level of analysis in which each of two tasks is assumed to be executed by a corresponding process. If one considers the level of subprocesses or stages, however, the interpretation might change. Assuming that each process (C and P) is composed of several stages, for example, the classical 4 stages supposed in the methods section above, one can imagine a partial overlap model that would be compatible with the present findings. For instance, one can easily imagine that both processes overlap during the encoding stage. Since there is convincing evidence for a capacity limited stage at the comparison and/or decision level that can service only one task element at a time (Welford, 1952, 1967; see Kantowitz, 1985, or Schweickert & Boggs, 1984, for recent reviews), one can further imagine that the central stimulus reaches this "bottleneck stage" first (the peripheral information arrives with an eccentricity-dependent delay) and blocks it for a time varying with task difficulty. Finally, one can add the assumption, made in the overlap model by Harris et al. (1979), that although stages may overlap for different stimuli, for a given stimulus, processing is always serial. This means that the encoding stage, for example, can process the central and peripheral stimuli simultaneously, but that the next stage (comparison) can only begin after encoding is completed, and so on. Thus, one can maintain the prediction of additive latency components compatible with the present findings without claiming a strictly serial model, in which even the encoding stage cannot process more than one stimulus at a time. The problem here is that the present experimental design and method used to analyse saccadic latency do not allow a conclusion as to whether such an overlap model is the most suitable and parsimonious of all possibilities. Other experiments are necessary.

First, a promising method for the analysis of the order of processing at the subprocess or stage level is Schweickert's (1978, 1983) generalization of the additive factors method. Use of this method in a slightly modified version of our dual-task should provide information on the structure and duration of combined parallel and serial subprocesses. Second, the present experiments could be redesigned to measure performance (% correct responses) and manual instead of saccadic reaction times. Thus, the absence of interference between the two tasks could be verified in a more general manner, e.g. also by use of performance operating characteristics (Navon & Gopher, 1979; Norman & Bobrow, 1975). Third, an experiment in which either the peripheral or the central stimulus appearance is delayed by some amount of time seems useful. By delaying either of the two sources of information and comparing the observed latencies to those obtained in the present experiments, one might gain further information concerning the exact order of processing (e.g. center-to-periphery), which could not be determined in the present study.

In conclusion, when information from central and peripheral vision has to be combined in order to program a correct saccade and when the central information has to be processed up to a relatively high level (e.g. memory search) while the peripheral information is processed on a lower level (letter discrimination), both the central and peripheral tasks contribute independently of each other to the total latency of a saccade. In addition, an inserted process which presumably combines the output from the processes operating on the central and peripheral stimuli yielding a single response decision also contributes to the total saccadic latency. The results indicate that neither at the level of processes (i.e. central vs. peripheral) nor at the level of subprocesses or stages (i.e. encoding, comparison etc.) can the information processing tasks in central and peripheral vision be executed totally in parallel. Whether, at the level of subprocesses, a strictly serial or a mixed/concurrent model is the best one to account for the results is still to be determined.

It is important to note that the present findings can hardly be generalized to a reading situation. Reading involves highly automatised processes at different levels of which some, at least, go on in parallel. In addition, in reading, saccades are almost permanently (pre)programmed into the same direction. The present dual-task, however, requires a direction decision at each trial, thus maximizing spatial uncertainty. Furthermore, it also involves a (non-automatised) task which is prototypic for serial processing, i.e. the central memory search task. Thus, although the issues of saccade latency decomposition and serial/mixed/parallel processing studied here are important for the study of reading, the present interpretations do not directly apply to reading.

Finally, like others, the present study seems to lead to more questions than to answers. However, besides the introduction of a dual-task useful for decomposing saccadic or manual reaction times, the present paper has merit in that it poses a certain number of open questions concerning information processing during a single eye fixation. Thus, it tries to attract the attention of the researchers working on eye movements to those problems, models and methods central to other fields of cognitive experimental psychology, namely the issues "reaction time decomposition," "serial/parallel stages" and "capacity limitations." A theory of eye movement control in visual search and reading that ignores these issues will be hard to defend.

References

Becker, W., & Jürgens, R., *An analysis of the saccadic system by means of double step stimuli*, Vision Research **19** (1979), 967-983.

Coltheart, M. (Ed.), "Attention & Performance XII: The psychology of reading," Erlbaum, Hillsdale, N.J., 1987.

Davis, R., *The human operator as a single channel information system*, Quarterly Journal of Experimental Psychology **9** (1957), 119-129.

Donders, F.C., *On the speed of mental processes*, in "W.G. Koster (Ed. & Transl.) Attention & Performance II," North-Holland, Amsterdam, 1969. (Original Dutch version published in 1868).

Eriksen, C.W., & Schultz, D.W., *Retinal locus and acuity in visual information processing*, Bulletin of the Psychonomic Society **9** (1977), 81-84.

Eriksen, C.W., & Schultz, D.W., *Information processing in visual search: a continuous flow conception and experimental results*, Perception & Psychophysics **25** (1977), 249-263.

Gough, P., *One second of reading*, in "J.F. Kavanagh & I.G. Mattingly (Eds.), Language by ear and eye," MIT Press, Cambridge, 1972.

Gould, J.D., *Eye movements during visual search and memory search*, Journal of Experimental Psychology **98** (1973), 184-195.

Harris, J.R., Shaw, M.L., & Bates, M., *Visual search in multicharacter arrays with and without gaps*, Perception & Psychophysics **26** (1979), 69-84.

Harvey, L.O., & Gervais, M.J., *Internal representation of visual textures as the basis of judgement of similarity*, Journal of Experimental Psychologie: Human Perception & Performance 7 (1981), 741- 753.

Holmes, D.L., Cohen, K.M., Haith, M.M., & Morrison, F.J., *Peripheral visual processing*, Perception & Psychophysics **22** (1979), 571-577.

Jacobs, A.M., *Eye movement control in visual search: how direct is visual span control?*, Perception & Psychophysics **39** (1986), 47-58.

Jacobs, A.M., *Towards a model of eye movement control in visual search*, in "J.K. O'Regan & A. Lévy-Schoen (Eds.), Eye movements: from physiology to cognition," North-Holland, Amsterdam, 1987a, pp. 275-284.

Jacobs, A.M., *On the role of blank spaces for eye movement control in visual search*, Perception & Psychophysics **41** (1987b), 473- 479.

Jacobs, A.M., *On localization and saccade programming*, Vision Research **27** (1987c), 1953- 1966.

Jacobs, A.M., & Lévy-Schoen, A., *Le contrôle des mouvements des yeux dans la lecture: questions actuelles*, Année Psychologique **37** (1987), 55-72.

Jacobs, A.M., & O'Regan, J.K., *Spatial and/or temporal adjustments of scanning behavior to changes in visibility*, Acta Psychologica **65** (1987), 133-146.

Kantowitz, B.H., *Channels and stages in human information processing: a limited analysis of theory and methodology*, Journal of Mathematical Psychology **29** (1985), 135-174.

Luce, R.D., "Response times," Oxford University Press, Oxford, N.Y., 1986.

Mackworth, N.H., *Visual noise causes tunnel vision*, Psychonomic Science **3** (1965), 67-68.

McClelland, J.L., *On the time relations of mental processes: an examination of processes in cascade*, Psychological Review **86** (1979), 287-330.

McLeod, P., *Parallel processing and the psychological refractory period*, Acta Psychologica **41** (1977), 381-396.

Miller, J., *Discrete versus continuous stage models of human information processing: in search of partial output*, Journal of Experimental Psychology: Human Perception & Psychophysics **8** (1982), 273-296.

Navon, D., & Gopher, D., *On the economy of the human information processing system*, Psychological Review **86** (1979), 214- 255.

Nazir, T.A., Heller, O., & Jacobs, A.M., *Eine Buchstabendiskriminationsmatrix für das periphere Sehen: zeitliche Faktoren*, in "Bericht über die 29. Tagung der experimentell arbeitenden Psychologen," Aachen, 1987, p. 181.

Norman, D.A., & Bobrow, D.G., *On data-limited and resource-limited processes*, Cognitive Psychology **7** (1975), 44-64.

O'Regan, J.K., Lévy-Schoen, A., & Jacobs, A., *The effect of visibility on eye movement parameters in reading*, Perception & Psychophysics **34** (1983), 457-464.

Poffenberger, A.T., *Reaction time to retinal stimulation with special reference to the time lost in conduction through nerve centers*, Archives of Psychology **23** (1912), 1-73.

Rayner, K., Inhoff, A.W., Morrison, R.E., Slowiaczek, M.L., & Bertera, J.H., *Masking foveal and parafoveal vision during eye fixations in reading*, Journal of Experimental Psychology: Human Perception & Performance **7** (1981), 165-179.

Rayner, K., & Fisher, D., *Letter processing during eye fixations in visual search*, Perception & Psychophysics **42** (1987), 87-100.

Sanders, A.F., *Stage analysis of reaction processes*, in "G.E. Stelmach & J. Requin (Eds.), Tutorials in Motor Behavior," North-Holland, Amsterdam, 1980.

Schiepers, C., *Response latency and accuracy in visual word recognition*, Perception & Psychophysics **27** (1980), 71-81.

Schweickert, R., *A critical path generalization of the additive factor method: analysis of a stroop task*, Journal of Mathematical Psychology **18** (1978), 105-139.

Schweickert, R., *Latent network theory: scheduling of mental processes in sentence verification and the stroop effect*, Journal of Experimental Psychology: Learning, Memory and Cognition **9** (1983), 353- 383.

Schweickert, R., & Boggs, G.J., *Models of central capacity and concurrency*, Journal of Mathematical Psychology **28** (1984), 223- 281.

Smith, E.E., *Choice reaction time: an analysis of the major theoretical positions*, Psychological Bulletin **69** (1968), 77-110.

Sperling, G., & Melchner, M.J., *Visual search, visual attention and the attention operating characteristic*, in "J. Requin (Ed.), Attention & Performance VII," Erlbaum, Hillsdale, N.J., 1978.

Sterling, J.J., & Salthouse, T.A., *Retinal location and visual processing rate*, Perception & Psychophysics **30** (1981), 114- 118.

Sternberg, S., *High speed scanning in human memory*, Science **153** (1966), 652-654.

Sternberg, S., *The discovery of processing stages: extensions of Donder's method*, Acta Psychologica **37** (1969), 139-154.

Taylor, D.A., *Stage analysis of reaction time*, Psychological Bulletin **83** (1976), 161-191.

Tolkmitt, F.J., *A revision of the psychological refractory period*, Acta Psychologica **37** (1973), 139-154.

Townsend, J.T., & Ashby, F.G., "Stochastic modeling of elementary psychological processes," Cambridge University Press, Cambridge, N.Y., 1983.

Welford, A.T., *The psychological refractory period and the timing of high speed performance - a review and a theory*, British Journal of Psychology **43** (1952), 2-19.

Welford, A.T., *Single channel operation in the brain*, Acta Psychologica **27** (1967), 5-22.

EFFECT OF PARAFOVEAL PREPROCESSING AND READING RHYTHM ON OPTIMAL LANDING POSITION IN WORDS OF DIFFERENT LENGTH AND FREQUENCY

FRANÇOISE VITU AND J. KEVIN O'REGAN

Groupe Regard, Laboratoire de Psychologie Expérimentale
C.N.R.S., Université René Descartes, E.H.E.S.S.
E.P.H.E., Paris

In reading, fixation durations vary between about 150 and 500 ms. This fairly large variability may be explained by factors such as frequency, length of words, syntax, context, and parafoveal preprocessing. However, in our opinion, a more important factor that has not been previously considered may actually be the main source of variability. This factor is the eye's first fixation position in a word. A recent series of experiments suggests the effect of this factor on fixation and gaze durations on a word.

The experiments (O'Regan, Lévy-Schoen, Pynte, & Brugaillère, 1984; Holmes & O'Regan, 1987; O'Regan & Lévy-Schoen, 1987), use the following paradigm. The subject sits in front of a computer screen wearing a photoelectric device that monitors horizontal eye movements. The computer displays a fixation mark on the screen. When the computer detects that the subject is fixating his eyes on the mark, it displays a group of words at the fixated position. The test word is the first of the group, and it is located at the position occupied by the fixation mark, with the remaining words on the right. The variable manipulated in these experiments is the position of the test word relative to the initial fixation mark. Thus, the test word may appear laterally displaced a few letters to the right or to the left relative to the fixation mark in such a way that on the word's appearence, the eye is fixating the word's first, second, third, etc., or last letter.

The experiments showed that an "optimal" or "convenient" landing position in a word exists: the eye must fixate this position first in order to recognize the word most efficiently. The effect is illustrated in Figure 1. The ordinate of this Figure gives the "gaze duration" on the test word, that is, the total time the eye spends on the test word before moving on to the next word. The gaze duration is plotted as a function of the position the eye initially was fixating relative to the word middle at the moment the word appeared. The different curves correspond to French test words of length 5, 7, 9 and 11 letters. Two graphs

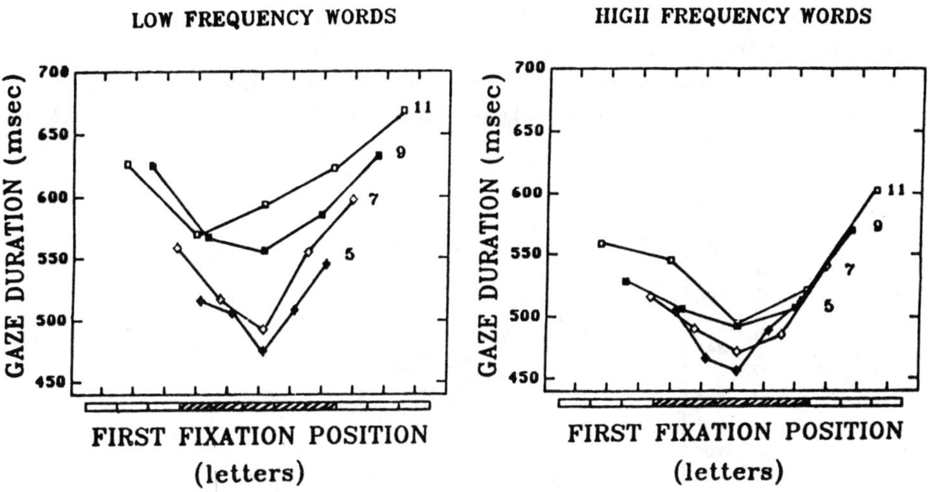

Fig. 1: Data from O'Regan and Lévy-Schoen (1987). Gaze duration (total time spent fixating a word before moving on to an adjacent word) is plotted as a function of the position the eye was fixating in the word when the word appeared on the computer screen (The blocks beneath the abscissa indicate letter positions in the words. Examples are given for 11-letter words (white blocks) and for 5-letter words (shaded blocks). Data are given for words of 5,7,9 and 11 letter length and either high or low frequency of occurrence in the language (French).

are shown, one for words of high frequency of occurrence (115 per million) in french, and one for low frequency of occurrence (2 per million).

It is evident from Figure 1 that the time it takes to recognize the word very strongly depends on the position the eye starts fixating on the word. There is an optimal viewing position where gaze duration is shortest. For example, for nine letter, low frequency words, this position is near the middle of the word. When the eye starts fixating to the left or to the right of this optimal position, gaze durations are considerably longer. We see that the penalty for not starting to fixate the word at the optimal position is 20 ms per letter of deviation from the optimal position. For other word lengths, similar penalties are found. Further analysis of the data showed that the penalty arises because, when the eye starts far from the optimal position, more fixations tend to be made on the word.

An important point concerning this and previous work is the fact that the optimal viewing position phenomenon has been demonstrated in a situation in which subjects read an *isolated* word which appears "underneath" the eye at different positions. The question arises whether a similar phenomenon can be demonstrated in normal, continuous reading. Some unpublished data of Blanchard and McConkie (presented in O'Regan & Lévy-Schoen, 1987), replotted in Figure 2, speak to this issue. In this experiment, subjects read long texts under fairly normal reading conditions while their eye movements were monitored. The graph shows the gaze duration on words of different lengths, (but not controlling for word frequency), as a function of the initial position where the eye landed in the word.

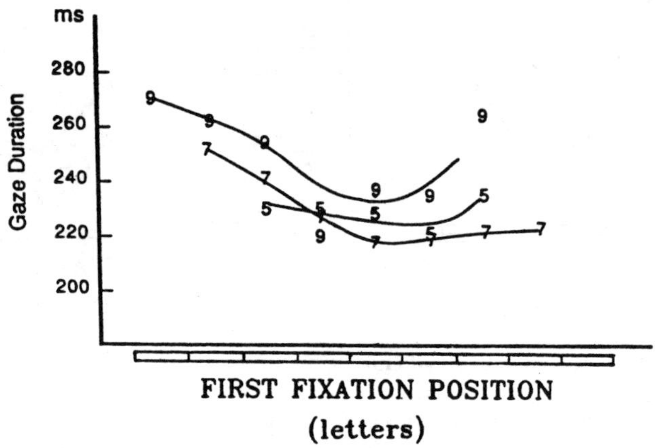

Fig. 2: Data replotted from O'Regan and Lévy-Schoen (1987), giving the results of Blanchard and McConkie's experiment on continuous reading. Total gaze duration, (time spent until leaving the word), is plotted as a function of the position upon which the eye first landed in the word (measured relative to the word's middle). Data are given for words of different length. Note that in this experiment, contrary to Figure 1, the frequency of the different word lengths was not controlled for.

As was the case for our data on recognition of isolated words, the Blanchard and McConkie data show that even in normal reading, there is an optimal viewing position in words. But there is an important difference: the penalty for not starting to fixate the optimal viewing position is much smaller in normal reading than in reading isolated words. Instead of being 20 ms per letter of deviation from the optimal viewing position, as found earlier, it is now only 9 ms per letter of deviation.

EXPERIMENT

The present experiment's purpose is to determine why the optimal viewing position phenomenon is weaker in normal reading. The difference between normal reading and recognizing isolated words may be due to additional factors that intervene in reading. Here we investigated two such factors, namely, reading rhythm and parafoveal preprocessing.

Reading rhythm may diminish the effect of first fixation position in the word: some kind of forward-moving reading strategy might prevent within-word refixations from occuring even if the eye lands in a non-optimal position. The average gaze durations would thus depend less strongly on the eye's initial fixation location in words.

Parafoveal preview might also modify the phenomenon of optimal viewing position. If a word has been partially preprocessed in the parafovea, then the need to make additional fixations in the word when the eye lands in a non-optimal position, may be reduced. This amounts to decreasing the penalty for not starting to fixate at the optimal viewing position.

To test if reading rhythm and/or preview contribute to the diminution of the phenomenon of optimal viewing position observed in continuous reading, we used the following method.

To introduce a reading rhythm, we simulated left-to-right reading conditions. Subjects had to read the test word after sequentially fixating two spaced-out asterisks and before moving to a comparison word placed at the test word's right. The task was to decide whether the test word was identical to the comparison word (Figure 3). If reading rhythm is an important factor, we expect that the penalty for not starting to fixate on the optimal viewing position will be smaller than in isolated word studies.

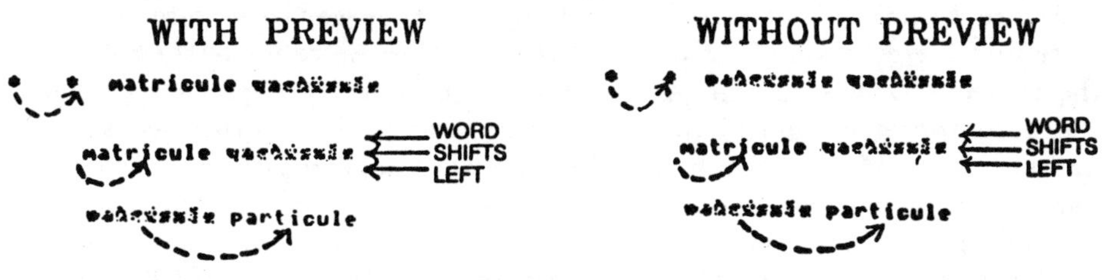

Fig. 3: Sequence of events for the experiment "with" and "without" preview conditions. The eye is fixating on the left asterisk and moves to the next asterisk. The eye then moves into the test word. During the saccade, the computer may shift the test word laterally so that the eye arrives at a different position from where it would normally arrive. In the example shown here, the word shifts two letters leftwards. After fixating on the word, the eye moves into the comparison word. The "with preview" condition is shown on the left, for which, when the eye is on the second asterisk, the word is visible in the parafovea. The "without preview" condition is shown on the right, for which the test word is masked by random dots while the eye is on the second asterisk. The random dots disappear and the word becomes visible only during the saccade leading to the test word.

To examine the role of parafoveal preview, we chose two parafoveal word presentation conditions: one in which the word was visible in the parafovea before being fixated and so could be preprocessed, and another in which the word in the parafovea was masked and so could not be preprocessed.

A further manipulation was necessary. The eye normally lands near the middle of words. Thus, in order to have data for other initial fixation positions in the word, we used the following technique. After the subject had successively fixated two asterisks and before he moved on to the test word, when the computer detected a saccade in the direction of the test word, the computer displaced the test word laterally to the right or to the left by a few letters (Figure 3).

Finally, note that the test word was masked out by random dots when the eye moved into the comparison word. This was done so that the word could not be further visually processed when the eye had left it.

We used words of two lengths (5 and 9) and of two frequencies (high and low). We used these lengths and frequencies for comparison with our previous work, in which we also had used a variety of frequencies and word lengths.

Results

The purpose of this experiment was to see if the optimal viewing position phenomenon became weaker in the present conditions in which we induced a reading rhythm, and whether the phenomenon was also weaker when there was a parafoveal preview than when there was not.

Figure 4 shows the results, plotted in the same way as Figure 1. Consider first the question of reading rhythm. For this, we compare the results of the previous experiment, in which there was no parafoveal preview (because the word appeared "under" the eye) and no reading rhythm (because the eye had been fixating a fixation mark when the word appeared), to the "without" parafoveal preview condition of the present experiment, in which there was again no parafoveal preview but, this time, a reading rhythm induced by successive fixation of the asterisks prior to the test word's appearance. The results for this condition are shown as solid lines in Figure 4. Due to the way the test word shifted as the eye saccaded into it, data is unfortunately not available for landing positions near the very end of the word.

The solid curves in Figure 4, for 5 and 9-letter words as well as for high and low frequency words, are remarkably similar to the data from the earlier experiment in Figure 1. In particular, there is an optimal viewing position in both experiments. In addition, the penalty for not starting to fixate this position is of the same order in both experiments, about 20 ms per letter of deviation from the optimal position. Therefore, reading rhythm appears not to diminish the strength of the phenomenon of optimal viewing position.

The effect of parafoveal preview on the optimal viewing position phenomenon can be ascertained by comparing the solid "without preview" lines in Figure 4 to the dashed "with preview" lines. First, it can be seen that the solid lines are above the dashed lines. There is a global 50 ms time saving obtained from

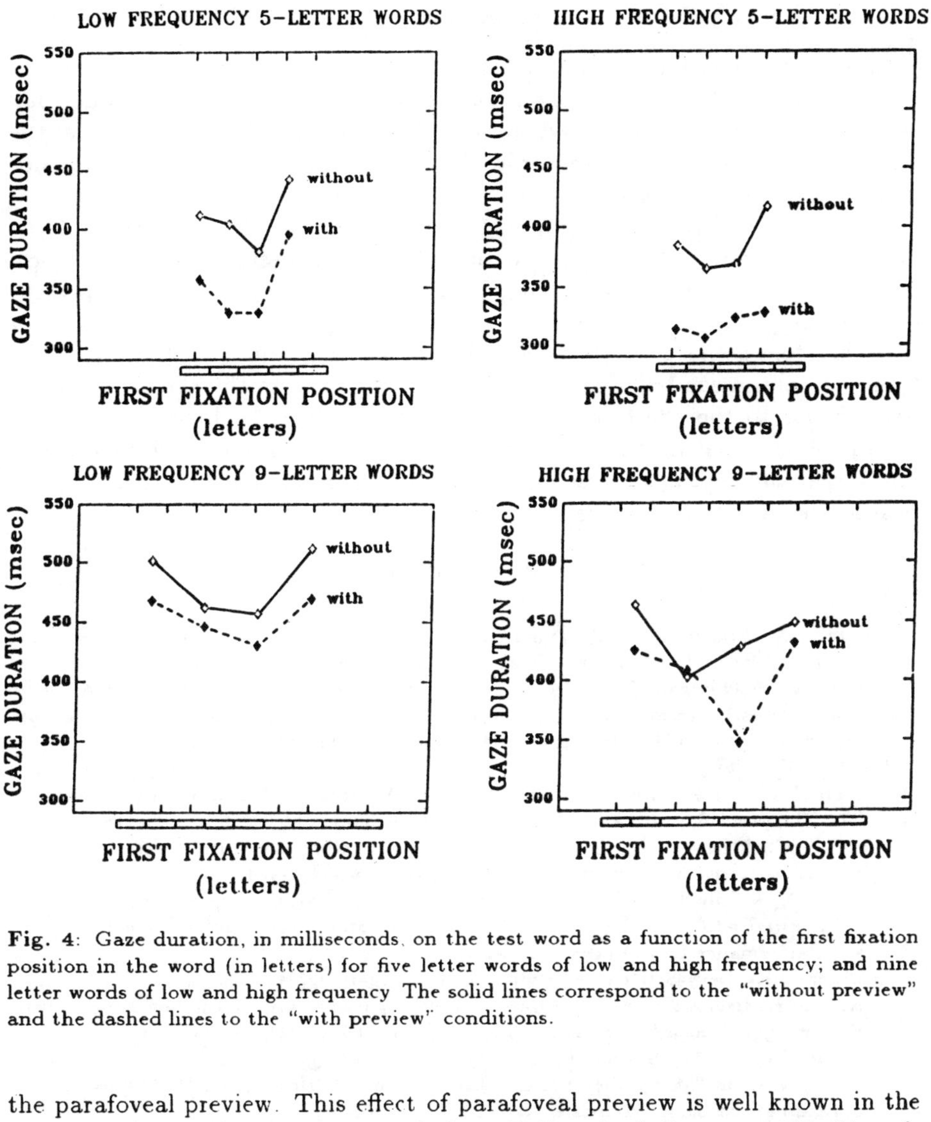

Fig. 4: Gaze duration, in milliseconds, on the test word as a function of the first fixation position in the word (in letters) for five letter words of low and high frequency; and nine letter words of low and high frequency. The solid lines correspond to the "without preview" and the dashed lines to the "with preview" conditions.

the parafoveal preview. This effect of parafoveal preview is well known in the literature (Inhoff & Rayner, 1980; Balota, Pollatsek, & Rayner, 1985; Lima & Inhoff, 1985; Inhoff, 1987). But, second and more interesting for the question raised by the present experiment, there is still an optimal viewing position in the "with preview" condition and the penalty for not starting to fixate it is as pronounced as in the "without preview" condition: 20 ms per letter of deviation. The data for the other word lengths and frequencies show similar results.

Conclusion

As was true for Blanchard and McConkie's data, the present data confirm the existence of the optimal viewing position in a situation similar to normal, continuous reading. However, whereas in Blanchard and McConkie's data, the strength of the effect was weaker with a penalty of 9 ms per letter for not fixating the optimal position, here, the penalty was 20 ms per letter, similar to findings in earlier experiments using isolated words. This was true both in experimental conditions with and without parafoveal preview of the test word, and despite the fact that a reading rhythm had been induced in the present experiment.

It therefore seems that the weakness of the penalty in Blanchard and McConkie's continuous text reading data is neither due to the effect of reading rhythm nor to the effect of parafoveal preview. This leads to the interesting hypothesis that it may be the case that it is *linguistic context*, facilitating parafoveal and central processing, that makes fixation at the optimal viewing position less critical in normal reading.

References

Balota, D.A., Pollatsek, A., & Rayner, K., *The interaction of contextual constraints and parafoveal visual information in reading*, Cognitive Psychology **17** (1985), 364-390.

Holmes, V., & O'Regan, J.K., *Decomposing french words*, in "J.K. O'Regan & A. Lévy-Schoen (Eds.), Eye movements. From physiology to cognition." Elsevier Science Publishers B.V., North Holland, Amsterdam, 1987, pp. 459-466.

Inhoff, A.W., *Parafoveal word perception during eye fixations in reading: Effects of perceptual salience and word structure*, in "M. Coltheart (Ed.), Attention and Performance XII. The psychology of reading," Erlbaum, Hillsdale, N.J., 1987, pp. 403-418.

Inhoff, A.W., & Rayner, K., *Parafoveal word perception: A case against semantic preprocessing*, Perception and Psychophysics **27** (5) (1980), 457-464.

Lima, S.D., & Inhoff, A.W., *Lexical access during eye fixations in reading: Effects of word-initial letter sequence*, Journal of Experimental Psychology. Human Perception and Performance **11** (3) (1985), 272-285.

O'Regan, J.K., Lévy-Schoen. A., Pynte, J., & Brugaillère, B., *Convenient fixation location within isolated words of different length and structure*, Journal of Experimental Psychology: Human Perception and Performance **10** (1984), 250-257.

O'Regan, J.K., & Lévy-Schoen, A., *Eye movement strategy and tactics in word recognition and reading*, in "M. Coltheart (Ed.), Attention and Performance XII: The psychology of reading," Erlbaum, Hillsdale, N.J., 1987, pp. 363-383.

6
Eye Movement Research in Perception and Cognition

EYE MOVEMENTS, ATTENTION AND VISUAL INFORMATION PROCESSING: SOME EXPERIMENTAL RESULTS AND METHODOLOGICAL CONSIDERATIONS

RUDOLF GRONER

Psychologisches Institut, Universität Bern

INTRODUCTION

One might start with an apparently naive question: why are eye movements with corresponding shifts of attention necessary? The functional significance of eye movements is closely related to the anatomy of the retina. The foveola, a small central region of less than 0.5 degree of visual angle, is composed of densely packed cone receptors, allowing for much higher resolution as compared with the peripheral visual field. It has also been shown (Spillman, 1971) that the size of the perceptive fields, as well as the size of the receptive fields, strongly increase from the center to the periphery. The same holds with the size of the cortical areas associated with central and peripheral regions of the visual field (Rovamo & Hirsu, 1979). Therefore, spatial resolution can be increased by projecting an image on different retinal areas via body locomotion and/or eye movements.

However, in addition, several researchers proposed that there is a qualitative difference between central and peripheral vision, involving two different systems. For example, focal versus ambient vision (Trevarthen, 1968), identifying versus locating mode (Held et al., 1967; see also Ungerleider & Mishkin, 1982), sustained versus transient mechanisms (Breitmeyer & Ganz, 1976), feature extraction versus object identification (Treisman, 1979; Treisman & Gelade, 1980), or attentive versus preattentive vision (Julesz, 1984).

Due to the space restrictions only a selective review is presented in the following sections. First we will consider the current usage of the term attention and then look at those studies relating it to saccadic eye movements. In the last section, the scope of the review will be extended from studies with single saccades or fixations as a dependent variable to those with several fixations (scanpaths).

THE NOTION OF "ATTENTION" IN EXPERIMENTAL PSYCHOLOGY

For earlier generations of experimental psychologists (e.g. Düker, 1955), the concept of attention was very dubious because of its circularity between empirical phenomenon and theoretical construct. For example, if a subject recalls an element of a learning-list, one can describe the result as an empirical finding.

However, one can not simultaneously describe the results in terms of behavior by stating that it is dependent on "attention." From this perspective, the question of attention eliciting a saccadic response is nonsensical or tautological.

I think, there were at least two reasons for the popularizing of the term attention in psychology. First, there was a change from the behavioristic to the cognitivist paradigm, allowing for a more functionalist view on psychological phenomena. Second, some experimental demonstrations became very well-known (Posner et al., 1980; Jonides, 1976), showing that the precueing of the location of a stimulus leads to an advantage in detection performance and reaction latency. Subsequently, the term attention came very much into fashion, although I think, one has to be careful of an unreflected use of this concept.

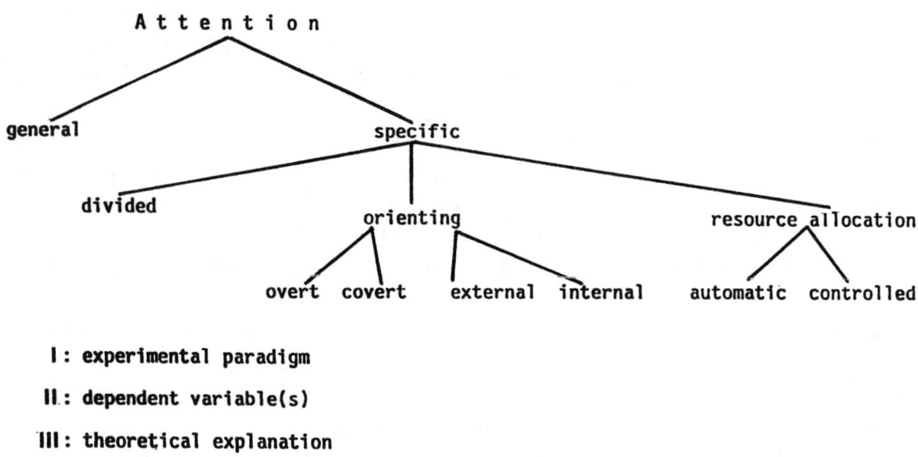

Fig. 1: Some fields of research in attention.

Figure 1 gives an outline of some of the usages of the term attention in current psychology. First, one should note attention in the sense of general state of wakefulness or alertness in an organism (more accurately described by the term "arousal"). Attention in the sense of arousal level was investigated in the late fifties and early sixties (Magoun, 1963; Duffy, 1962) in connection with the study of the reticular activation system which serves as a regulatory control mechanism over brain activity. Although there are some studies relating saccadic activity to arousal level (e.g. Hinton, 1982), we will not cover this aspect but rather focus on issues of selective attention. Although no general definition exists, Posner's (1980) description of attention, as an alignment of the sensory input, is closest to the gist of most recent studies. We can distinguish between paradigms with divided attention, that is, those in which information is presented simultaneously on competing channels, from paradigms with orienting attention. Dependent on what causes the orienting, we can distinguish between overt and covert orienting attention. Overt orienting refers to a change in the alignment of the sensory receptors (e.g. eye and/or head movements). Jonides (1981) defined covert attention as "the control of the mind's eye movement." The difference between these two categories lies in the kind of dependent variabe used. In overt orienting attention experiments, the dependent variables are behavioral measures, such as saccades. Experiments investigating covert orienting attention have to rely on indirect performance measures. A further distinction has been drawn between externally and internally controlled orienting. This distinction is very close to the characterization of data-driven (bottom-up) versus stimulus-driven (top-down) processing (e.g. Kahneman, 1973; Norman & Bobrow, 1975). A final issue concerning attention is the notion of resource allocation or limited capacity (Shiffrin & Schneider, 1977; Navon & Gopher, 1979; Wickens, 1984). While automatic processing is assumed to tap less from the pool of resources, controlled processing requires much more from the hypothetical resources' pool.

The above categorization of attention (after Johnston & Dark, 1985) could be criticized for two reasons: (1) the aspects involved are not independent of each other. (For example, divided attention can be conceived as a consequence of a particular resource allocation.) (2) This categorization mixes different aspects in an uncontrolled manner (theoretical or explanatory principles are mixed with different experimental paradigms). These shortcomings could be avoided by a three-dimensional classification with the factors (I) experimental paradigm, (II) dependent variable, and (III) theoretical explanation (see bottom of Fig. 1).

In the following, a brief review of some relevant findings in attention research will be presented, first focusing on studies with dependent variables other than eye movements, and then on issues of attention and its relation to the control of eye movements.

Studies of Shifts of Covert Attention

It has been an old question in psychology whether it is possible to shift attention independent of eye movements. For instance, Helmholtz (1909) stated that "it is possible, simply by an conscious and voluntary effort, to focus attention on some definite spot in a field," as was also argued by Wundt who claimed that it is possible to separate the line of fixation from the line of attention. However, until the mid-seventies, most experimental studies (e.g. Mowrer, 1941; Mertens, 1956; Grindley & Townsend, 1968; Shiffrin & Gardner, 1972) failed to demonstrate this claim. After 1972, a number of studies appeared with evidence which demonstrated that shifts of attention occurred in the absence of eye movements (Eriksen & Hoffman, 1973; Jonides, 1976; Posner, Nissen, &

Ogden, 1972; Posner, Snyder, & Davidson, 1980, etc.). The following example is typical of its genre and greatly influenced research in this area: A visual target appeared either to the right or left of a fixation point. It was preceded by a cue which was either a plus sign or an arrow pointing to the right or left. If the plus sign was presented, the target was equally likely to occur to the left or right of the fixation point. If an arrow was presented, the probability was 80% that the detection stimulus would occur on the indicated side (i.e. the cue was most often a valid one) and 20% that it would occur on the other side (most often an invalid one). Thus, it was possible to examine both the benefits from knowing where in space the stimulus will occur, and the cost when it occurs at the position other than the expected position. Compared with the control condition (with only a plus sign), it was shown, that a decrease of manual reaction time occurred under the valid cue condition and an increase under the invalid condition (Posner et al., 1978). A trivial explanation of this phenomenon would be that the difference in reaction time is due to the latency of an eye movement saccade which is produced when target and cues are on opposite sides, but not if they are on the same side. I do not intend to seriously maintain this alternative explanation, not only because it seems too simple, but also because it was explicitely discarded by Posner who, however, did not always control fixation by means of an eye movement monitor.

One might expect that attention should also correlate with retinal eccentricity. However, Posner (1978) found that costs and benefits from attention did not vary much with stimuli ranging from 0.5 to 25 degrees eccentricity, which is especially astonishing for the within-fovea condition and in disagreement with Engel (1971). Engel required subjects to locate a single form (two lines converging) embedded in a complex visual field. He provided both a fixation point and a point away from fixation where attention was to be concentrated. He found the field of highest acuity (in Engel's terms: conspicuity) for the ability to identify the target included the fovea but elongated in the direction of the subject's attention.

The difference between Engel's and Posner's results might be due to the fact that Engel's task required high visual acuity and Posner's conditions are simple detection tasks well above threshold where there is still enough spatial resolution of the receptors far in the periphery. According to Posner, although attentional orientation to the periphery allows detection to occur more quickly, it will not provide an increase in the retinal resolution and therefore does not produce any changes in acuity. According to Posner et al. (1980), attention represents a system for routing information and for control of priorities; it provides an alignment and not a sensitization. (For another perspective on this question, see Groner, Groner, & Hofer, 1986.)

Posner's view of attention is compatible with Norman's (1968) metaphor referring to attention as a kind of spotlight with an adjustable beam. There is even some evidence that the beam can be split. For example, Egly and Homa (1984) instructed subjects to fixate at the center of a grid consisting of 3 concentric rings with diameters of 2, 4, and 6 degrees of visual angle. Two letters were presented for 30-60 ms and then followed by a pattern mask. One letter was displayed in the center of the diplay and the other, the displaced letter, appeared in one of 8 positions on one of the rings. Subjects had to report which letter was in the center (which they did with 95% accuracy) and then to localize the displaced letter. As in Posner's experiments, accuracy of localization of the displaced letter was facilitated by valid precueing of the ring on which it appeared and inhibited by invalid precueing. The most relevant result was found with invalid precueing. Let us consider the case in which the middle ring is precued but the displaced letter actually is on either the inner or the outer ring. If precueing of the middle ring causes the attentional spotlight to expand just enough to contain the middle ring, then the miscued letter is going to fall either inside or outside the spotlight, and accuracy of localization of the letter should change accordingly. In fact, the cost of miscueing was just as great when the letter was on the inner ring as when it was on the outer ring. These data indicated that attention could be split. Analogous results of "splitting the attentional beam" into more than one sensitive area have been reported by Lambert (1987) and Müller and Findlay (in press).

The spotlight metaphor was also extended to movements in space and time. Shulman, Remington, and McLean (1979) investigated the temporal properties of movement of the attentional spotlight across a visual field. They asked whether a visual detection stimulus (that occurred on less than 10% of the trials at a position between the fixation point and a target), would show facilitation in latency at a time intermediate between leaving the home position and reaching the target. They expected reaction time at this position first to improve relative to the target, as attention moved through it, and then to increase. Each trial started with an arrow which cued subjects to move attention to a visible target 18 degrees from the fixation point. At varying intervals following this cue, detection stimuli were presented. The detection stimuli occurred on 75% of the trials. The remainder served as catch trials. On trials in which there was a detection stimulus, it occurred at the designated target 70% of the time (for expected position). At each other location, at either the intermediate position on the cued side (near expected), or at a position opposite the target, or at an intermediate point on the side opposite the target (near unexpected), it appeared with a probability of 10%.

Figure 2 shows the results of the Shulman et al. study. On the abscissa, the stimulus onset asynchrony (SOA), that is, the interval between cue and target, is plotted, on the ordinate the manual reaction time. All curves are u-shaped with a minimum latency of 350 ms (which represents the most efficient warning time). A surprising result is that the lowest line with the shortest reaction times

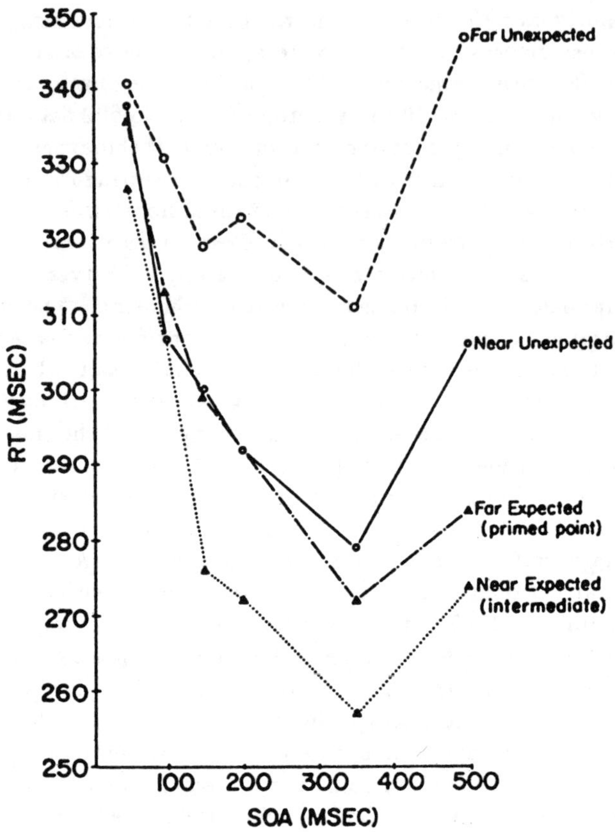

Fig. 2: Reaction time as a function of stimulus onset asynchrony (SOA) for the expected and unexpected locations. Source: Shulman, Remington, & McLean, 1979. Copyright 1979 by the American Psychological Association. Reprinted by permission.

comes from the near expected condition intermediate between fixation point and target. The primed point or far expected condition was the one which was attention directed, and follows next with a somewhat longer reaction time. This time course was interpreted as evidence for the temporal movement of attention from the fixation to target position. Not fully compatible with this hypothesis, is the result of the near unexpected condition which coincides (up to an SOA of 350 ms) with the primed point condition, although its spatial distance from the attended target is relatively large. Although not in line with Posner's hypothesis, this effect could be accounted for in terms of foveal eccentricity, that is, reaction time is faster for stimuli closer to the fovea.

In their experimental series, Remington and Pierce (1948) used as a precue an arrow that appeared above a fixation point, and targets occurred at a precueing validity of 80% either to the right or to the left along a horizontal meridian at eccentricities of 2 or 10 degrees, consisting of small dots to which the subjects had to respond as quickly as possible. The onset of the precue was separated from the target by SOAs ranging from 16 to 600 ms. However, since eye movements were not controlled in this study, the main conclusions were based on SOAs of less than 250 ms. In order to estimate the effect of retinal eccentricity on attention shifts for each SOA, reaction times to the cued-near-location were subtracted from those of the cued-far-location. They concluded that the findings were not compatible with a fixed velocity analog model and interpreted the data to indicate that the attentional focus either moved at a speed proportional to the distance to be traveled, or, as an alternative interpretation, that the attentional focus moved in a discrete shift independent of the distance to be traversed.

With a similar experiment, Tsal (1983) arrived at quite different conclusions. The subjects were given a choice reaction time task in which they had to discriminate the letter X from the letter O at eccentricities of 4, 8, and 12 degrees. As a precue, a small dot appeared close to the subsequent target location at an SOA between 50 and 183 ms. Correlating the functions of reaction times at different SOAs and target locations, it was concluded "that the SOA facilitated performance via movements of attention at a constant velocity" (p. 526). This was estimated to be approximately 8 ms per degree of visual angel.

The conclusions of Tsal, Shulman et al., and Remington and Pierce, have been questioned by Eriksen and Murphy (1987). They argued that in most of these studies, at least, five variables have been neglected that determine the shape and parameter of the reaction time - SOA function: (1) the time required to perceive the cue and its location, (2) the latency of initiating the attentional relocation, (3) the time required for the relocation to occur, (4) individual differences and (5) general signal- or warning effects. The authors conclude with a caveat: "How attention shifts from one locus to another in the visual field is still an open question. Not only is the experimental evidence conflicting, but the experiments are based on a string of tenuous assumptions that render interpretations of the data quite problematic. This reflects not so much on the design of the experiments as on the uncertain state of our knowledge of the phenomena of attention." (p. 305)

The Relation between Attentional Processes and Eye Movements

Goldberg and Wurtz (1972), by performing single cell recordings in the superior colliculus of monkeys, showed an increase in firing rate whose receptive field was to be the target for an eye movement when the eyes began to move.

Initially, Goldberg and Wurtz brought this system into connection with a general attention mechanism. Wurtz and Mohler (1976) demonstrated that other methods of producing attention did not produce an increase in firing rate of collicular cells. These and similar findings led Wurtz and Mohler to propose that attention shifts were programs for the movement of the eyes.

The results already reported have shown that attentional processes could be elicited without any concomitant eye movements. However, that attentional processes and the elicitation of concomitant eye movements are two completely independent systems is quite unlikely. For example, Gopher (1973) observed that subjects, during dichotic listening tasks, made large saccades followed by long fixations in the direction of the attended ear. This result was interpreted that subjects were utilizing eye movements to emphasize the desired direction of attention.

A more moderate view, already mentioned in connection with Wurtz and Mohler, assumes that attention shifts are programs for eye movement (facilitation hypothesis). Klein (1980) states this position as follows: "When attention to a particular location is desired, the observer prepares to make an eye movement to that location; the oculomotor readiness, via as yet unknown feedforward pathways, has the effect of enhancing processing in or from sensory pathways dealing with information from the target location." He asked the following questions: (1) Whether allocating attention to a position would facilitate making an eye movement to that position, and (2) whether making an eye movement would facilitate manual responses to stimuli at the target position for the eye movement. The subjects were given a cue as to where to shift attention and then were commanded either to move their eyes or to report a detection stimulus by pressing a key. Each trial began with a cue. There were two kinds of trials: On eye movement trials, an asterisk appeared to the left or right of fixation. On detection trials, the subject had to respond to a luminance increment by pressing a key. Klein's results did not support either hypothesis: Subjects moved their eyes equally fast in the direction and away from the directions of attention. Furthermore, the detection task was totally unaffected by the direction in which the subjects moved their eyes. These results clearly showed that, under certain conditions, there was no relationship between spatial attention and eye movement latencies. However, these experiments involved a relatively unnatural discrimination which resulted in very long saccade latencies and reaction times. Under more normal conditions, one might get different results.

This experimental design was used by Remington (1980) in order to study the mutual interaction between covered attentional processes and overt saccadic behavior. Using a display consisting of five illuminated squares (subtending a total of 20 degrees of visual angle), subjects had to detect a luminance increase in one of the squares. In addition, a fixation cross appeared on either the middle or one of the outermost squares. Independent variables were: (1) the SOA between the onset of the fixation cue and luminance change which could range from 0 to 500 ms and (2) the position where the luminance change took place, which could be either the target location of the fixation cross (the outer squares) the inner squares or the one in the middle. As a dependent variable, Remington used the hit rate. However, a better measure would have been the difference between hits and false alarms, but that was impossible since the position of responses could not be detected.

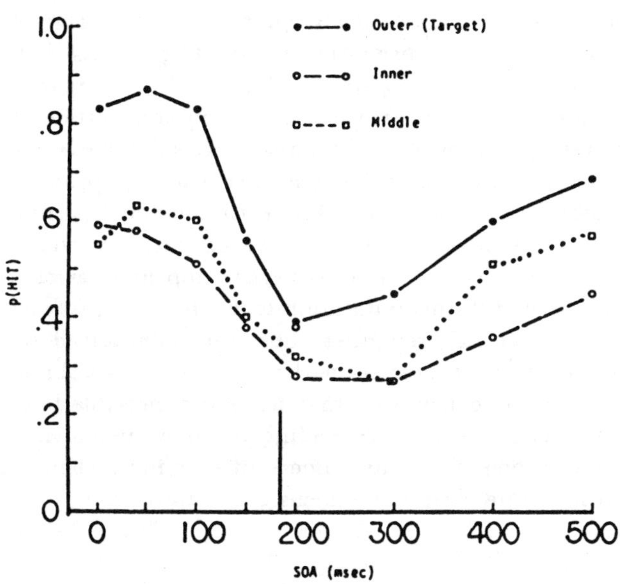

Fig. 3: The probability of a correct probe detection, p(HIT), for Experiment 1 as a function of stimulus onset asynchrony (SOA) for each position, averaged over subjects. (Mean eye movement latency, indicated by the vertical bar, is 185 ms.) Source: Remington, 1980. Copyright 1980 by the American Psychological Association. Reprinted by permission.

As shown in Figure 3, the highest performance level correlated with the target followed by the middle and inner positions. With respect to SOA, performance was best if the fixation cue and detection task appeared simultaneously, then decreased until 200/300 ms (indicated by the vertical bar on the abscissa). These results were interpreted to indicate that attention precedes the eye movement to the target location. The decrease between 100 and 200 ms can be attributed to saccadic suppression which begins to affect vision 100-150 ms after the movement cue or 35-85 ms prior to the movement. Attention effects, on the other hand, are pronounced at all SOAs, including the simultaneous onset condition. The lack of a statistical interaction between SOA and position was interpreted as evidence of independent processes within one system. Saccadic suppression and attention are separate processes and affect vision prior to the saccade. Whenever a peripheral event is used to trigger an eye movement, attentional shifts occur. It is hypothesized that there is a common mechanism that links both attention and eye movements to the onset of a peripheral event but separate mechanisms that control the two movements.

Shepherd, Findlay, and Hockey (1986) used a technique which avoided peripheral stimulation. If attention is always "captured" by the peripheral stimulus, it is difficult to distinguish between attention effects due to peripheral stimuli and those due to eye movements. Shepherd et al. manipulated spatial attention by varying the probability that a peripheral probe stimulus would appear in different positions. At the same time, saccades were directed by a central arrow, thus avoiding peripheral stimulation. The probe stimuli had the following effect on saccade latencies: Probe stimuli which appeared before the saccade, shortened saccade latencies if they appeared at the saccade target, and they lengthened saccade latencies if they appeared at the opposite side of fixation. These facilitatory and inhibitory effects were shown to occur at different stages of saccade preparation and were interpreted to indicate that attention plays an important role in the generation of voluntary eye movements. Shepherd et al. concluded "that while it is possible to make attention movements without making corresponding eye movements, it is not possible to make an eye movement (in the absence of peripheral stimulation) without making a corresponding shift in the focus of attention."

Studies of Saccadic Latencies

In this section emphasis will be placed on the time preceeding a visually guided saccade, i.e. the saccadic reaction time, which presents a wealth of possibilities for studying attention. The basic idea of these studies is that any change in the attentional system which is necessary to execute an eye movement requires a certain time which is included in the saccadic reaction time. The process is serial and not parallel in nature (Fischer & Breitmeyer, 1987). The underlying assumption of this approach is that mechanisms of attention regulate the preparation and execution of a saccade.

The modal value of the reaction time of a saccade in response to the onset of a peripheral target is in the order of 200 ms. However, only a minor part of this time is needed for afferent neural transmission (about 30 ms) and for efferent oculomotor delay (approximately 25 ms). What goes on in the brain during the rest of the time? Morgan (1978) called this surplus delay "the oculomotor procrastination."

Saslow (1967) was one of the first who reported that the introduction of a temporal gap between the offset of a central fixation point and onset of a peripheral target light decreased the human saccadic reaction time to about 150 ms as compared to 250 ms when the fixation point remained visible (called overlap condition). Using the gap task with monkeys, Fischer and Boch (1983) reported goal-directed saccadic eye movement characterized by their extremely short reaction times in order of about 70 ms. The task of the monkey was to fixate a fixation point. The fixation point then was turned off, and after 200 ms, a peripheral target appeared to which the animal was required to make a saccade in order to detect a small reduction of the target's luminance. In the frequency distribution of the saccadic reaction times, a separate peak occurred at about 70 ms besides a second peak at about 140 ms. Saccades being centered around the first peak were called "express saccades," those around the second peak were named "fast regular saccades."

Using the gap paradigm with human subjects, Fischer and Ramsperger (1984) again demonstrated the occurrence of express saccades. Humans were somewhat slower than monkeys; their corresponding peak in the saccadic reaction time distribution occurred at 100-120 ms.

Figure 4 shows the frequency distributions of saccadic reaction times, obtained from one human subject (Fischer & Breitmeyer, 1987). In panel A, the gap paradigm was used, that is, the fixation point switched off 200 ms prior to the peripheral target. In panel B, the overlap paradigm was applied with the instruction to the subject that he/she should direct attention to the fixation point. One can clearly see two peaks in A and B. The part of the distribution around the first peak in A, however, representing the express saccades, is much larger than in B. In panel C, the results are shown under a condition in which the subject was asked to gaze on a fixation point without paying attention to it. Many more express saccades occurred under this condition as compared to the second condition.

As we have seen, the disappearance of the fixation point (gap paradigm) or the ignoring of the fixation point (in the overlap paradigm) facilitate the occurrence of express saccades. As a logical consequence, the direction of gaze and attention were to be dissociated in space in the next experiments (Mayfrank et al., 1986). Subjects were instructed to direct their gaze straight ahead towards the center of a screen, however, without providing them with a fixation point (Figure 5). In Figure 5 they were in addition instructed to direct their attention to a light source located in the periphery. When the target appeared 4 deg to the right or left, they had to move their eyes from the center of the screen to the target. Again, the same two conditions were used: (1) The attention target remained visible when the saccade target appeared (overlap).

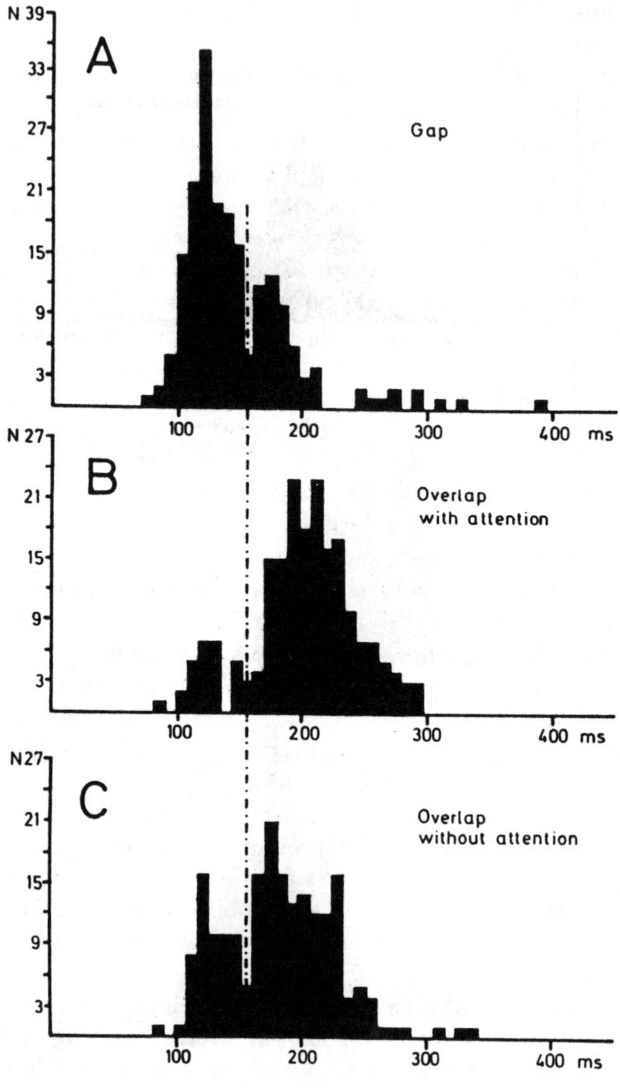

Fig. 4: Distributions of saccadic reaction times of a single human subject. In **A** the fixation point went off 200 ms (gap) before the saccade target was turned on. Saccadic reaction times (horizontal axis) are measured from target onset (bin width 10 ms). In **B** and **C** the fixation point remained visible (overlap). In **B** the subject was instructed to pay attention to the fixation point, in **C** the instruction was not to pay attention to it. The peaks of express saccades occur to the left of the vertical broken line. Source: Fischer & Breitmeyer, 1987. Reprinted with permission from Neuropsychologica, Vol. 25, Copyright 1987 by Pergamon Journals Ltd.

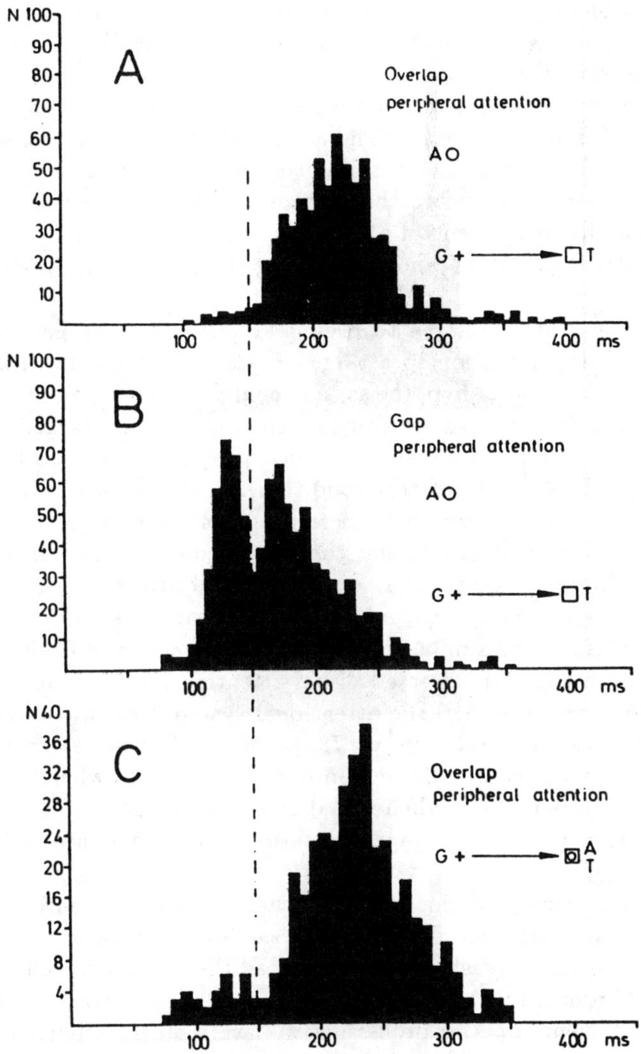

Fig. 5: Effect of peripheral attention on the occurrence of express saccades. In **A** the overlap paradigm was used with the instruction to pay attention to a peripherally located stimulus (A). Express saccades are virtually absent. In **B** the peripheral attention target (A) was turned off before the saccade target (T) occurred randomly at the right or left. In **C** the peripheral attention target was located just above the saccade target and remained visible (overlap). In all three conditions the subjects were required to keep their direction of gaze (G) in the middle of the screen without providing them with a fixation point. Source: Fischer & Breitmeyer, 1987. Reprinted with permission from Neuropsychologica, Vol. 25, Copyright 1987 by Pergamon Journals Ltd.

(2) The attention target disappeared 200 ms before the saccade target appeared (gap) In panel A, one can see the saccadic reaction time distribution under the overlap condition with the attention target located 5 deg above the center of the screen There are hardly any express saccades. In panel B, the distribution in the gap condition is presented: There is a large number of express saccades. One hypothesis compatible with this result would be that a disengagement of attention is necessary before the saccade can be initiated. In the overlap condition, this disengagement of attention needs some extra-time, whereas in the gap condition, this shift can occur during the gap interval prior to saccade onset.

These findings can be related to Klein's (1980), discussed earlier, who suggested that shifting attention to a target location does not facilitate saccadic reaction time. Under this hypothesis, one could expect a large number of express saccades in the overlap condition when the attention target is located at the saccades's target location, since attention does not have to be shifted on that occasion. The results of this condition are shown on the bottom panel C. Surprisingly, only a very small percentage of express saccades occurred, although the subject's attention was constantly concentrated on the target location. This finding suggests that directed visual attention, wherever in the visual field it might be engaged, inhibits express saccades.

The result of these and similar experiments led Fischer and Breitmeyer (1987) to the conclusion that "(i) directed visual attention largely reduces the occurrence of express saccades; (ii) the attentional system has two states (a) disengaged and (b) engaged" (Klemp, p. 78, p. 80). "If visual attention is disengaged, express saccades are allowed. In contrast, in cases where the command to make the saccade is given when visual attention happens to be angaged, the change from engaged to disengaged attention takes time thus, adding to the saccadic latency."

An important aspect of this model is that - unlike the earlier hypotheses about the relation between attention and saccades generation - it focuses on an aspect which is, at least, as important as the eye movement, that is the eye fixation. From a functional point of view, it is important that the visual system has sufficient time for processing the available information.

It is interesting to see how Fischer (1987) implemented this basic mechanism of attentional control of eye movements into a larger model of information processing and saccade generation. The visual centers in the central nervous system are distributed through three different processes, all of which send their output to the oculomotor center (M). A, denotes attentional mechanisms; D, decision making; and C, computation of the coordinates of the next fixation. As well as the functional considerations, there is empirical evidence for a three-loop concept; perhaps the weakest among this evidence is the observation that the frequency distribution of saccadic reaction times exhibits at least 3 differ-

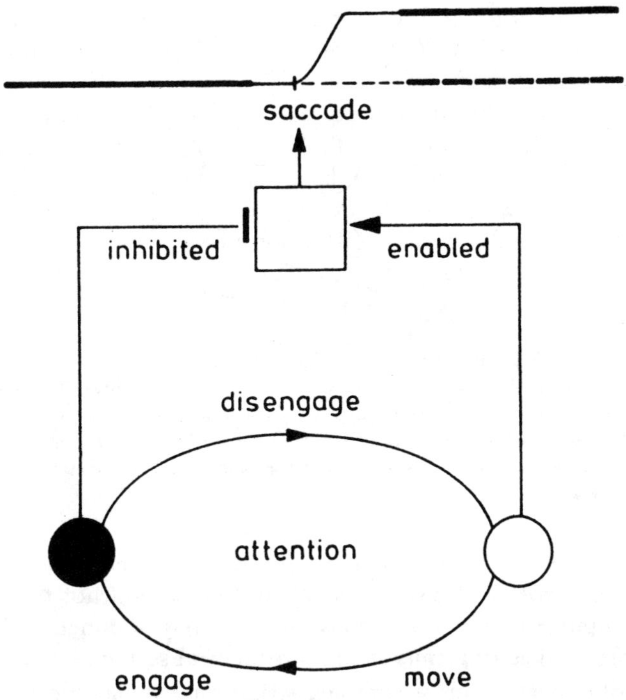

Fig. 6: Schematic diagram of the mechanisms in visual attention and their coordinating relationship to the generation of saccades. The upper trace shows eye position during engaged attention (heavy line) and during disengaged attention (thin line). If no saccade occurs (broken line) attention may be moved and engaged again resulting in a situation of directed peripheral attention. Engaging attention (solid circle) inhibits saccades; disengaging attention (open circle) enables saccades. Source: Fischer & Breitmeyer, 1987. Reprinted with permission from Neuropsychologica, Vol. 25, Copyright 1987 by Pergamon Journals Ltd.

ent peaks (although embedded in considerable statistical noise). The three-loop concept is also based on experiments using electrical stimulation to elicit saccades and lesion experiments which demonstrated that the saccadic system can be activated through different pathways.

Although this model well integrates neurophysiology and psychophysics, it is incomplete in the sense that evidence is lacking for the so-called higher functions. How can the contents of memory or motivational aspects be fed into this model? There is hardly any other possibility than the attentional system to incorporate the effects of higher functions such as memory and motivation. It becomes apparent that the concept of attention in information processing terms is similar to an interface between higher processes and elementary visual information processing. It also serves the function of a multiplexing device

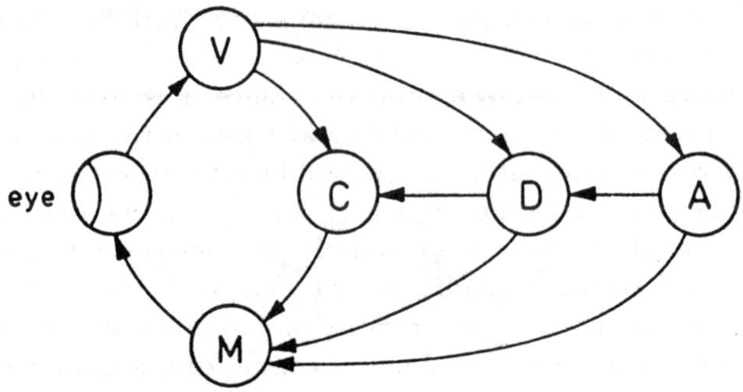

Fig. 7: Scheme of the three-loop concept of preparation of visually guided saccades. Visual information (V) from the retina of the eye is distributed to three different processes - A, D, and C - all of which send their output to the oculomotor center (M). A, attentional mechanisms; D, decision making; and C, computation of coordinates. The three loops are interconnected: A with D and D with C. Source: Fischer, 1987. Reprinted with permission of Springer-Verlag.

which coordinates simultaneous or competing demands from other centers into one executable process. However, we should be careful not to be carried away by these computer metaphors as long as they are just functional analogies and not workable models implemented in a biological software.

Before going over to more complex situations, we should have a brief look back at the questions asked and their tentative answers. The fundamental question about the relation between attention and saccadic responses could not be answered in an unambiguous way. While there appears consensus that it is possible to dissociate attention from spatial orientation in gaze, the converse relationship is less clear, i.e. whether there are saccadic eye movements without a corresponding shift of attention. The difficulty in investigating this relation lies in the fact that there is difficulty in measuring attention in a direct way. In the experiments reported earlier, attention was manipulated as an independent variable in one of the three following ways: (1) by means of expectations (typically by varying the probability of stimulus occurrence in different positions); (2) by instruction (simply telling the subject where to direct the attention), or (3) by stimulus saliency. In information processing terms, the first two manipulations would be characterized as top-down processes, whereas the third one would constitute a bottom-up process. We also should note that the dependent variables of the experiments were simple performance measures, such as manual reaction times or detection probabilities in those experiments where the effect of attention was to be evaluated, and saccadic reaction time of the first saccade following the experimental condition.

In connection with a more complex task, such as, reading or looking at pictures, these experimental conditions are too simple for a straightforward application. Scanpaths of considerable complexity must be observed. With respect to the attentional processes, one has to expect a mutual interaction between bottom-up and top-down processes, since it is most likely that the control modes operate at the same time or at least, in rapid succession. It is clear, that the more complex situations pose difficult methodological questions. First, there is the problem of experimental control. As we have seen, even a relatively simple question led to quite complicated designs with multiple tasks and quite unnatural stimulus conditions. Second, with respect to the dependent variable, reaction times or performance probabilities are one-dimensional, but looking at eye movements in their full complexity, a data point must be characterized by three dimensions in their spatio-temporal coordinates.

Since the studies by Buswell (1935), Berlyne (1958) and Yarbus (1967), there had hardly been any study systematically exploring the attentional value of different stimuli in competing situations (stimulus saliency). One could think, for instance, of an illumination change on one location of the visual field competing with motion simultaneously elicited at another location. Another interesting question would be the comparison between experimentally induced bottom-up versus top-down conditions.

With complex pictures, there was one feature which attracted most fixations according to Berlyne (1958), Yarbus (1967) and Mackworth and Morandi (1967): *informativeness*. In Yarbus' complex paintings, the informative parts were the persons depicted (as opposed to furnitures), the eyes, mouth and nose of faces, etc., but explicitly neither the very darkest or the very brightest regions of the picture nor regions with the greatest details or contours. However, Mackworth and Morandi (1967), (using the same term "informativeness" independently of Yarbus), report contours as regions of a high information content in contrast to regions composed largely of unbounded textures (with a supposedly low information content). Although the term "informativeness" is possibly the lowest common denominator one can find between the widely different stimulus aspects, we should keep in mind that it is highly circular in the sense that it is a word for what it should explain. Even though Mackworth and Morandi assessed ratings of informativeness of different regions of a picture, one could argue that these subjects rated as informative just what captured their eyes. This, of course, could be called attention, but then we are back again at the stage of the early experimental psychology critizing the tautological usage of the term attention. In those contexts where it does not have a precise operational and non-tautological meaning, it probably should be avoided.

Thus, avoiding the word "attention" and replacing it by the notion of "control" let us go briefly through some classes of eye movement control models for complex cognitive tasks.

Classes of Models of Eye Movement Control

One can distinguish between two general classes of models. The first one postulates a direct moment-to-moment control. It is assumed that the decision of how long the eye is to remain at a fixation and where to move it next is controlled by the information extracted from the current fixation (Rayner & McConkie, 1976; Rayner, 1977; O'Regan, 1979; Lévy-Schoen & O'Regan, 1979; Just & Carpenter, 1980; O'Regan, 1983; Carpenter & Just, 1983, this volume). Probably the most radical formulation of a direct moment-to-moment-control model has been advanced by Just and Carpenter. Their assumptions are (i) the *immediacy assumption*: It is assumed that the reader tries to interprete each word immediately upon encountering it; and (ii) the *eye-mind assumption*: The reader continues to fixate a word until all cognitive processes initiated by that word have been completed.

According to Carpenter and Just (1983; see also Fisher & Shebilske, 1985), these assumptions are supported by evidence that the time spent looking at a word (1) is strongly influenced by the characteristics of that word (the word n-effect) and (2) the time spent looking at the word is not influenced by the length or frequency of the preceding word (the word (n-1)-null result). It was suggested that encoding and lexical access "begin on the word that enables them, as immediacy posits, and that they tend to be completed before the next word is fixated, as the eye-mind assumption posits" (Carpenter & Just, 1983, p. 280). However, it should also be made clear that Carpenter and Just's assumption did not relate to single fixations and saccade *anywhere* in the visual field, but to "gazes," i.e. transitions between larger meaningful areas. In their view, a process that influences a gaze may have its effect on the number of fixations, their duration, or both.

The second class of models assumes a more delayed or indirect control of later saccades and fixation times by cognitive processes such as a memory buffer (Bouma & deVoogd, 1974; Shebilske, 1975) or by means of a pre-programming of eye movements (Vaughan & Graefe, 1977; Vaughan, 1979; Zingale & Kowler, 1987). Probably the earliest proposal of such an indirect control model was offered by Buswell (1935). This model compares the control system with a device consisting of two impulses with a gain control. The eye movements are created by a "kicker" given by the two impulses bumping the eye around with a constant force on each kick. The gain control can adjust the distance achieved by each impulse according to the force required (which would correspond to picture complexity or text difficulty). This system is similar to a gearshift in a car that can adjust the speed or force to suit the environmental conditions. It is a nice analogy taken from an age where the car was the important vehicle for providing a metaphor, which today is provided by the computer.

With respect to the two classes of models, no clear decision in favour of one or the other alternative has yet been achieved. In order to arrive at a conclusion, more experimentation will be needed. It already was mentioned that a single or the first saccade in a complex stimulus setting is certainly not the whole story and one should analyze a whole sequence of them in order to arrive at some empirical evidence about the processes of saccade planning. Therefore, as a last review topic of this paper, the issue of scanpaths will be briefly presented.

The Analysis of Scanpaths and Models of their Regulation

Buswell (1935) and Yarbus (1967) among others, had noted that under certain conditions the sequence of successive fixations appeared as a relatively regular, lawfull pattern. This observation was followed up and formulated by Noton and Stark (1971) as the "scanpath hypothesis." They suggested that when confronted with a new stimulus, a particular sequence of fixations, called scanpaths, will occur which will reoccur when the same stimulus causes recognition. The scanned information is stored as a sequence of foveal details, linked by traces of the eye movements which would restore their original position in space. This memory scheme was called a "feature ring."

No subsequent researcher ever found as clear-cut a result as Noton and Stark's (1971). However, some tendency towards scanpath-like patterns was also found by other authors (for a review see Stark & Ellis, 1981; Ellis, 1985).

In some of our own studies, we tried to analyse the fixation data of several subjects in a facial recognition task with respect to scanpaths (Groner, Walder, & Groner, 1984). The within-subject correlation between the learning and recognition of the faces with the between-subject correlations were compared. For four out of six subjects, there was a statistical significant correlation between their own scanpaths in learning and recognition and this correlation was in most cases also higher than their corresponding between-subjects correlation. It was concluded that, with these subjects, elements of individual scanpaths could be found. Subsequently, we called these idiosyncratic fixation patterns "local scanpaths," local in the sense that the fixations follow each other in an immediate local succession. In addition to those, we also found interesting statistical patterns on a larger time scale, which we called "global scanpaths." Global scanpaths can be obtained in the following way: First divide the total inspection period in different parts. Our usual division was a threefold one: into start, middle, and end. Next, compare the frequency distributions at different inspection periods. Thus, local scanpaths reflect the spatio-temporal organization of eye fixations on a local scale of successive events, while global scanpaths reflect the distribution of eye fixations when taking into account the entire inspection process. Therefore, it is not unreasonable to assume that local scanpaths are controlled by the momentary fixation and the associated peripheral information in a moment-to-moment control mode, and that global scanpaths are regulated by some top-down process such as search plans or cognitive strategies. As one can imagine, such an easily made claim is much more difficult to test empirically. Some evidence in this direction could be found in an experiment in which European subjects had to learn a set of Japanese Kanji symbols which were previously completely unknown to them (Koga & Groner, in press). While the initial scanpaths of the subjects were rather irregular and hardly displayed any local scanpaths, the learning process was described as a large scale global scanpath. It should be noted that the scanpath analysis was applied a posteriori and is therefore difficult to serve as a test in this experiment.

A more systematic attempt towards the identification of local and global scanpaths was undertaken by Groner and Menz (1985). By using a complete factorial design, the relative contribution of the stimulus, task and subject as well as their mutual interactions were investigated with respect to local and global scanpaths. Since the experiment involved two stimuli, three tasks and twelve subjects, and each of these combinations was to be replicated within the same individual five times, a problem arises with respect to habituation effects. This problem was solved by using random dot patterns in which the gross characteristics could be kept constant but the small details or fine-grain structure changed.

The upper part of Figure 8 shows two different stimuli. They are constructed (lower part) by means of a three-by-three grid of subsquares within which only the point density was defined, but not their small details. This design resulted in an equivalent peripheral stimulation, but left the foveal details different over the replication trials of the same stimulus.

The results of this study were quite complex. The factorial design allowed the test of all possible interactions between the factors, and many of them reached statistical significance. With respect to both local and global scanpaths, it was shown that they were subject-specific. It was also demonstrated that different tasks (free inspection, a search and a concept identification task) produced specific global scanpath patterns. This is in accordance with the hypothesis that global scanpaths reflect a top-down mode of information processing. However, this experiment also demonstrated the limits of experimental control in complex tasks in which individual differences come in. This situation apparently allowed the subjects to make up for their own strategies. With respect to the importance of individual differences for the analysis of eye movements in a comlex setting, I agree with Carpenter and Just (this volume) and Putz-Osterloh and Lüer (1979). They had demonstrated that different information processing strategies occur in high and low ability subjects in spatial ability tests which were measured by means of an eye movement analysis.

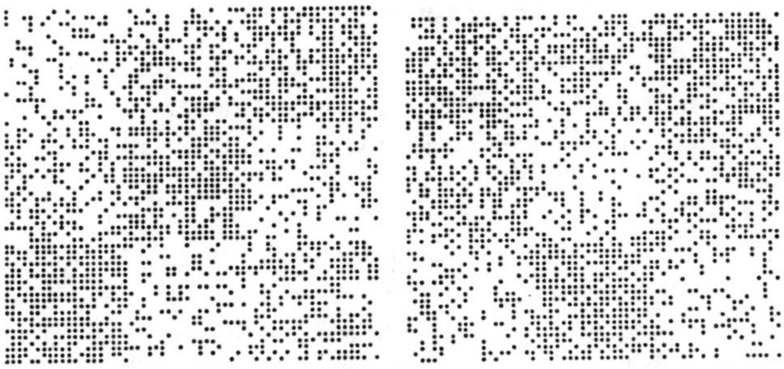

Fig. 8a: Two examples of random dot patterns as they were used in our experiments. The relative size of dots compared with the interdot spaces was actually smaller. (For details of size and how the stimuli were constructed see Fig. 8b). Source: Groner & Menz, 1985. Reprinted with permission of Elsevier Science Publishers B.V., Amsterdam.

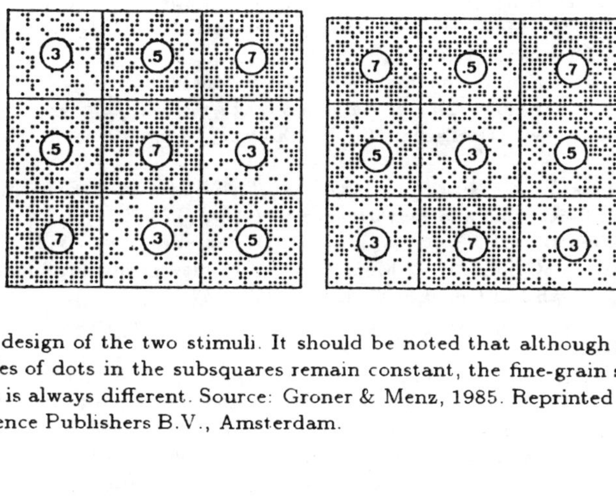

Fig. 8b: The design of the two stimuli. It should be noted that although for all instances the probabilities of dots in the subsquares remain constant, the fine-grain structure within the subsquares is always different. Source: Groner & Menz, 1985. Reprinted with permission of Elsevier Science Publishers B.V., Amsterdam.

Concluding Remarks

While it seems possible to direct visual attention to parts of the visual field without associated eye movements, it has been argued - although without convincing experimental proof - that saccadic eye movements always elicit an attentional response. The attentional and the saccadic system seem to be regulated by different, although closely interrelated control systems which serve as some kind of interface and multiplexer between motivational states, memorized events and expectations, interconnected with a system that monitors new incoming stimuli. The way top-down and bottom-up processes interact with each other is still an open question which should be approached by ingenious experiments and explicit information processing models.

Acknowledgement

Supported by the Swiss National Science Foundation, grants 1.187.85 and 3.940.84. - I would like to thank Bruno Breitmeyer for reading an earlier version of the manuscript and providing some valuable suggestions.

References

Berlyne, D.E., *The influence of complexity and novelty in visual figures on orienting responses*, Journal of Experimental Psychology **55** (1958), 289-296.

Bouma, H., & deVoogd, A.H., *On the control of eye saccades in reading*, Vision Research **14** (1974), 273-284.

Breitmeyer, B.G., & Ganz, L., *Implications of sustained and transient channels for theories of visual pattern masking, saccadic suppression, and information processing*, Psychological Review **83** (1976), 1-36.

Buswell, G.T., "How people look at pictures," University of Chicago Press, 1935.

Carpenter, P.A., & Just, M.A., *What your eyes do while your mind is reading*, in "K. Rayner (Ed.), Eye Movements in reading: perceptual and language processes," Academic Press, New York, 1983.

Duffy, E., "Activation and behavior," Wiley, New York, 1962.

Düker, H., *Untersuchungen über die sogenannte Aufmerksamkeit.*, in "Bericht 20. Kongress der Deutschen Gesellschaft für Psychologie, Berlin 1955," Hogrefe, Göttingen, 1956.

Egly, R., & Homa, D., *Sensitization of the visual field*, Journal of Experimental Psychology: Human Perception and Performance **10** (1984), 778-793.

Ellis, S.R., & Smith, J.D., *Patterns of statistical dependency in visual scanning*, in "R. Groner, G.W. McConkie, & C. Menz (Eds.), Eye movements and human information processing," North Holland, Amsterdam, 1985.

Engel, R.L., *Visual conspicuity, directet attention and retinal locus*, Vision Research **11** (1971), 563-576.

Eriksen, C.W., & Hoffman, J., *The extent of processing of noise elements during selective encoding from visual displays*, Perception and Psychophysics **14** (1973), 155-160.

Eriksen, W.W., & Murphy, T.D., *Movements of attentional focus across the visual field: A critical look at the evidence*, Perception & Psychophysics **42** (1987), 299-305.

Fischer, B., *The preparation of visual guided saccades*, Reviews of Physiology, Biochemistry and Pharmacology **106** (1987), 1-35.

Fischer, B., & Breitmeyer, B., *Mechanisms of Visual Attention revealed by Saccadic Eye Movements*, Neuropsychologia **25** (1987), 73-83.

Fischer, B., & Boch, R., *Saccadic eye movements after extremely short reaction times in the monkey*, Brain Research **260** (1983), 21-26.

Fischer, B,. & Ramsperger, E., *Human express-saccades: extremely short reaction times of goal directed eye movements*, Experimental Brain Research **57** (1984), 191-195.

Fisher, D.F., & Shebilske, W.L., *There is more that meets the eye than the eyemind assumption*, in "R. Groner, G.W. McConkie, & C. Menz (Eds.), Eye movements and human information processing," North Holland, Amsterdam, 1985.

Goldberg, M.H., & Wurtz, R.H., *Activity of superior colliculus in behaving monkey. II. Effect of attention on neuronal responses*, Journal of Neurophysiology **35** (1972), 560-574.

Gopher, D., *Eye movement patterns in selective listening taskes of focused attention*, Perception and Psychophysics **14** (1973), 259-264.

Grindley, D.G., & Townsend, V., *Voluntary attention in peripheral vision and its effects on acuity and differential thresholds*, Quarterly Journal of Experimental Psychology **20** (1968), 11-19.

Groner, R., "Hypothesen im Denkprozess. Grundlagen einer verallgemeinerten Theorie auf der Basis elementarer Informationsverarbeitung," Huber, Bern, Stuttgart & Wien, 1978.

Groner, R., & Groner, M., *Towards a hypothetico-deductive theory of cognitive activity*, in "R. Groner & P. Fraisse (Eds.), Cognition and eye movements," North Holland, Amsterdam, 1982.

Groner, R., & Groner, M., *Hypothesis theory - a review*, in "E.v.d. Meer & J. Hoffmann (Eds.), Knowledge aided information processing in human beings," North Holland, Amsterdam, 1987, pp. 193-219.

Groner, R., Groner, M., & Hofer, D., *The role of anticipation in the encoding of motion signals - sensitization or bias*, in "F. Klix & H. Hagendorf (Eds.), Human memory and cognitive capabilities: Mechanismus and performances," North Holland, Amsterdam, 1986.

Groner, R., & Menz, C., *The effects of stimulus characeristics, task requirements and individual differences on scanning patterns*, in "R. Groner, G.W. McConkie, & C. Menz (Eds.), Eye movements and human information processing. Proceedings of the XXIII. International Congress of Psychology," North Holland, Amsterdam, 1985.

Groner, R., Walder, F., & Groner, M., *Looking at faces: Local and global aspects of scanpaths*, in "A.G. Gale & F. Johnson (Eds.), Theoretical and applied aspects of eye movement research," North Holland, Amsterdam, 1984.

Held, R., Ingle, D., Schneider, G.E., & Trevarthen, C.B., *Locating and identifying: two modes of visual processing*, Psychologische Forschung **31** (1967), 42-62.

Held, R., Ingle, D., Schneider, G.E., & Trevarthen, C.B., *Locating and identifying: two modes of visual processing: A symposium*, Psychologische Forschung **31** (1968), 299-348.

Helmholtz, H. von, "Handbuch der physiologischen Optik," Voss, Hamburg & Leipzig, 1909.

Hinton, J.W., *Ocular Responses to Meaningful Visual Stimuli and their Psychological Significance*, in "R. Groner & P. Fraisse (Eds.), Cognition and eye movements," North Holland, Amsterdam, 1982.

Johnston W.A., & Dark, V.J., *Selective attention*, Annual Review of Psychology **37** (1986), 43-75.

Jonides, J., *Voluntary versus reflexive control of the mind's eye's movement*, Paper presented at the Psychonomic Society meeting, St. Louis, Mo, 1976.

Julesz, B., *Toward an "axiomatic" theory of preattentive vision*, in "G.M. Edelman, W.E. Gall, & W.M. Cowan (Eds.), Dynamic aspects of neocortical function," Wiley, New York et al., 1984.

Just, M.A., & Carpenter, P.A., *A theory of reading: From eye fixation to comprehension*, Psycholgical Review **87** (1980), 329-354.

Kahnemann, D., "Attention and Effort," Englewood Cliffs, New Jersey: Prentice-Hall, 1973.

Klein, F., *Does oculomotor readiness mediate cognitive control of visual attention?*, in "R. Nickerson (Ed.), Attention and performance VIII.," Erlbaum, Hillsdale, New York, 1980, pp. 259-276.

Koga, K., & Groner R., *Intercultural experiments as a research tool in the study of cognitive skill acquisition: Japanese character recognition and eye movements in non-Japanese subjects*, in "H. Mandl & J. Levin (Eds.), Knowledge acquisition from texts and pictures," North Holland, Amsterdam (to appear).

Lambert, A.J., *Expecting different categories at different location and selective attention*, Quarterly Journal of Experimental Psychology **39A** (1987), 61-76.

Lévy-Schoen, A., & O'Regan, J.K., *The control of eye movements in reading*, in "P.A. Kolers, M.E. Wrolstad, & H. Bouma (Eds.), Processing to visible language," Plenum Press, New York, 1979.

Mackworth, N.H., & Morandi, A., *The gaze selects informative details within pictures*, Perception and Psychophysics **2** (1967), 547-552.

Magoun, H.W., "The waking brain," Thomas, Springfield, Ill, 1963.

Mayfrank, L., Mobashery, M., Kimmig, H., & Fischer, B., *The role of fixation and visual attention on the occurrance of express saccades in man*, European Journal of Psychiatry and Neurological Science **235** (1986), 269-275.

Maylor, E.A. et al., *Facilitatory and inhibitory components of orienting in visual space*, in "M.I. Posner & O.S.M. Marin (Eds.), Attention and performance XI," Erlbaum, Hillsdale, 1985.

Mertens, J.J., *Influence of knowledge of target location upon the probability of observation of peripherally observable testflashes*, Journal of the Optical Society of America **6** (1956), 1069-1070.

Mowrer, O.H., *Preparatory set (expectancy) - Further evidence of its central locus*, Journal of Experimental Psychology **28** (1941), 116-133.

Müller, H.J., & Findlay, J.M., *Sensitivity and criterion effects in the spatial cueing of visual attention*, Perception and Psychophysics (to appear).

Navon, D., & Gopher, D., *On the economy of the human processing system*, Psychological Review **86** (1979), 114-255.

Norman, D.A., *Towards a theory of memory and attention*, Psychological Review **75** (1968), 522-536.

Norman, D.A., & Bobrow, D.G., *On data-limited and resource-limited processes*, Cognitive Psychology **7** (1975), 44-64.

O'Regan, J.K., *Eye guidance in reading: Evidence for the linguistic control hypothesis*, Perception and Psychophysics **25** (1979), 501-509.

O'Regan, J.K., *Elementary perceptual and eye movement control processes in reading*, in "K. Rayner (Ed.), Eye movements in reading: Perceptual and language processes," Academic Press, New York, 1983.

Posner, M.I., "Chronometric explorations of mind," Erlbaum, Hillsdale, NJ, 1978.

Posner, M.I., Nissen, M.J., & Ogden, W.C., *Attended and unattended processing modes: The role of set for spatial location*, in "H.L. Pick & E.J. Saltzman (Eds.), Modes of perceiving and processing information," Erlbaum, Hillsdale, NJ, 1978, pp. 137-157.

Posner, M.I., Snyder, C.R.R., & Davidson, B.J., *Attention and the detection of signals*, Journal of Experimental Psychology: General **109** (1980), 160-174.

Putz-Osterloh, B., & Lüer, G., *Wann produzieren Probanden räumliche Vorstellungen beim Lösen von Raumvorstellungsaufgaben?*, Zeitschrift für Experimentelle und Angewandte Psychologie **26** (1979), 138-156.

Rayner, K., & McConkie, G.W., *What guides a reader's eye movements?*, Vision Research **16** (1976), 829-837.

Rayner, K., *Visual attention in reading: Eye movements reflect cognitive processes*, Memory and Cognition **4** (1977), 443-448.

Remington, R.W., *Attention and saccadic eye movements*, Journal of Experimental Psychology: Human Perception and Performance **6** (1980), 726-744.

Remington, R., & Pierce, L., *Moving attention: Evidence for time-invariant shifts of visual selective attention*, Perception & Psychophysics **35** (1984), 393-399.

Rovamo, J., & Virsu, V., *An estimation and application of the human cortical magnification factor*, Experimental Brain Research **37** (1979), 495-510.

Saslow, M.G., *Effects of components of displacement-step stimuli upon latency of saccadic eye movement*, Journal of the Optical Society of America **57** (1967), 1024-1031.

Shebilske, W., *Reading eye movements from an information processing point of view*, in "D. Massaro (Ed.), Understanding language," Academic Press, New York, 1975.

Shepherd, M., Findlay, J.M., & Hockey, R.J., *The relationship between eye movements and spatial attention*, The Quarterly Journal of Experimental Psychology **38A** (1986), 475-491.

Shiffrin, R.M., & Gardner, G.T., *Visual processing capacity and attentional control*, Journal of Experimental Psychology **93** (1972), 72-82.

Shiffrin, R.M., & Schneider, W., *Controlled and automatic human information processing: II. Perceptional learning, automatic attending and general theory*, Psychological Review **84** (1977), 127-190.

Shulman, G.L., Remington, R.W., & McLean, J.P., *Moving attention through visual space*, Journal of Experimental Psychology: Human Perception and Performance **5** (1979), 522-526.

Spillmann, L., *Foveal perceptive fields in the human visual system measured with simultaneous contrast in grids and bars*, Pflügers Archiv **326** (1971), 281-299.

Stark, L., & Ellis, S.R., *Scanpaths revisted: cognitive models direct active looking*, in "D.F. Fisher, R.A. Monty, & J.W.Senders (Eds.), Eye movements: Cognition and visual perception," Erlbaum, Hillsdale, NJ, 1981.

Treisman, A., *The psychological reality of levels of processing*, in "L.S. Cermak & F.I.M. Craik (Eds.), Levels of processing and human memory," Erlbaum, Hillsdale, NJ, 1979.

Treisman, A., & Gelade G., *A feature-integration theory of attention*, Cognitive Psychology **12** (1980), 97-136.

Trevarthen, C.B., *Two mechanisms of vision in primates*, Psychologische Forschung **31** (1968), 299-337.

Tsal, Y., *Movements of attention across the visual field*, Journal of Experimental Psychology. Human Perception & Performance **9** (1983), 523-530.

Ungerleider, L.G., & Mishkin, M., *Two cortical visual systems*, in "D.J. Ingle, M.A. Goodale, & R.J.W. Mansfield, (Eds.), Analysis of visual behavior," MIT Press, Cambridge, Massachusetts, 1982.

Vaughan, J., *Control of visual fixation duration in search*, in "J.W. Senders, D.F. Fisher, & R.A. Monty (Eds.), Eye movements and the higher psychological functions," Erlbaum, Hillsdale, NJ, 1979.

Vaughan, J.,& Graefe, T.M., *Delay of stimulus presentation after the saccade in visual search*, Perception and Psychophysics **22** (1977), 201-205.

Wickens, C.D., *Processing Resources in attention*, in "Parasuraman & E.A. Davis (Eds.), Varieties of Attention.," Academic Press, Orlando, Florida, 1984.

Wurtz, R.H., & Mohler, C.W., *Enhancement of visual responses in monkey striate cortex and frontal eye fields*, Journal of Neurophysiology **39** (1976), 766-772.

Yarbus, A.L., "Eye movements and vision," Plenum Press, New York, 1967.

Zingale, C.M., & Kowler, E., *Planning sequences of saccades*, Vision Research **27** (1987), 1327-1341.

HOW CAN WE KNOW THE VERIDICAL VELOCITY OF A MOVING OBJECT?

KAZUO KOGA [1], TATSURO MAKINO [2], KATSUAKI SAKATA [3], AND NOBUKO TAKAHASHI [4]

[1] Department of Aerospace Psychology, The Research Institute of Environmental Medicine, Nagoya University
[2] Department of Educational Psychology, Waseda University, Tokyo
[3] Japan Color Research Institute, Tokyo
[4] Department of Psychology, Waseda University, Tokyo

INTRODUCTION

Recording techniques for eye movements can be categorized into two types: head free and head fixed recording methods. When a head free recording device is used, the head position has to be recorded independently of the eye movements; or, both the amount of head and eye position must be recorded simultaneously in order to identify the net amount of eye movements.

Almost all research has been aimed at obtaining the exact measurement of eye movements independent of head or body movements or the measurement of constancy or visual stability without recording eye movements precisely. These studies fail to take into account the relative displacement of an object on the retina when the head or body moved or even when only the eyes moved.

Static visual stimuli can be more suitable than kinetic ones when identification of the scanning path of the subject's eye to an object is of main interest. Even when a stimulus was presented dynamically, only the spatial data analysis, such as the fixation duration, its latency, number of fixations and so on, have been studied without taking into account the temporal characteristics of the eye movement.

A very rare exception was the study of saccadic suppression, that is, the relationship between eye movements and the change of visual perception. Another example is the research on pursuit eye movement in which the relative moment between eyes and object based on the temporal characteristics of the object motion has been described (Bridgeman et al., 1976). The investigation of pursuit eye movement, however, has not been related to the relationship between perception of temporal velocity and eye movements (Mack, 1986). There have been numerous studies concerned with the perception of relative motion or induced motion perception. The strong affection of the perception of temporal velocity of moving objects comes from the eye movement itself (Mack, 1986).

We will present some evidence as to how eye movement modifies temporal velocity perception under slit view conditions as well as then examine it under much more general conditions.

If a pattern is moved behind a stationary narrow slit or aperture, we can recognize the whole pattern although only a part of it is visible at any moment. This phenomenon was first observed by Zoellner (1862) and was experimentally investigated and confirmed by Parks (1965). Parks explained the phenomenon using a theory referred to as *post-retinal visual storage*, and his findings were supported by several researchers (Rocks & Sigman, 1973). Results were interpreted from the standpoint of cognitive function. One of the important arguments supporting a cognitive hypothesis was the fact that the decay time of iconic memory (0.5 s) is suitable to explain the storage of the fragments seen through a slit. A study by Casco and Morgan (1984) showed that even the apparent movement through a slit cannot be recognized in individual fragments, but only as a whole. This perceptual processing had occurred prior to temporal velocity perception because the perception occurred only after the completion of feature perception. More recent research by Shimojo and Richards (1986) proposed a computer simulation model in which the hidden parts of the moving figure behind the slit were predictable.

Parks also observed that the perceived object (in his experiment, a camel), was foreshortened depending on the velocity with which the object passed behind the slit. This finding posed a problem related to the uncertain relation between pattern cognition and temporal velocity perception in the human visual system. In a discussion of these results Anstis and Atkinson (1976) hypothesized that the distortion was caused by eye movements. They showed that there was a linear relationship between perceived size and the size of eye movements. This suggests the possibility that visual perception can be modified at the retinal level. This explanation is referred to as *retinal painting theory*. Morgan, Findlay, and Watt (1982) did some "aperture viewing" experiments and found that they could strictly discriminate the process of post retinal storage from the portion which can be modified by eye movements based on the various aperture viewing conditions. They found that eye movements could modify or affect the perception of a moving figure within a specific range of the stimulus motion.

On the other hand, McCloskey and Watkins (1978) denied the possibility of eye movement contributing to the perception of a complete figure. They presented two different figures moving in opposite directions behind a slit. Subjects could recognize both figures simultaneously, demonstrating that eye movements could not contribute to the figural generation on the retina. However, there are two difficulties with their experiments. First, eye movements were not monitored. Subjects were only instructed to fixate their eyes on a position of the slit. It is thus impossible to deny the existence of eye movement contributions since eye movements could have occurred, moving in both directions alternately. It is indeed possible that two different total feature perceptions might have been completed. Second, they discussed only the discrepancy in size perception between the two different experimental conditions. That is, the moving slit over the stationary figures and the moving figures observed through a stationary slit. When a figure was moved behind a stationary slit, perceived size of the figure was shorter than when a stationary figure was seen through the moving slit.

This observations have long been a point of critical discussion (Haber & Nathanson, 1968; Haber, 1968; Parks, 1968; Hochberg, 1968; Rock & Halper, 1969; Parks, 1970; Rock & Sigman, 1973; Rock, 1983). Again according to Morgan (1981), the two different problems to be explained are visual perception for feature completion and motion recognition.

How is it that we can recognize the veridical velocity of the moving outer world even when eyes and head move or to raise the question another way, how can we confirm temporal motion velocity of the object when both eyes and objects are moving since the retinal images are always unstable? The experiments reported here will help clarify the role of eye movements in the perceived temporal velocity of the target at an early stage of visual perception and indicate the important role of eye movements in feature and motion recognition. We think that eye movements, particularly, smooth pursuit eye movements, contribute to the latter.

Experiment 1

Methods

The visual stimuli were similar to Park's. In our experimental situation, we generated the same type of camel and slit on a CRT display controlled by an Apple-II computer with a movement from right to left. The only difference was that a vertical grid was added to the original picture used by Parks in order to identify the retinal slip or blur. The subjects themselves could easily report when the eyes did not pursue the camel or grid. Figure 1 shows a schematic example of the visual stimulus used. The distance between the subject's right eye and the display was 425 mm. The height and the width of the camels were 35 x 35 mm. The inter-camel-distance was the same as the width of the camels. The width between grid lines was either 5 or 7 mm.

The moving velocity of the camel was fixed at 40 mm/s (5.4 ° /s) from right to left. The slit was overlaid on the moving camels using another picture frame (buffer memory on the Apple-II). The width of the slit was either 5, 6, 7 or 65 mm. In the case of the slit width of 65 mm, the condition was called "slit-off condition" and the rest were called "slit-condition." In both, slit and slit-off

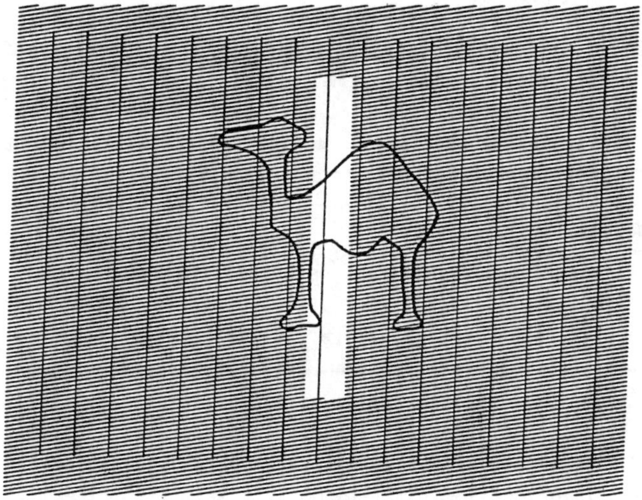

Fig. 1: The line drawings of the camel and vertical grids were generated on the CRT display under the control of an Apple-II computer. Both the camel and grids moved from right to left at a velocity of 5.4 ° /s. Using a second frame memory, the slit overlapped the camel. A hatched area in the figure indicates the invisible part of the display.

conditions, a grid was displayed together with the camel moving at the same velocity. The stimuli were observed for 90 seconds in each condition.

Eye movements were recorded using an auto-tracking first Purkinije technique aided by a minicomputer system (Koga & Osaka, 1983) for both horizontal and vertical eye positions. The spatial resolutions was 6' of visual angle and the temporal resolution was 16.7 ms. The eye movement data were calibrated with respect to magnitude and linearity prior to the recording. All data were linearized after the experiments and reconverted to analogue output using a MELCOM-70/10 minicomputer system.

Three subjects HA, JS and KI (two male and a female) with normal vision participated in the experiment. They were all uninformed about the purpose of the experiment.

Results

All subjects showed a characteristic horizontal eye movement pattern in every experimental condition including the slit-off condition. No characteristic vertical eye movements were observed. Figure 2 shows a typical horizontal eye movement pattern. Eye movements could be categorized into fixations, smooth pursuit movements and saccade. Sequences of small saccades, relatively short fixations and smooth pursuit eye movements were seen in every subject. One can easily recognize the successive eye movement components. The subject's

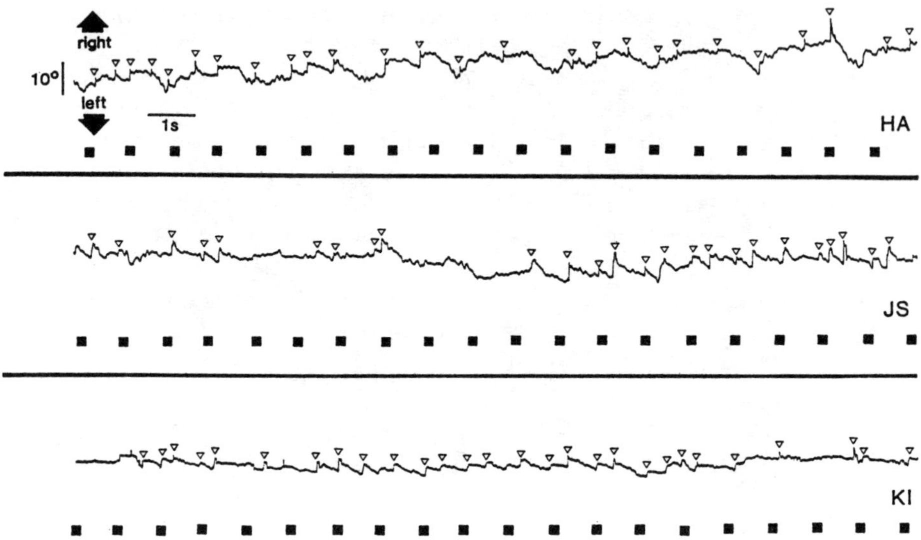

Fig. 2: Horizontal eye movements of each of the three subjects in the slit (5 mm) and grid (7 mm) condition are shown. The open triangle indicates the occurrence of a saccade and the filled square indicates the appearance of the camel's head at the right side edge of the slit. Codes HA, JS and KI in the figure indicate the individual subject.

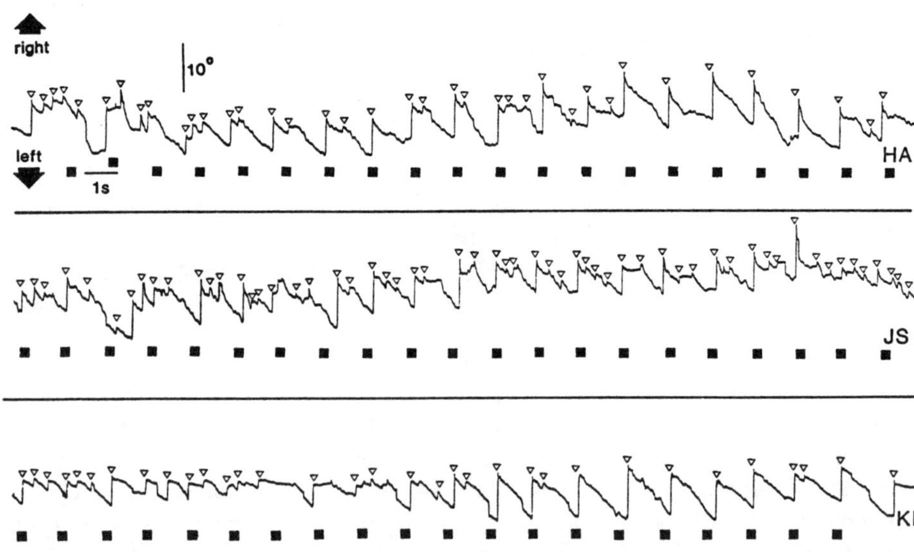

Fig. 3: Horizontal eye movements in the slit-off and grid (7 mm) condition are shown. Open triangle and filled square indicate the occurrence of a saccade and the appearance of a camel.

eye was fixated until the head of a camel appeared (fixation phase) on the right edge of the slit. When the subject recognized the camel's head, the eyes began to pursue it (smooth pursuit movement phase). The smooth pursuit eye movements were repeated several times when a camel, with grid, was passing behind the slit. On the contrary, when no camel was seen and only a grid passed behind the slit, subjects fixated their eyes around the slit edge. Figure 1 indicates the phasic correspondence between the fixations and the constant delay between the appearances of the camels (filled square).

As soon as the camel had disappeared on the left hand side of the slit, a saccadic eye movement from left to right occurred to the opposite side of the slit edge followed by a fixation phase while waiting for the next camel to appear. In the slit-off condition, the velocity of the smooth pursuit eye movement was almost equal to the physical movement of the camel. In this situation, eye movement patterns seemed to be typical optokinetic nystagmus (OKN) and could be categorized into two components, smooth pursuit and saccadic eye movement phase. The timing of saccades corresponds to the appearance of the camel's head at the right side edge of the slit. Typical OKN patterns are shown in Figure 3.

Tab. 1: Saccadic latency in seconds measured from an appearance of the camel's head at the right edge of the slit and its magnitude are shown in each slit and grid condition. The duration and magnitude of smooth pursuit eye movement are also shown. The mean velocity of the smooth pursuit eye movement is shown The numbers in the first column indicate the total frequency of the saccades in each experimental condition

	experimental condition		fast phase			slow phase	
n	slit size (mm)	distance between grids (mm)	latency (s)	magnitude (deg.arc)	duration (s)	magnitude (deg.arc)	velocity (deg.arc/s)
139	7	5	0.49±0.34	1.68±0.70	0.39±0.27	1.77±1.08	4.54
94	6	5	0.56±0.35	1.86±1.02	0.38±0.19	1.78±0.64	4.68
69	5	5	0.56±0.35	1.83±1.19	0.32±0.17	1.53±0.92	4.78
94	7	7	0.61±0.35	1.67±0.69	0.37±0.19	1.52±0.60	4.11
85	6	7	0.59±0.34	1.69±0.94	0.39±0.24	1.52±0.87	3.90
68	5	7	0.42±0.35	1.58±0.84	0.30±0.16	1.26±0.92	4.20
108	off	5	0.52±0.36	3.72±2.27	0.58±0.36	3.40±2.19	5.86
91	off	7	0.59±0.38	4.65±2.53	0.76±0.41	4.30±2.41	5.65

Table 1 shows the mean latency and magnitude of each saccade after a camel appeared in the slit. The duration, magnitude, and velocity (magnitude/duration) of the smooth pursuit eye movements are also shown in the same table. There were no significant differences among the slit conditions. The spatial distance traveled by smooth pursuit eye movements was always recovered by a saccade. However, the maximum width of the slit was only 0.94 degree of visual angle over all conditions. Thus, the size of saccadic and smooth pursuit eye movement exceeded the slit width but not the camel width. There were two or three saccades during the appearance of a single camel. And one more important result was that there was no fixation phase in the slit-off condition. Subjects continued the pursuit eye movements. Large and fast saccades interrupted them rhythmically. This will be discussed later on.

Discussion

Only a few saccades were observed while a camel moved behind the slit. This indicates that the retinal image of the camel is subdivided into several image fragments because the saccadic suppression inhibits an image exposure for a very short time. It is possible that a very small part of the visual image information is lost during that time. Each image fragment may be recognized only by smooth pursuit eye movements. It is thus possible that the total perceptual image of the camel is foreshortened compared to the physical image, as a result of saccadic suppression. However, this hypothesis was not fully supported in the experiment since the saccadic suppression was not measured. Further, it is difficult to explain why saccadic suppression should lead to a foreshortening of perceived camel size. As we will argue later, retinal error caused by smooth pursuit movement can also lead to elongation of perceived size when pursuit velocity of the eyes is slower than that of the target.

There was a velocity difference between v1 and v2. Smooth pursuit eye velocity (v2) was slightly slower than that of the camel (v1). This should have caused a retinal blur and also enlarged the image because the difference between v1 and v2 was negative against the moving direction of the camel. The effect would be true if the difference were positive. The image of the camel would have overlapped successively and elongated the image in the opposite direction. On the other hand, one or more saccades occurred as a camel moved through the slit and the saccades intercepted not only the smooth pursuit eye movement but also the image generation.

Saccadic suppression could have the effect of foreshortening the length of the camel image. Negative velocity differences between the eyes and the camels and saccadic suppression could prevent size identification of the objects passing behind the slit. Although there was no control for the size of the camels in the present experiment, one of the three subjects reported in the slit condition the impression of small camel size as compared with the perceived size of camels in the slit-off condition. Therefore, we could not pursue the problem of size perception under the slit viewing situation.

The perceived temporal velocity of the grid "with camel" was slower than "without camel" situations in all subjects. When the subject pursued the camel, they perceived slower motion perception of the grids. The pattern of eye movement can reasonably explain the perceptual motion sensation. The grid had a constant physical velocity (v1 = 5.4 ° /s). The velocity of the grid (v1) is perceived by comparison with the (stationary) edge of the slit when the eye was fixated. On the other hand, during the smooth pursuit eye movement which was triggered by the moving camel, the eye moved with a slightly slower velocity (v2 = 4.3 ° /s): mean velocity in the slit condition) than the physical velocity of the grid (v1). A slippage or retinal error could thus occur on the retina as the result of the velocity difference between v1 and v2.

Roughly speaking, the image of the camel could be fixed on the retina during the pursuit eye movement phase. On the other hand, it could be argued that the image of the camel moved on the retina with almost physical velocity (v1) during the fixation phase. Both the camel and grid were fixed on the retina during the pursuit phase, and only the image of the grid traversed the retina during the fixation phase. Thus, the phase difference of the eye movement made for the velocity difference of the grid, and this could cause the different motion perceptions alternatively in the phase of "with camel" and "without camel" as to the grid.

Subjects could recognize the camel and grid by rotating the eyes in accordance with the camel movement in the slit-off condition. In this condition, the velocity of the smooth pursuit eye movements was almost equal to the physical movement of the camel (v3 = 5.7 ° /s: mean velocity throughout the slit-off condition). A more important difference between slit and slit-off conditions was that there was no fixation phase in the slit-off condition. The velocity difference v1-v3 was nearly zero in this situation. Subjects could pursue the camel as exactly as when fixating an immobile camel. They also could fix the image of the grid on the retina, that is, no retinal error was there. Thus, they reported no different motion perception of the grids. Subjects could recognize the entire shape of the camel with the grid throughout the observation period. No change in the perception of the moving grid was reported. Subjects always perceived the camel with grid as moving at a constant speed. However, if the eye rotated in the same direction and approximately at the same velocity as the camel, how can one perceive the velocity of the camel? After all, there is no image displacement of the camel on the retina. There are several different cues to recognize the movement of the camel. One of them is the cue from the stationary aperture which can be recognized as the frame of reference for the moving camel.

Experiment 2

If it were true that eye movements which are elicited by the camel contribute to the perceived motion of the grid, a grid with a camel would produce a much faster motion perception than a grid without a camel, if the grid has equal but reversed velocity against the camel.

Methods

Methods were identical with the previous experiment. The only exception was that the movement direction of the grid was reversed against the direction of the camel Camels appeared from right to left at a constant velocity of 5.4 ° /s The grid line appeared from left to right at the same velocity as the camel Only the 7 mm slit condition was tested for a duration of 90 seconds. The same three subjects (from Experiment 1) participated in this experiment. They were requested to observe the visual stimuli as naively as possible.

Results

We observed complicated eye movement patterns. A typical eye movement pattern which contains the rhythmical alternative saccade and smooth pursuit eye movements (OKN) is shown in Figure 4.

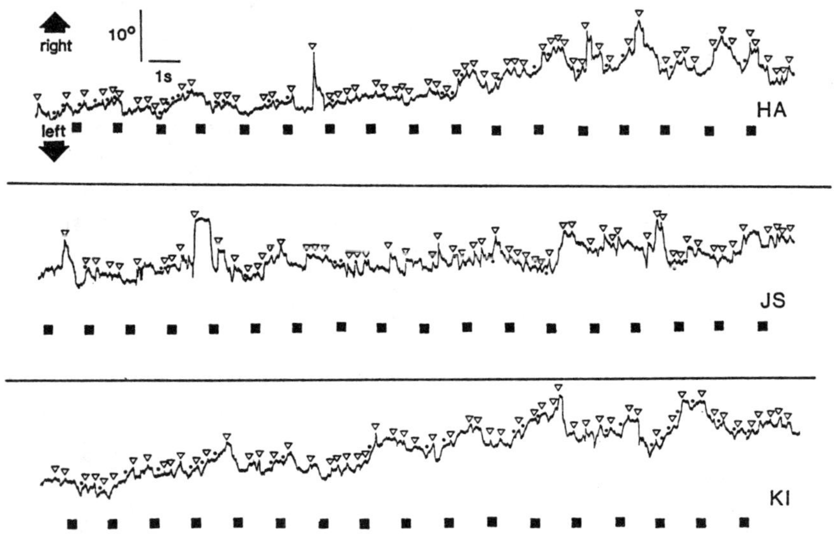

Fig. 4: Horizontal eye movements when the movement direction of both camel and grid were antagonistic are shown. The open triangle. filled square and code name indicate the same as shown in the previous figure. The small dot indicates the smooth pursuit eye movements from left to right which may be triggered by the movement of the grid

The frequency of the saccades, that is, the fast phase in OKN, were relatively small but more frequent when compared to the previous experiment. The eye movement patterns were irregular and not as simple as in the first experiment. Instead of the smooth pursuit eye movement from right to left as observed in Experiment 1, small but frequent pursuit eye movements from left to right were observed.

Discussion

Small saccades from left to right against the camels movement are most likely caused by the antagonistic grid movement which traversed from left to right against the camel. Main OKN, i.e. large saccades triggered by the camel, and small OKN, i.e. small saccades triggered by the grid were mixed in this situation. However, all subjects reported that the perceived velocity of the grid with a camel was much faster than the grid without a camel. The difference between perceiving the grid motion in the grid-with-camel and the grid-without-camel phase was completely opposite to that of Experiment 1, as was expected.

The entire shape of the camel behind the slit was also identified. However, the perceptual difference between perceived and physical size of the camel's body was not clearly discriminated as in Experiment 1. Our research was focused on velocity not size perception. The latter problem requires further investigation.

EXPERIMENT 3

The possibility of the modification of perceived velocity due to changes in eye movement was observed in the slit view condition in the previous two experiments. The present experiment is an attempt to confirm the contribution of eye movement to temporal velocity perception. In the earlier part of this paper, perceived velocity change was always reported under the slit view situation. If the motion perception change is affected due to fixation or pursuit eye movements, the slit view condition might be redundant. We will examine this here. If the mode of eye movement is specific to the perceived velocity changes, this should still occur under the no-slit situation. The no-slit condition was different from the slit-off condition in terms of the slit size. In the no-slit condition, slit size was elongated to the virtual size of the CRT display, that is, 380 mm.

Methods

Methods were changed compared with the previous two experiments. We used a more powerful graphic display system, a COMTEC/2555 in order to generate more complicated motion of the object. Although the image generation procedure was different from the previous experiments, the physical parameters of the stimuli remained the same as the previous ones. The 21-inch display had a resolution of 1280 x 1024 pixels and drawing speed was 200,000 short vector/s. The graphic display was controlled by a MELCOM-70/10 computer (Mitsubishi) through an IEEE488 interface.

Visual stimuli were a) single recurrent target movement from left to right with velocities of 15.8 ° /s, 31.6 ° /s, and 45.0 ° /s and, b) continuous grid movements from left to right with velocities of 1.8 ° /s, 2.8 ° /s, and 3.7 ° /s.

The observation period was 90 seconds. Eye movements were measured in the same way as in the previous experiments.

The subjects were five graduate students who had normal vision. They were asked to press a button when a motion perception change of the stimuli occurred. Motion perception change was defined as the temporal velocity changes of the moving stimuli, that is, of a simple target or grid. A timing mark of the button pressing was also recorded simultaneously with the eye movements.

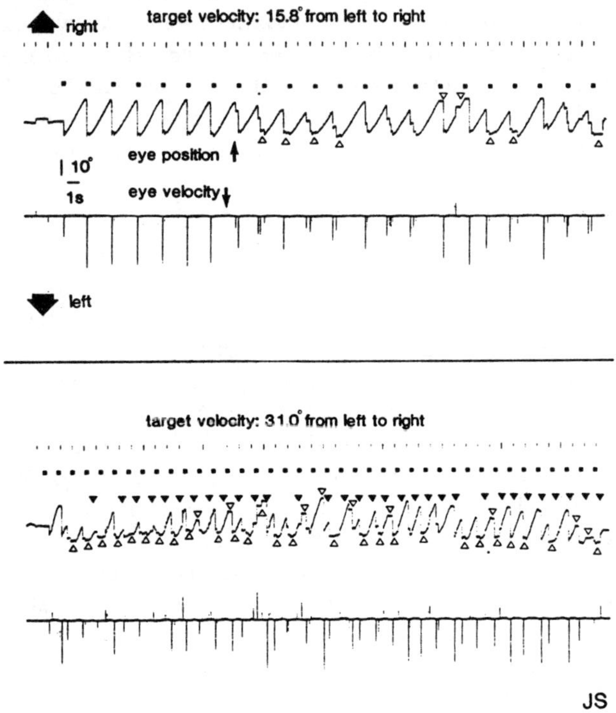

Fig. 5a: Horizontal eye position and its velocity are shown when the single recurrent target moved from left to right with a velocity of 15.8 ° /s and 31.0 ° /s. An open triangle indicates the fixation phase and a filled square indicates the appearance of the target at the left side edge of the CRT display. Filled triangles indicate the occurrence of perceived temporal velocity change which is marked by the subject's pressing a button.

Results

Figure 5a shows the correspondence between the perception changes of the velocity and the saccadic eye movements under the condition of single recurrent target movement from left to right at a velocity of 15.8 ° /s and 31.0 ° /s. Figure 5b shows the same data obtained from another subject under the condition of 15.8 ° /s, 31.0 ° /s, and 45.0 ° /s target movement from right to left. Only the horizontal components of the eye position and eye velocity are shown. When the visual stimuli moved with the lowest velocity of 15.8 ° /s, the eye could pursue it perfectly, and even when no subject reported any change of motion perception, the saccade and fixation phase were observed. On the other hand, when the target velocity was 31.0 ° /s or 45 ° /s, the motion perception change coincided with the end of the fixation phase after the saccade. Unrhythmical fixation phases always led to a motion perception change as indicated in Figure 5a but not so clear in Figure 5b. In Figure 5a, the subject's perception change of the target motion (filled triangle) was synchronized with a short delay of the fixation phase (open triangle).

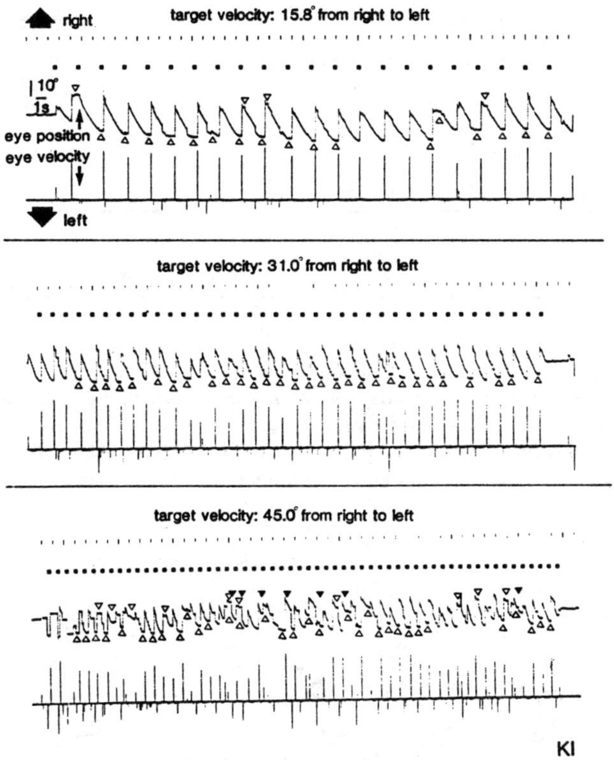

Fig. 5b The same data as Figure 5a except that the three different target velocity conditions, 15.8 ° /s, 31.0 ° /s, and 45.0 ° /s, are shown. Two target velocities are the same as in Figure 5a. An open and filled triangle indicate the fixation phase, a filled square indicates the appearance of the target and the subject's percept change.

Figure 6a and 6b show the eye movements and perceived velocity change when a subject looked at the continuous uni-directional grid movements. Subjects followed the grid movements with perfectly smooth pursuit eye movement.

Particularly in the case of subject MY (Figure 6b), pursuit eye movement continued for a relatively longer period than other subjects, and a relatively big saccade followed. On the contrary, with subject HA (Figure 6a), there were relatively short alternations of the fixation and pursuit phases. In both cases, the fixation phase was always observed at the end of the smooth pursuit eye movement phase and a big saccade occurred immediately after the end of the fixation phase. Faster motion perception as to the physically constant target movement always occurred just after the beginning of the fixation.

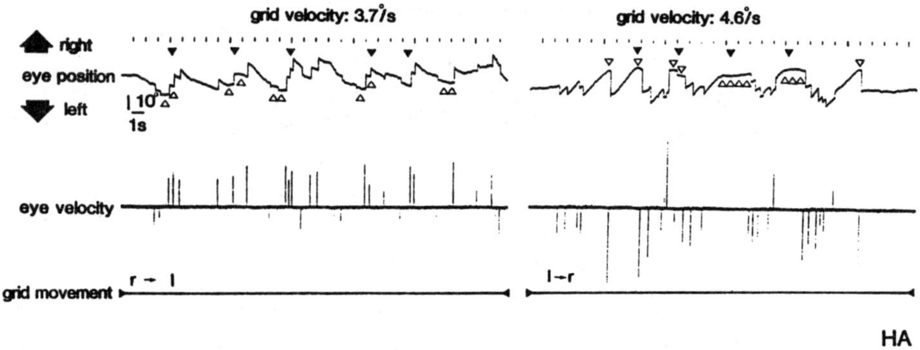

Fig. 6a Horizontal eye position and its velocity are shown when the continuous grid pattern was moved from left to right with the velocity of 3.7 ° /s and from right to left with the velocity of 4.6 ° /s. Open triangles indicate the fixation phase and filled triangles indicate the subject's response when the change of motion perception occurred.

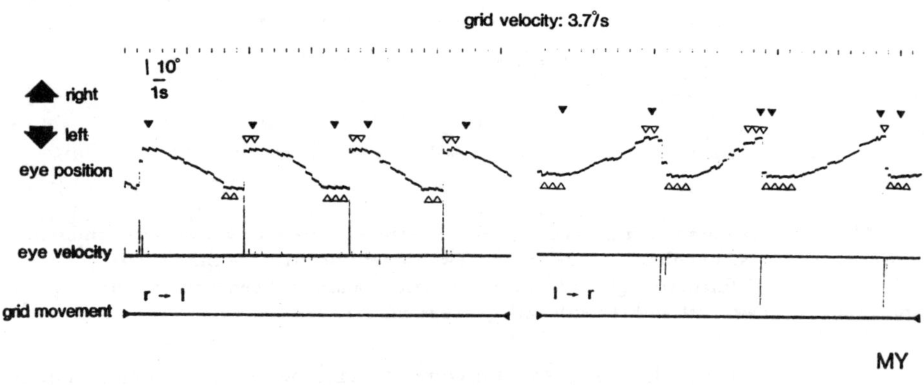

Fig. 6b: The same data as Figure 6a but only in a single grid velocity condition; 3.7 ° /s is shown.

Discussion

The synchronization between velocity perception change and the phase difference of the eye movements were observed under the slit view condition in the previous two experiments. This was again confirmed in the present experiment. The relationship between eye movement patterns and temporal velocity perception change was again observed even under the no-slit condition. Therefore, it is possible to say that the motion perception change occurred not only under the slit view condition but also in a usual object moving situation, that is, the no-slit condition. The change of velocity perception always occurred when the pattern of eye movement changed. That is, the phase shift from pursuit eye movement to fixation, or from saccade to fixation always corresponded to changes of perceived velocity. When the subject pursued a target with a constant velocity, the image was fixed on the retina and during the fixation period the image moved on the retina. Thus, the physical velocity of the image on the retina appears to directly determine changes in perceived temporal velocity.

Conclusion

We believe that absolute velocity perception can be modified by eye movements in several ways. Smooth pursuit eye movements strongly affect visual perception. Findings concerning the perceived velocity change in the grid with and without camel phase in Experiment 1 and 2 support our hypothesis, namely that perceived velocity perception can be modified by relative velocity differences between an object and the eyes. For example, if something such as an automobile moved behind a grid-type fence, we can easily recognize the automobile but do not attend to the fence when the eyes pursue the car, or we can discriminate the vertical grid lines of the fence but cannot recognize the moving car when fixating a position on the fence. Figure 7 symbolizes the retinal image of the moving objects when eyes are fixated on the fence or pursue the moving objects.

We believe it is much more likely that this kind of primitive perception should occur at a peripheral perceptual level than at a central level. The results of the characteristic eye movements obtained in Experiment 1 and 2 are likely to explain the different motion perception of the grid. However, there is less direct evidence that the complete retinal painting is due to the eye movements. It might be possible to conclude that a part of it is performed by the small smooth pursuit eye movements. It is enough to explain the shrinkage of the camel from the results obtained here in Experiment 1 und 2. We suppose that a lesser contribution from the eye movements produces this kind of illusory sensation, and it is much more reasonable to hypothesize a cognitive functioning in this situation.

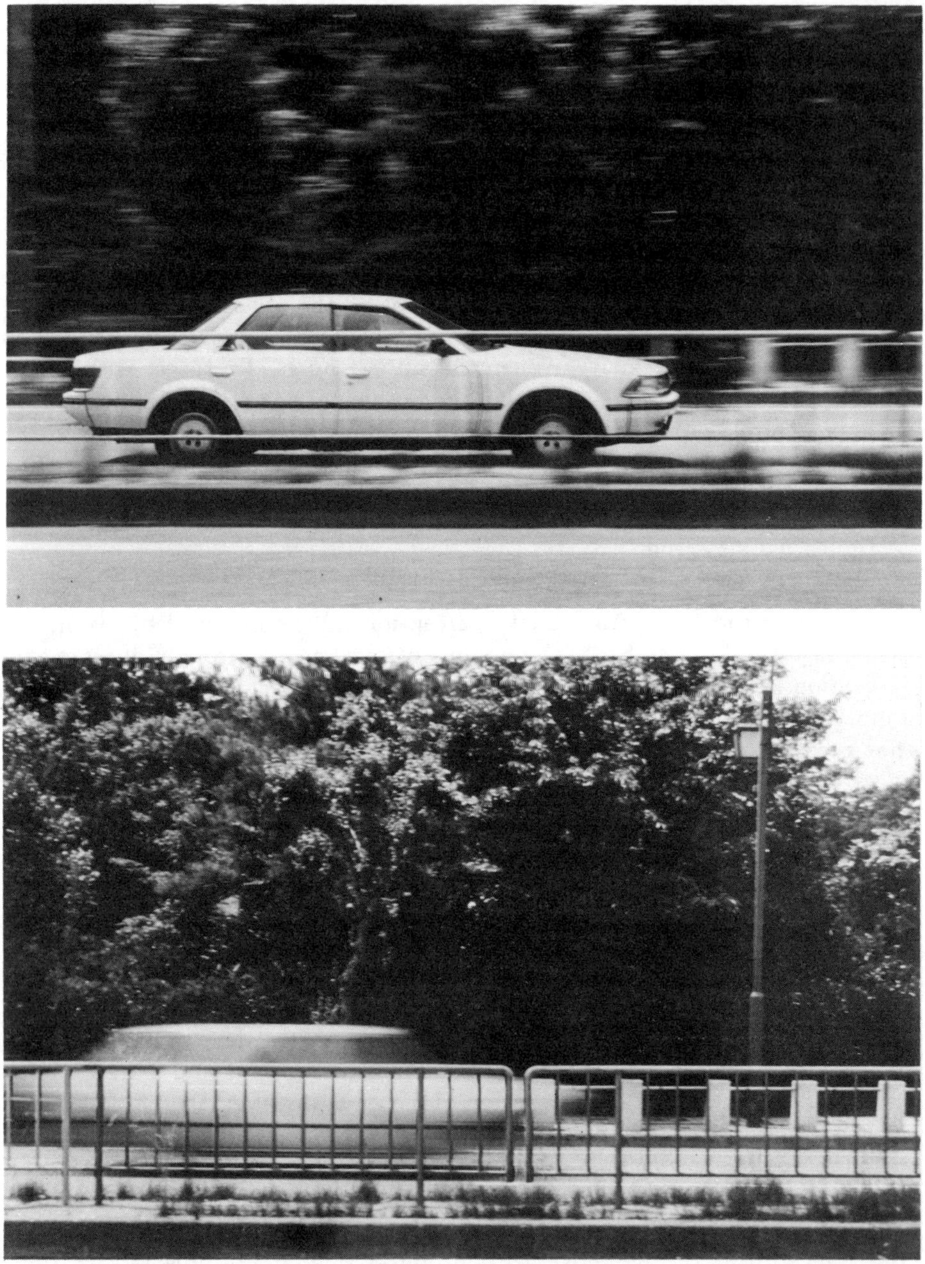

Fig. 7: The moving automobile behind the fence was photographed from two persepctives. The upper panel symbolizes the retinal image when the eye pursues the moving object but not the fence and the lower panel symbolizes the same scene when the eye fixates somewhere on the fence but does not pursue the moving object.

From the results of Experiment 3, we believe that the contribution of the eye movements to perceived temporal velocity is greater than we originally expected. However, it has been said that our visual stability, i.e. when the eye moves and retinal image displacement occurs, we perceive that the eye moves and surrounding objects are immobile. We suppose that such a percept comes from the higher cortical function done by the comparison between extraocular muscle afferent signals and visual image signals. If this is true, how could motion perception changes be perceived in this situation, the same as in the usual visual stability model? Does the visual stability model contain motion perception? We hardly know the afferent information from extraocular muscle in a psychological sense. As a result we have a tendency to trust our own visual experience without knowing how fast or how far the eye has moved. It has already been indicated that there is the possibility that even the retinal image can be distorted by eye movement.

Judgement of shape, size, depth, distance and motion must be done at a higher cortical level mainly based on the constancies. The environment is always moving around us and we are also moving ourselves in a way of body movement, neck bending or rotation, head and eye movements. The retinal image can be affected by these mutually independent movements. Here we provide evidence that eye movements can modify perceived temporal velocity.

Acknowledgment

This research was partly supported under the aids of Grant-in-Aid for Scientific Research (category-B, 6145001) by the Ministry of Education, Science and Culture of Japan in 1986 and 1987. The authors are grateful to Dr. Walter F. Bischof at the University of Alberta for his advice and help in the preparation of the manuscript. We are also grateful to our research colleague Dr. S. Ikumatsu at Cyuukyo University for his help. The photographs used were taken by him.

References

Anstis, S.M., & Atkinson, J., *Distortions in moving figure viewed through a stationary slit*, American Journal of Psychology **80** (1967), 572-585.

Bridgeman, B., & Mayer, M., & Glenn, L., *Figural distortion accompanying smooth pursuit eye movement*, Vision Research **16** (1976), 431-433.

Casco, C., & Morgan, M., *The relationship between space and time in the perception of stimuli moving behind a slit*, Perception **13** (1984), 429-441.

Haber, R.N., & Nathanson, L.S., *Post-retinal storage? Some further observations on Park's camel as seen through the eye of a needle*, Perception and Psychophysics **3** (1968), 349-355.

Haber, R.N., *Perceptual reports vs recognition responses: A reply to Parks*, Perception and Psychophysics **4** (1968), p. 374.

Hochberg, J., *In the mind's eye*, in "R.N. Haber (Ed.), Contemporary theory and research in visual perception," Holt, Rinehart, & Winston, New York, 1968, pp. 309-331.

Koga, K. & Osaka, R., *A comparison of triple recording methods of eye movement*, Japanese Psychological Research **25** (1983), 181-190.

Mack, A., *Perceptual aspects of motion in the frontal plane*, in "K.R. Bofl, L. Kaufman, & J.P. Thomas (Eds.), Handbook of perception and human performance, Vol. I, Chap. 17," J.W. & Sons, New York, 1986, pp. 1-38.

Matin, L., *Visual localization and eye movements*, in "K.R. Boff, L. Kaufman, & J.P. Thomas (Eds.), Handbook of perception and human performance, Vol. I, Chap. 20," J.W. & Sons, New York, 1986, pp. 1-45.

McCloskey, M., & Watkins, M., *The seeing-more-than-is-there-phenomenon: Implications for locus of iconic storage*, Journal of Experimental Psychology: Human Perception and Performance **4** (1978), 533-564.

Morgan, M.J., *How pursuit eye movements can convert temporal into spatial information*, in "D.F. Fisher & J.W. Senders (Eds.), Eye movements: Cognition and visual perception," Erlbaum, Hillsdale, N.J., 1981, pp. 110-133.

Morgan, M.J., Findlay, J.M., & Watt, R.J., *Aperture viewing: A review and a synthesis*, Quarterly Journal of Experimental Psychology **34A** (1982), 211-233.

Parks, T.E., *Post-retinal visual storage*, American Journal of Psychology **78** (1965), 145-147.

Parks, T.E., *Further comments on the evidence for post-retinal storage*, Perception and Psychophysics **4** (1968), p. 373.

Parks, T.E., *A control for ocular tracking in the demonstration of post-retinal visual storage*, American Journal of Psychology **82** (1970), 425-440.

Rock, I., & Halper, F., *From perception without a retinal image*, American Journal of Psychology **82** (1968), 425-440.

Rock, I., & Sigman, E., *Intelligent factors in the perception of form through a moving slit*, Perception **2** (1973), 357-369.

Rock, I., "The logic of perception," MIT Press, Cambridge, Massachusetts, 1983.

Shimojo, S., & Richards, W., *"Seeing" shapes that are almost totally occluded: A new look at Park's camel*, Perception and Psychophysics **39** (1986), 418-426.

Zoellner, F., *Über eine neue Art anorthoskopischer Zerrbilder*, Annalen der Physik **117** (1982), 477-484.

IDENTIFYING COGNITIVE STRUCTURES THROUGH EYE MOVEMENTS

WERNER KRAUSE

Sektion Psychologie, Friedrich Schiller Universität, Jena,
and Centre National de la Recherche Scientifique,
Laboratoire de Psychologie Expérimentale, Paris

Effective cognitive structuring of given information is essential for human perception, concept formation, comprehension and problem solving. The aim of this paper is to verify the symbolic-distance-effect (SDE) method used in problem-solving tasks through eye movement recordings.

IDENTIFYING COGNITIVE STRUCTURES IN SOLVING ORDERING PROBLEMS BY MEANS OF THE SDE

We proceeded with the intention to bridge the gap between complex and elementary problem solving tasks. We tried to find a relationship between the two tasks in order to define the performance in the complex problem-solving tasks in terms of performance in elementary problem-solving tasks (Krause, 1987).

In a first experiment of this study, the ability to solve complex problems was judged in terms of how successful one was in making a technical device in a mechanical engineering course. Elementary problem solving refers to the inference processes used to solve ordering problems.

We proceeded from the idea that problem solving is characterized by cognitive structure transformation. In an earlier study, we reduced phenomena in problem solving into elementary mechanisms used in structure transformations. We hypothesized that there are three basic components: integrating, selecting and structuring (Krause, Seifert & Sommerfeld, 1987). This study, however, concentrates on structuring as a basic component in problem solving.

We assume that complex and elementary problem solving is dependent on evaluated (i.e. effective or uneffective) cognitive structures. Mental load is one of the criteria of the effectiveness reached in human problem solving; obviously for elementary as well as complex problem solving. In our first experiment we determined, for each single subject, the cognitive structure in an elementary problem solving task. The cognitive structure in the elementary problem solving task was determined in the course of solving an ordering problem only for those subjects who were able to solve the complex problem. Each cognitive structure was evaluated by means of a mathematical model described by Sommerfeld (1987) The evaluated cognitive structures in complex problem solving tasks were not directly measured; but performance was indicated by the subjects marks given in a mechanical engineering course for making a technical device (in cooperation with G. Hoehne and H. Sperlich at the Technical College of Ilmenau). We were interested in correlating the evaluated performance in a complex problem solving task with the evaluated cognitive structures used in solving elementary problems.

Measuring cognitive structures. The ordering problem solving task was to comprehend and remember given information and in consequence, to answer questions on given and inferrable information. The time taken to make a decision was registered. The experimental material selected was of such a nature that improvement of information storage and processing could be achieved by way of an adequate formation of definite hierarchical structures. The given information consisted of a set of structural information units of the type element - comparative relation - element, presented on a terminal.

Figure 1 illustrates a given set of structural information units and their transformation into different cognitive structures connected with an improvement in retention and processing of information during the solution of ordering problems. Obviously, it is more difficult to answer the question: Is C r i, when the given set of structural information units is used, than when the structural information units are hierarchically ordered. The information that elements are members of different classes is useful to answer the question, whereas in the first case, the ordinal position difference has to be determined.

In this paper we describe experiments on the abilities of problem solvers to classify and hierarchically structure unknown information. That is, we investigated the ability to structure information by way of the minimal mental load needed to perform the task. The elements used in the experiment were geometrical patterns and their relation to each other (see Figure 2). The structural information units were given separately, step by step, and were stochastically ordered. Additionally, four possible cognitive structures were shown which were characterized by different numbers of classes. Figure 2 shows the different internal representations.

The SDE method was used in the following manner to measure individual cognitive structures (Figure 3). If the subject did not structure the given information hierarchically and if he/she used only one of the ordered elements to cope with the task, this situation was characterized by the existence of the SDE between two elements. If the subject structured the given information hierarchically and used more than one class to cope with the task, no SDE occurred between elements from different classes. In this case, the reaction time (t) was not a function of the distance (d) between these elements, i.e. the slope of $t=f(d)$ was not significantly different from zero. On the basis of the minimum difference of the slope from zero, we determined the cognitive structure for each single subject by calculating the slope for all possible combinations of three

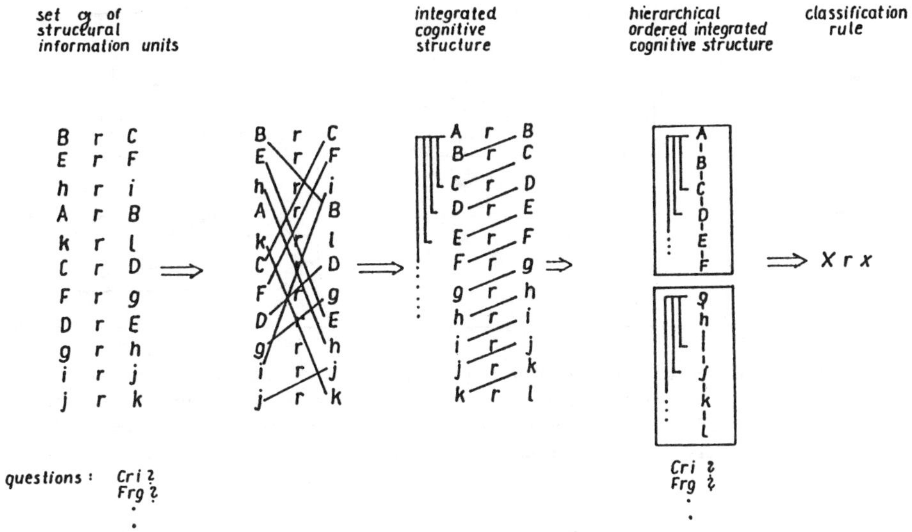

Fig. 1: An illustration of the improvement in solving ordering problems through hierarchically ordered structures.

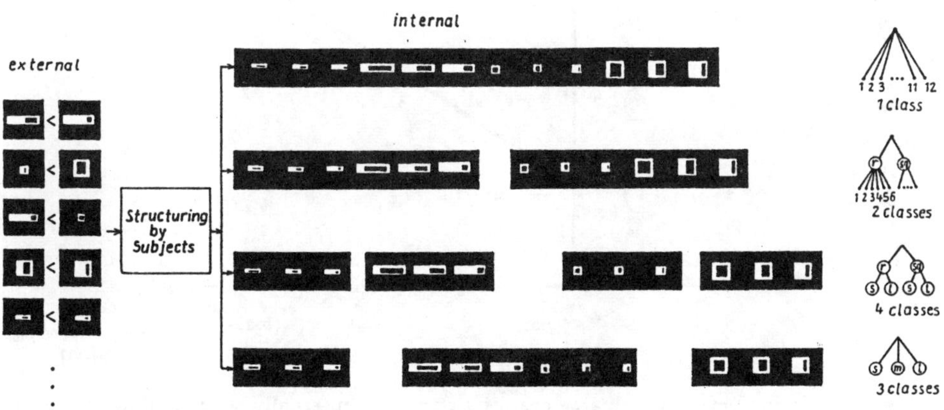

Fig. 2: The given unknown information and any possible cognitive structures. The structural information units are given separately step by step ($<$ means to the left of).

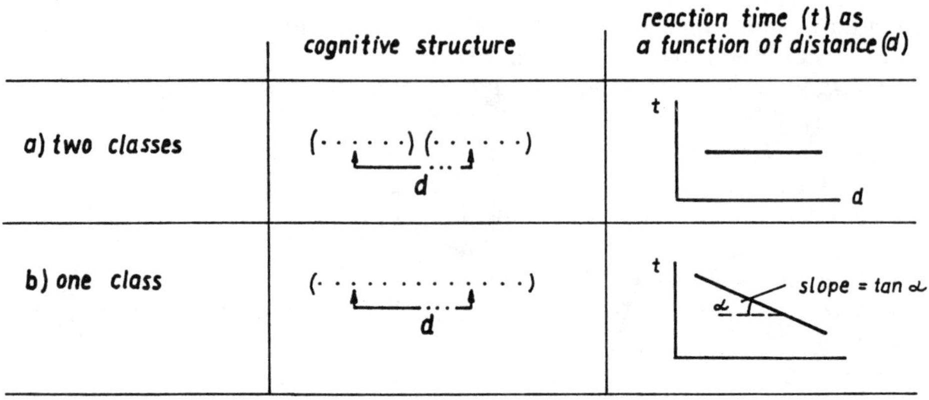

Fig. 3: Method to measure the individual cognitive structures: (a) Subjects use classes (the absence of the SDE is expected, because the subjects compare two elements as members of different classes. That means, the reaction time is independent of their distance d). (b) Subjects do not use classes (the existence of the SDE is expected).

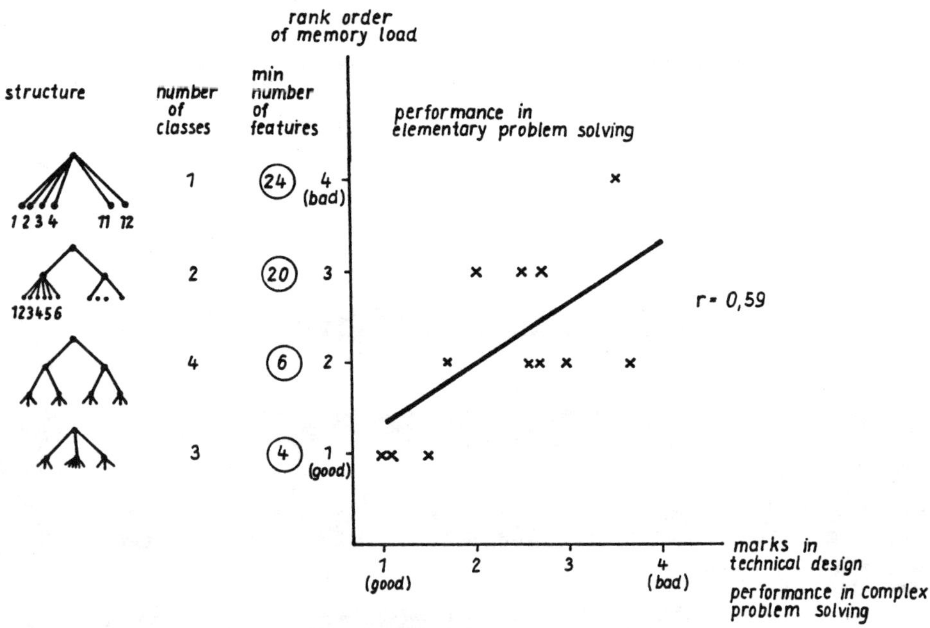

Fig. 4: Relation between evaluated cognitive structures internally acquired during elementary problem solving task and the performance of the subjects in solving complex tasks characterized by marks in mechanical engineering (12 Ss, students of mechanical engineering at the Technical College of Ilmenau).

boundaries (boundary M1, M2, M3 = 2,3,...,11 for four classes) and by seeking those combinations of boundaries having a minimum slope.

Results and conclusions. Figure 4 demonstrates the different cognitive structures characterized by the minimum number of features objectively necessary to describe the correspondent structures used to cope with the task by students having different marks in the design of an instrument. Results showed that good students in mechanical engineering used an internal representation with a minimal number of features. This finding implies that good problem solvers transform unknown information which is conducive to information storage and processing, in order to reduce the mental load. Essential is the reduction of the complexity of a problem (Klix, 1983).

In summary, we hypothesize that the ability to structure unknown information is one of the basic components in human problem solving. In order to verify this, a study of eye movements during problem solving tasks was conducted.

Basis Assumptions for Using Analysis of Eye Movements in Relation to the Performance on Problem Solving Tasks

Hypothetically, we distinguish between two cases:

(1) After the acquisition of information, the solving process is independent of the exposition time:

$$t_{proc} \neq f(t_{exp}). \tag{1}$$

In this case any eye movement analysis for problem solving would be irrelevant.

(2) After the acquisition of information, the solving process depends on the exposition time:

$$t_{proc} = f(t_{exp}). \tag{2}$$

In this case, eye movement analysis in problem solving may be very informative.

Let us assume that the total time t_{tot} in solving a problem is determined by the time to acquire t_{acq} the information plus the time to process t_{proc} the information.

$$t_{tot} = t_{acq} + t_{proc}, \tag{3}$$

with $t_{acq} \ll t_{proc}$, nearly equal to

$$t_{tot} = t_{proc} \tag{4}$$

and allowing for the assumption that the analysis of eye movements can be correlated with an analysis of problem solving, it follows, that (5) can be derived from (4) and (1):

$$t_{tot} = f(t_{exp}). \tag{5}$$

We assumed that the total time as well as other behavioral parameters in problem solving would be dependent on the variation of the exposition time. Table 1 shows the results of our second experiment. The procedure is the same as described in the first experiment. Results show a dependency of the total time used to solve the problem, errors and boundaries of classes upon the exposition time implying that eye movement analysis in problem solving may be very informative.

Tab. 1: Time total, errors, and boundaries of classes for different exposition times for 3 subjects (Ss).

Ss	time total (ms)		errors		boundaries of classes	
	texp=ttot	texp<70ms	texp=ttot	texp<70ms	texp=ttot	texp<70ms
K	642	370	9	20	3/9	9
F	1508	493	95	51	6/9	9
W	710	446	9	14	3/6/9	3

Analysis of Cognitive Structures Based on Eye Movements

To verify the SDE method for cognitive structure analysis, we determined the eye fixation frequency during the solving of ordering problems. We used the eye movement equipment and method from the Laboratory of Prof. Ariane Lévy- Schoen (cf. Jacobs and Lévy-Schoen, this volume). Subjects were seated in a chair without a head rest. Each structural information unit was presented on a screen 50 cm from the subject's eye. Eye movements were recorded by a photo- electric mechanism linked to a micro computer (Acorn BBC). This recording procedure was developed by Y. Barbin (1982) and the researchers of the Groupe Regard (Coeffe, Humbert, Jacobs, & O'Regan, 1985). This system processes horizontal eye movements and records the direction and size of saccades and the position and duration for each structural information unit.

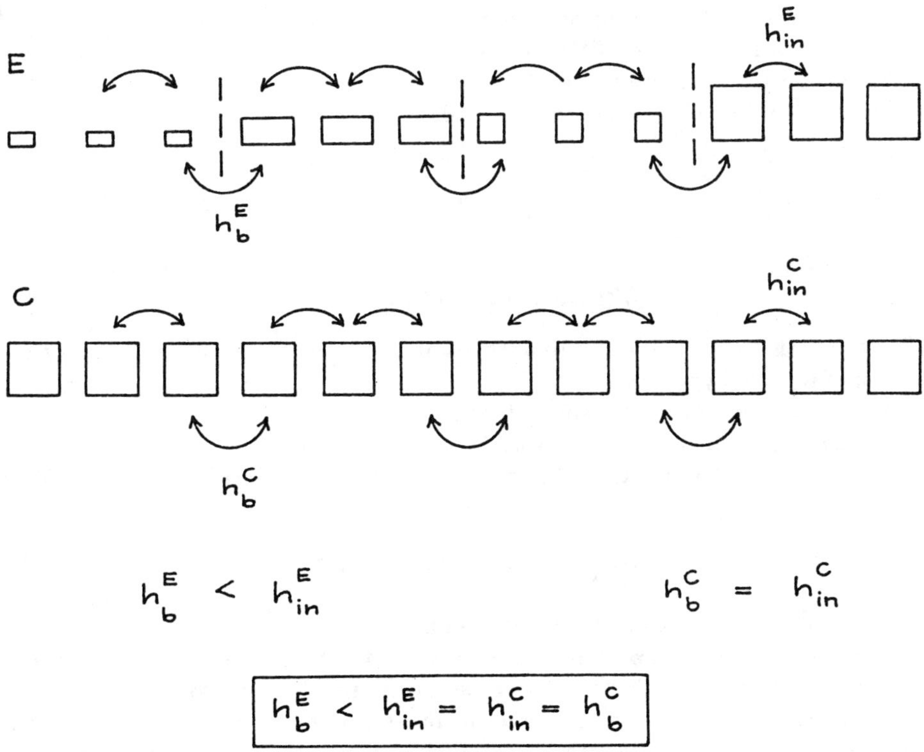

Fig. 5: Comparison of eye fixation frequencies between two series: the experimental situation (E) with a given structure and the control situation (C) without any given structure (h = eye fixation frequency for pairs of elements, b = fixation between different classes, in = fixation in a class, d = distance, t = time).

Registrations were made of the number of fixations for two series at the boundaries of classes of a cognitive structure

(a) a structure condition (experimental, E) and
(b) a no structure condition (control, C) (Figure 5).

The assumption was made that in condition E, the fixation frequency $h^E b$ between different classes would be smaller than the fixation frequency $h^E in$ within a class:

$$h^E b < h^E in.$$

A comparison of the fixation frequencies at the same positions used in condition E was made in condition C. Since there were no objective boundaries in condition C, an assumption of no differences in the fixation frequencies of "within" and "between" classes was made.

$$h^C b = h^C in.$$

Our hypothesis was:

$$h^E b < h^E in = h^C in = h^C b.$$

The prediction of eye fixation frequencies in different situations is necessary to corroborate our hypothesis.

We proceeded from the results obtained in two experiments with (SDE) (no classification of information in solving ordering problems, see Figure 3) and without (SDE) (classification of information in solving ordering problems). The reaction time

$$t^{SDE}1,\ t^{SDE}2,\ t^{0SDE}1\ and\, t^{0SDE}3$$

for the distance d=1 and d=3 is given (Figure 6).

Furthermore, we know from the analysis of the SDE that a decrease in reaction time is attributable to a decrease in the number of fixations as well as to a decrease in fixation time per element as a function of distance between elements which have to be compared. However, there was a preference for the first case: The longer reaction time in the case of small distances was caused by a higher number of fixations. Krause (1985) determined the average number of eye fixation frequencies (h) for the distance (d=1) and (d=3):

$$h^{SDE}1 = 2.7\, and\, h^{SDE}3 = 0.9.$$

Based on this data, together with the above (Figure 6), we expected:

$$h^E b < h^E in = h^C in = h^C b$$

$$0.9 < 2.7.$$

The *results* found in solving ordering problems confirm our assumption (Figure 7, Table 2): Group I showed significantly fewer fixation frequencies in accompanying elements from different classes in contrast to those from the same class (0.90 fixations/two elements vs 1.65 fixations/two elements) (Mann-Withney-Test, $p < .05$). For this group, we found exact boundaries by means of the SDE method to measure the cognitive structures, described in the first experiment.

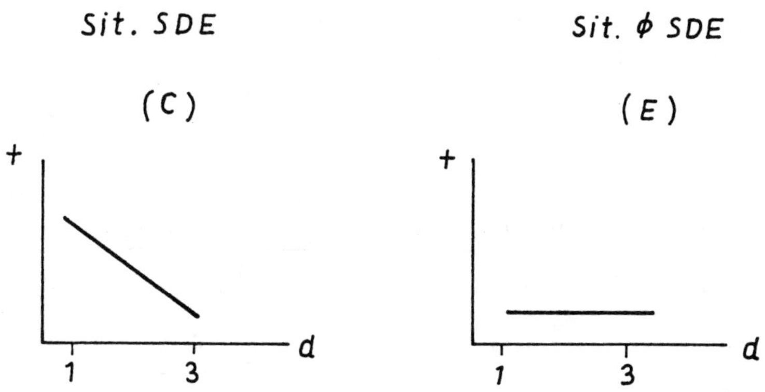

given : $t_1^{SDE},\ t_3^{SDE},\ t_1^{\phi SDE},\ t_3^{\phi SDE}$

$h_1^{SDE} = 2.7,\ h_3^{SDE} = 0{,}9,\ h_1^{SDE} = h_b^C$

searched: $h_1^{\phi SDE} = h_b^E$?

$$(h \mathrel{\hat{=}} t) \wedge (t_1^{\phi SDE} < t_1^{SDE}) \Rightarrow h_1^{\phi SDE} < h_1^{SDE} = 2.7$$

$$(h \mathrel{\hat{=}} t) \wedge (t_1^{\phi SDE} = t_3^{\phi SDE}) \Rightarrow h_1^{\phi SDE} = h_3^{SDE} = 0.9$$

expected : $\boxed{h_1^{\phi SDE} = h_b^E = 0.9}$

$$h_b^E < h_b^C = 2.7$$

$$\boxed{\begin{array}{l} h_b^E < h_{in}^E = h_{in}^C = h_b^C \\ 0.9 < 2.7 \end{array}}$$

Fig. 6: The derivation of our hypothesis. We expected: $h^Eb = 0.9$ and $h^Eb < h^Ein$. Two experimental situations were assumed with (SDE) and without (0SDE). $t^{SDE}1$ = reaction time in the case of a SDE with distance (d) = 1; $h^{SDE}1$ = eye fixation frequency in the same situation; $h^{SDE}1 = 2.7$ and $h^{SDE}3 = 0.9$. See Krause (1985) for deviation of above values.

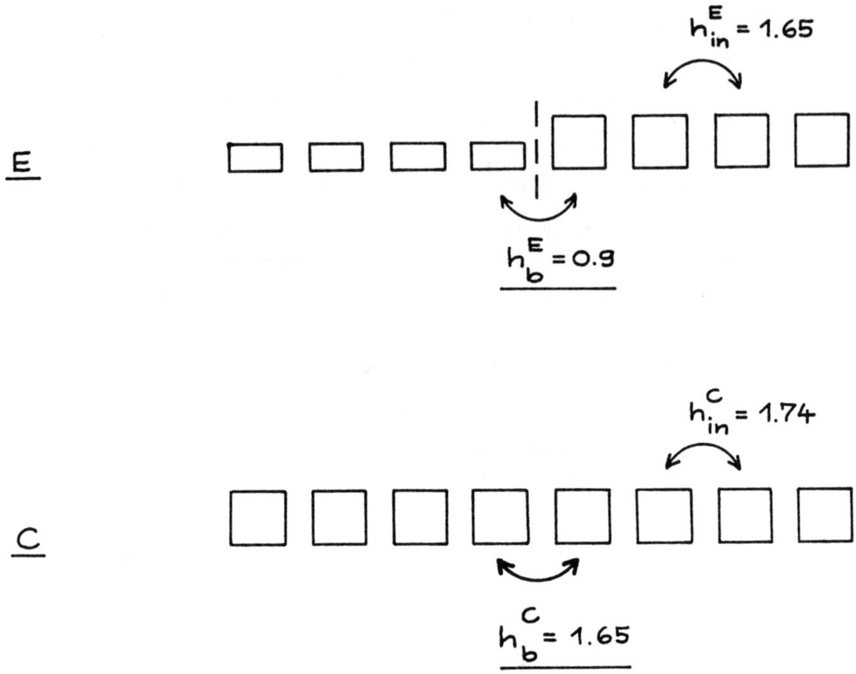

expected: $h_b^E < h_{in}^E = h_{in}^C = h_b^C$

observed

GI : $0.90 < 1.65 = 1.65 \approx 1.74$

GII : $2.81 \nless 2.87 \approx 2.25 \approx 2.61$

Fig. 7: Results for (E) and (C) conditions, G = group.

Strangely, group II, did not show this difference (2.81 fixations/two elements vs 2.87 fixations/two elements). For this group, we did not found exact boundaries by means of the SDE method, described in the first experiment. The cause for this finding lies in the representation. While the subjects in group I showed a hierarchical structure in accomplishing the task, that is, using the characteristics of the patterns leading to clear boundaries of class (discontinuous representation), group II subjects showed a rather linear, imaginative

Tab. 2: Number of fixations/picture in order to compare two elements for solving the ordering problems for the two groups

	structure is given		no structure is given	
	number of fixations		number of fixations	
Ss I.	at the boundaries of classes of a cognitive structure	within a class	"at the boundaries of classes of a cognitive structure"	"within a class"
K	1.07	1.74 s	0.85	1.02 ns
C	1.00	1.40 s	1.43	1.36 ns
T	0.63	1.81 s	2.67	2.86 ns
/3	0.90	1.65 s	1.65	1.74 ns
II.				
F	3.57	4.0 ns	2.08	2.72 s
W	2.33	1.98 ns	3.33	3.06 ns
A	2.53	2.64 ns	1.35	2.05 s
/3	2.81	2.87 ns	2.25	2.61 ns

order, which had no definitive boundaries (one of the patterns is more to the left, the other more to the right, etc.). This form of representation is, thus, more continuous (analogue representation).

Conclusion: Eye movement measurement is a useful method to analyze cognitive structures. Future experiments will focus on the determination of the fixation location in order to mathematically describe the ability of structuring information in terms of a low mental load required.

Acknowledgement

The data reported here were gathered as part of a study carried on in the Centre National de la Recherche Scientifique, Laboratoire de Psychologie Expérimentale, Paris, France. The author expresses his thanks to Ariane Lévy- Schoen, Arthur Jacobs and Kevin O'Regan for their assistance and most fruitful discussions.

References

Barbin, Y., *"Cybermérope": un système analogique de traitement du signal pour l'étude en temps réel des mouvements oculaires horizontaux dans des contextes d'éclairements ambiants variés*, D.E.A. Electronique Instrumentation, Université Paris VI (1982).

Coeffe, C., Humbert, R., Jacobs, A.M., & O'Regan, J.K., *Mesure des mouvements oculaires en temps réel*, Informatique et Sciences Humaines **65** (1985), 57-72.

Jacobs, A.M., & Lévy-Schoen, A., *Breaking down saccade latency into central and peripheral processing times in a visual dual-task*, (this volume).

Klix, F., *Begabungsforschung - ein neuer Weg in der kognitiven Intelligenzdiagnostik*, Zeitschrift für Psychologie **191** (1983), 360-387.

Krause, W., *Komponentenanalyse des Symbol-Distanz-Effektes mit Hilfe von Augenbewegungsmessungen*, Zeitschrift für Psychologie **193** (1985), 259-272.

Krause, W., *Structuring in problem solving*, WORKSHOP, Berlin 1987, Zeitschrift für Psychologie (to appear).

Krause, W., Seifert, R., & Sommerfeld, E., *Ausbildung und Transformation kognitiver Strukturen im Problemlösen*, ZKI-Informationen **2** (1987).

Krause, W., *Structuring in problem solving*, WORKSHOP, Berlin 1987, Zeitschrift für Psychologie (to appear).

O'Regan, J.K., & Lévy-Schoen, A. (Eds.), "Eye movements: From physiology to cognition," North-Holland, Amsterdam, 1987.

Sommerfeld, E., *Evaluation of cognitive structuring in elementary problem solving - a model approach*, WORKSHOP, Berlin 1987, Zeitschrift für Psychologie (to appear).

USING EYE MOVEMENTS TO STUDY DECISION MAKING OF RADIOLOGISTS

CALVIN F. NODINE, HAROLD L. KUNDEL, JAMES B. POLIKOFF, AND LAWRENCE C. TOTO

Temple University & University of Pennsylvania

Does the number of fixations that cluster on true targets detected during visual search for lung tumors in chest x-ray images differ from the number of fixations that cluster on non-target (normal) chest features? The purpose of this study was to answer this question by measuring and describing the way experts search for and detect inconspicuous targets in pictorial scenes. The experts were radiologists. The inconspicuous targets were lung tumors. The pictorial scenes consist of chest anatomy and pathology in the form of solitary lung nodules.

The inconspicuous targets were embedded or camouflaged by pictorial scenery in the present study. Therefore, detection was not automatic in the sense that the target did not typically "pop out" upon global or cursory examination of the image. Because of this fact, the viewer had to systematically search the image to uncover an inconspicuous target. Using eye-movement recordings, it is possible to identify when and where a viewer recognizes an abnormality on an x-ray image, but falsely rejects it as normal (False Negative decision= FN). If these FNs can be identified by eye-movement measurements, they can be fed back to the viewer for reconsideration, leading to an improvement in detection accuracy.

Automatic vs. Controlled Search and Detection

Nodine and Kundel (1987), and others cited below have distinguished between two types of visual information processing in search and detection tasks: automatic detection and controlled search and detection. Schneider and Shiffrin (1977) propose that in automatic detection, items of a scene are compared simultaneously, in parallel, with items stored in a memory set, whereas in controlled search, serial comparison of items with memory set is required for detection. This distinction has been incorporated into a model of visual search shown in Figure 1.

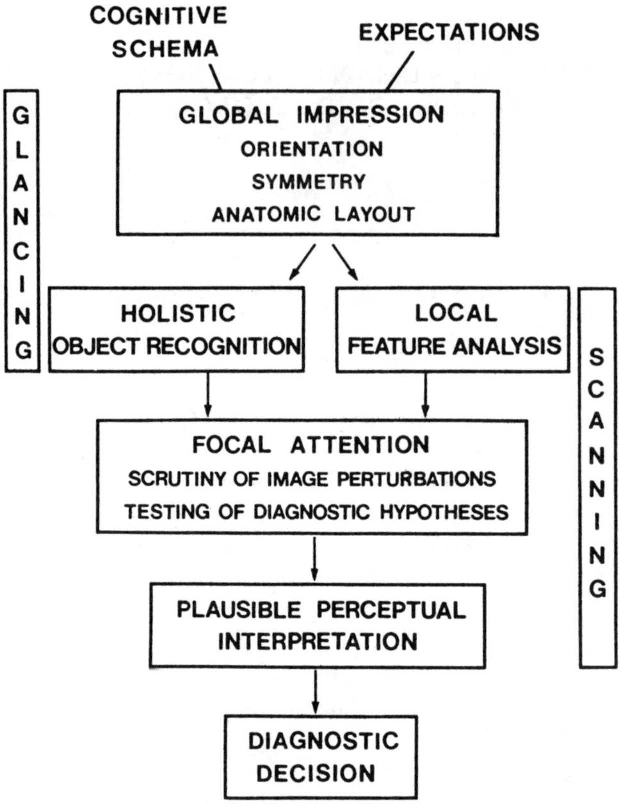

Fig. 1: Model of visual search. The initial glance results in a global impression that provide the viewer with information about image pattern. Scanning tests diagnostic hypotheses by scrutinizing suspected objects of image scenery. The evidence gathered from these tests is used to generate plausible perceptual interpretations that lead to diagnostic decisions.

Global Impression vs. Focal Attention

Visual encoding of the scene takes place in two phases. The first phase is a Global Impression. The second phase is Focal Attention. The scene is grasped globally in the first 200 ms of viewing (Kundel & Nodine, 1975). During the global impression image orientation, symmetry detection and the layout of objects of anatomic scenery is registered and compared, in parallel, with a memory set of scenery items based on the viewer's cognitive schema of human anatomy and pathology.

If targets or abnormalities do not "pop out" during the global impression because they are camouflaged by the anatomic scenery, controlled search and detection is initiated. Controlled search requires that the image be examined sequentially by focal attention in order to pick up inconspicuous targets. The controlled search process is interactive in nature being controlled, in part, by cognitive schema and expectations, and in part, by peripheral visual input. This peripheral input provides a local context for examining details of the image scenery. The detailed input is sifted and tested against the viewer's cognitive schema of the target object in memory.

Attending, Recognizing, Deciding

Since inconspicuous targets are characteristically embedded or camouflaged in anatomic scenery, parts of the target may be obscured by anatomy. Due to the fact that the target is a lung nodule composed of living cells, feature dimensions of the target will necessarily overlap with feature dimensions of the anatomic scenery in which it is growing. This means that the process of matching input against target features stored in memory set has built-in uncertainty attached to it, even when the viewer applies highly-specific target criteria. Thus, visual encoding of objects of image scenery during the controlled search process may reveal an anatomic ambiguity that the viewer may decide is a target, or may flag as a potential, but undecided target. The viewer's decision, positive or negative, is based on building up confidence in the decision-making process by serially matching local input at a focal attention node, defined by a fixation cluster, against his memory set of target features.

Consistent with Treisman and Gelade's feature-integration model of information processing (1980), we believe that the viewer's detection decision is based on the conjoining of input features with corresponding features in a memory set. Detection is usually based on anatomic or pathological evidence in the image. Target detection results when the target object is recognized outright, or, when input scenery features are recognized as embedded parts of a target object of search. The implication in this latter case is that since feature integration is required for detection, localized attention and its accompanying scrutiny precede detection. This means that inconspicuous target detection will be sensitive to information-processing load measures such as (a) number of serial comparisons, (b) number of conjunctions of features required for detection, and (c) ease of differentiation between target and background features (King et al., 1984). These information-processing load measures can be inferred from eye-fixation data.

Measuring Information-Processing Load

Two dependent variables have been used to measure information-processing load during visual search, fixation duration or dwell (Kundel, Nodine, & Carmody, 1978; Nodine, Carmody, & Kundel, 1978, Friedman & Liebelt, 1981) and number of fixations falling on features of image scenery (Loftus, 1972, 1981).

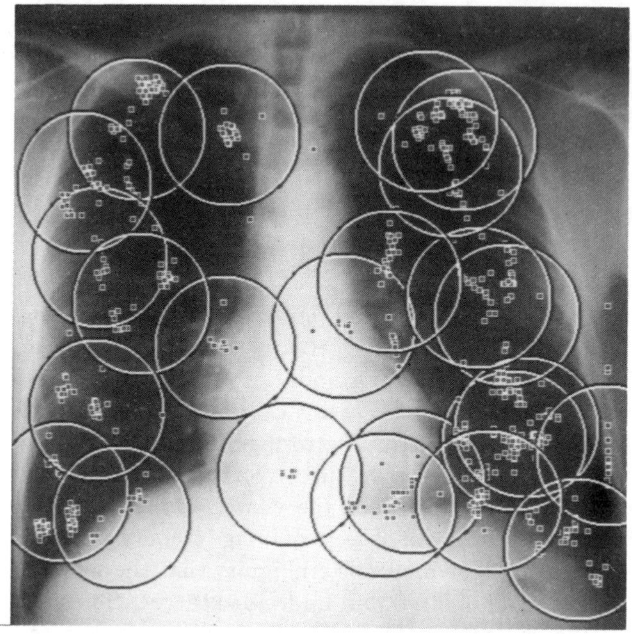

2A

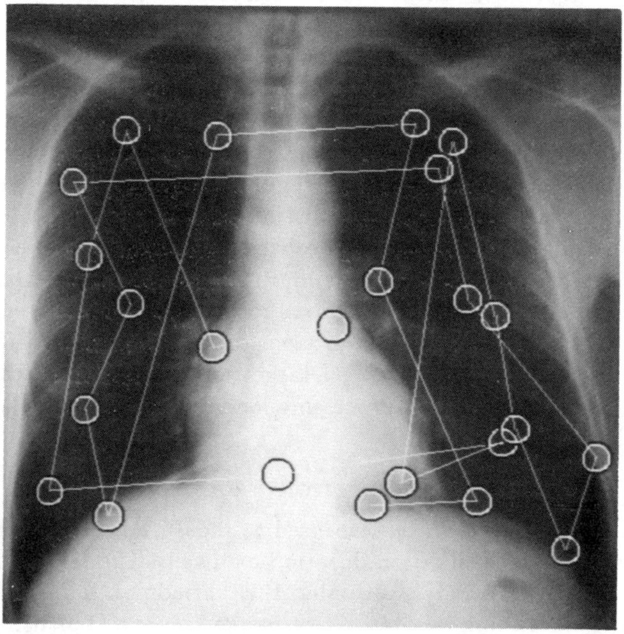

2B

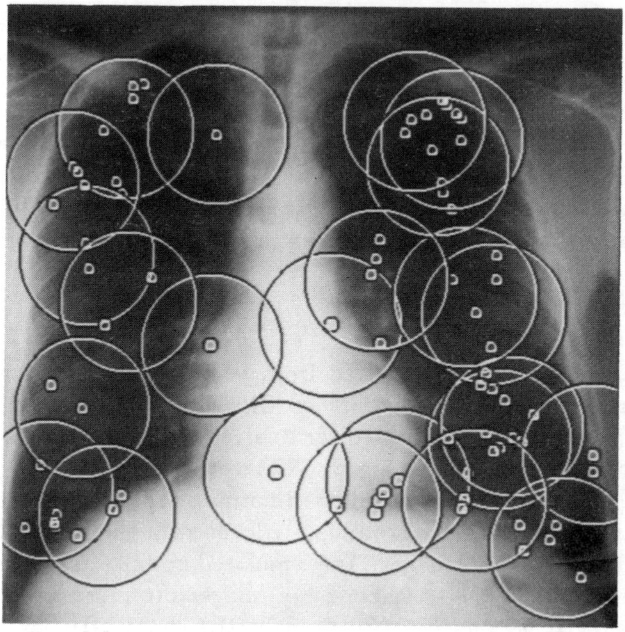

2C

Fig. 2: A series of eye-fixation records showing the locus of the axis of gaze during fixation and the path of the eye during movement. 2A: The raw eye-position data. 2B: The eye-fixation record showing the foveal field of view for each fixation. Circles have a radius of 5 °. 2C: The same fixation record showing fixation clusters. Circles have a radius of 2.5 °

The present study looks at both dependent variables. In order to compare the two dependent variables, we developed an algorithm for analyzing eye movements by grouping fixations into clusters on the basis of spatial and temporal parameters. The distance parameter limited fixation clusters to a range of $\pm$ 2.5 ° on the display which corresponds to a circular visual field size having a 90 percent average detection rate for inconspicuous (contrast value = 0.12) lung nodules (Kundel, Nodine et al., 1987). The minimum duration of a fixation was 33 ms. The parameter settings of our algorithm are within the range of settings explored by Karsh and Breitenbach in defining an eye fixation (1983). Using this clustering algorithm, we generated maps showing locations of fixation clusters as radiologists searched for lung nodules.

Figure 2 schematically shows the three stages of the eye-movement data analysis. First, the raw eye-movement record. Each small square represents 16 ms worth of x,y eye position. The circles (2.5 ° radius) drawn around groups of data points identify potential clusters of fixations. The sampling rate was 60 x,y data records per s. Second, the eye- fixation record in which x,y data have been grouped into fixations using a running mean having threshold values of 0.5 ° and, at least, 2 data records (33 ms). Lines connect the fixation points to show the sequence of fixations. Third, the same record showing fixation clusters. Fixations are grouped into clusters again using a running-mean, but this time with threshold values of 2.5 ° and 1 fixation or 33 ms. Circles having a radius of 2.5 ° have been drawn around each cluster. A cluster can have a minimum of one fixation.

METHOD

Eye-movement data were collected from two experiments. In Experiment 1, two experienced radiologists searched 240 chest images. Of the 480 eye-movement records, 93 were rejected for analysis because of poor calibrations. Results are reported on the remaining 387 records.

Half of the chest images were confirmed normals. A simulated solitary inconspicuous lung-nodule target was randomly located in the lungs of the remaining half of "normal" chest images. The simulated nodules are indistinguishable from most nodular shapes on chest x-ray images produced by solid spherical lumps of tissue. It is convenient to describe the characteristics of the nodule by its location, size (diameter), contrast, and edge sharpness (blur). We chose a gaussian function to define the edge sharpness of the nodule. Since a gaussian function is normally defined in terms of amplitude and standard deviation, we defined simulated nodules by measuring size and shape directly, and edge sharpness by the amplitude and standard deviation of the gaussian function. These simulated nodules were than rated for conspicuity.

The conspicuity of the nodule targets was judged subsequent to the search task by both radiologists. This was accomplished in two ways. First, each of the nodule images was shown and the search time to detect them was measured either by recording the elapsed search time until the viewer pointed to the nodule, or, a maximum time of 16 s was assigned if the nodule was not detected. Second, if the nodule was detected, it was rated for visibility using a scale from 1 (almost invisible) to 5 (highly visible), or, if it was not detected, the experimenter pointed to the nodule and asked the viewer to rate it. Fifty-five percent of the nodules were not detected in the alloted search time and required pointing out. The average rating of this subset of nodules was 1.40 (sd = .61). The remaining nodules were detected after an average search time of 8.37 s (sd = 5.40). The average rating of the detected nodules was 3.85 (sd = 1.20). Given these ratings, it can be assumed that a majority of the nodule targets were inconspicuous.

In Experiment 2, the same two radiologists searched 120 chest images, each for solitary lung-nodule targets. Half were normal, and the other half contained a single simulated nodule target. After the search task was completed, the viewer was shown the image again and asked to point out suspected nodule locations and areas that may have been ambiguous or troublesome. Results are reported on fixation clusters during the search and pointing task.

Cluster maps like the one described in Figure 2C above were produced for each radiologist's search of each image. Each cluster identified an aspect of the anatomic scenery of the chest that received attention as it was presumably being tested for the presence of a target. Thus, each fixation cluster could be thought of as a sub-decision leading up to an overall decision as to whether the image was normal or nodule containing. The fact that each fixation cluster represents the results of a psychophysical test of the presence or absence of a nodule target in the anatomic scenery falling within the radiologist's effective field of view, differs significantly from traditional Receiver Operating Characteristic (ROC) analysis (signal-detection theory) which assumes that a single overall decision represents the results of the psychophysical test. Subsequent analyses of the fixation cluster data will follow a multiple-decision-per-image model of detection rather than a single- decision-per-image model.

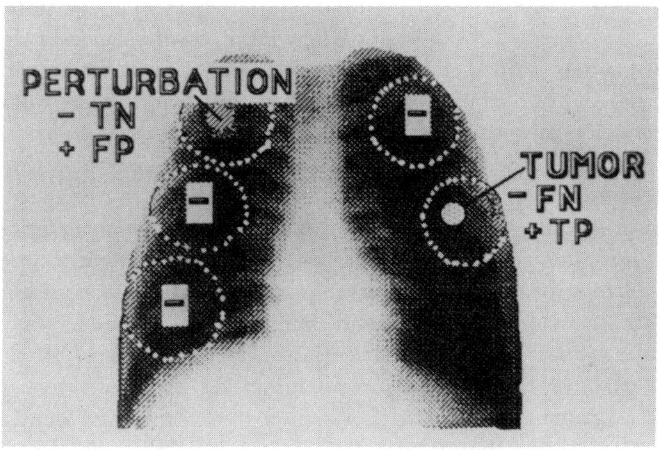

Fig. 3: Decision Nodes: Fixations clustering on objects of image scenery are indicated by circles. Each circle represents a decision node. The type of decision can be positive indicating the presence of a nodule target (+), or negative indicating the absence of a nodule target (−). The conjoining of the decision with either true nodule targets or false image targets results in four decision categories shown.

Eye-fixation clusters for each image resulting in positive decisions were classified as true or false positives; and, those resulting in negative decisions were classified as true or false negatives. A positive decision was true when a fixation cluster fell on a nodule target and false when a fixation cluster fell on a normal feature that was designated as nodule-containing. A negative decision was *true* when a normal feature was fixated by a cluster and no overt (positive) decision followed. Due to this default definition of true negative decisions, they occurred frequently on both normal chest images *and* chest images containing nodules. A negative decision was *false* when a nodule was fixated, but no overt positive decision followed Figure 3 shows the four types of decision schematically.

CHARACTERIZING FIXATION-CLUSTER DISTRIBUTIONS

The observed distributions of (a) number of fixations per cluster, and (b) cluster durations for each of the four decision categories were tested for chi square goodness of fit against normal, Poisson and negative binominal distributions. The negative binominal distribution produced the best chi square fits for the four decision categories.

THE FLOW OF PERCEPTUAL EVENTS LEADING TO A DECISION

We assume that the eye samples an area of the image and acquires a chunk of data during each fixation cluster. A number of information processing events accompany data acquisition: the data are analyzed; a decision is made to *supplement* the present data or *explore* new data; computation of the location of the new data is determined, local or distant; and, an eye movement is initiated. McConkie, Underwood et al., (1985), and Jacobs (1987) have outlined similar perceptual events that they assume are associated with a fixation during the reading of text. The decision to supplement the current fixation data which entails a local move, or, explore new data which entails a distance move can be considered a Bernoulli trial since the probability to move or explore is assumed to remain constant over trials, and, the trials are statistically independent. If the decision is to supplement the current fixation data by a local move, then the number of fixations in the cluster will increase until sufficient data is acquired to satisfy information- processing criteria for decision making. If the decision is to explore new data, the eye will jump beyond the range of the current fixation cluster, thus, initiating a new fixation cluster in a new image location. Just and Carpenter (1980) have shown that the durations of clusters of fixations called "gazes" increased directly with the syntactical importance of the word in the sentence being fixated. Thus, gaze duration, which is directly proportional to the number of fixations per cluster, reflects information-processing load in reading.

RESULTS AND DISCUSSION

Results of Experiment 1

A fixation cluster was classified according to the viewer's decision about the local image features at each fixation cluster. Each fixation cluster fell into one of four categories determined from a truth table that mapped the observer's decision, "normal" or "nodule" against the state of the image, either truly normal or nodule-containing. Positive decisions were relatively easy to classify because the viewer made an overt response which can be related to where and what he was fixating at the time of a decision. Negative decisions were more difficult to classify because each time a new fixation cluster was formed, the viewer may be making a decision about the presence of nodule features, but if none were recognized, the viewer's decision was deferred, resulting in a default normal decision, and the eye moved on.

For example, in a 15 s search period, a radiologist generates an average of 18 fixation clusters over a chest image. Each cluster has the potential to result in a decision, but if no nodule features were recognized, the decision was defaulted. Since defaulted decisions presumably do not require feature scrutiny, the number of fixations per cluster may enable us to differentiate defaulted from non-defaulted decisions. If nodule features were recognized, the viewer presumably scrutinized them in order to decide whether or not they meet his criteria of abnormal. The application of the viewer's decision criteria for abnormal sometimes resulted in positive decisions and sometimes resulted in negative decisions.

If it is assumed that the detection of a nodule consists of fixating, recognizing and decision-making, then these three components require information-processing of visual data that is reflected by multiple fixations leading to an increase in fixation-cluster durations. Kundel, Nodine, and Carmody (1978) differentiated between scanning, recognition and decision-making errors for false negative (FN) decisions on the basis of fixation dwell times. Twenty-five percent of the FNs were classified as recognition errors. These recognition errors were associated with a smaller difference between initial fixation dwell on the nodule target and total fixation dwell on the nodule target: 200-300 vs. 200-600 ms respectively; than the difference between initial fixation dwell and total fixation dwell for decision-making errors: 150-800 vs. 800-2100 ms respectively. Greater differences between initial and total fixation dwell suggest that decision-making requires longer fixations, or perhaps more fixations, to process visual data in order to make a decision once the eye fixates a target.

Just how many fixations clustering on image features are required for various decisions is shown in Figure 4. This figure shows the distributions of numbers of fixations clustering on decision areas of the chest image associated with true negative, false negative and true positive decisions in Experiment 1. False positive decisions were omitted because of so few data.

The curves are described by the mean and mode in Table 1. The mean and mode provide only an intuitive sense of the differences between distributions across categories since the distributions are not normal. Table 1 indicates that the mode for TPs is bimodal. This favors the interpretation that some targets

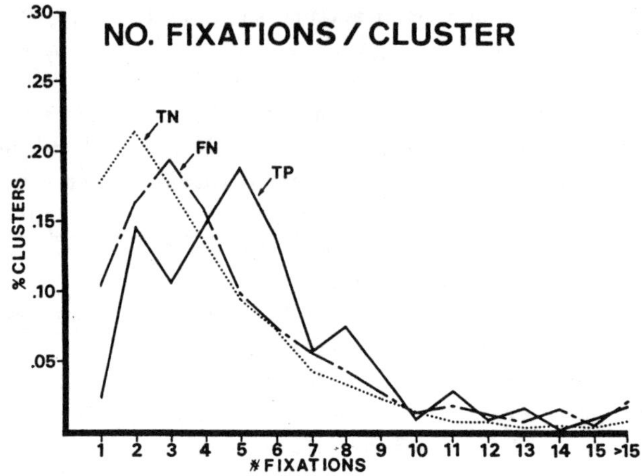

Fig. 4: The distributions of number of fixations per cluster for true negative (TN), false negative (FN) and true positive (TP) decisions. Because of the small numbers of false positive (FP) decisions, no distribution is shown. The three decision types were determined by measuring all fixation locations leading up to an overt decision by the viewer. If the decision is positive (nodule present), fixations clustering on truly abnormal image features are categorized as true positives (TP). If the decision is negative (nodule absent), fixations clustering on truly abnormal image features are categorized as false negatives (FN); fixations clustering on truly normal image features are categorized as true negatives (TN). The true negative decisions peak at 2 fixations per cluster, the false negatives at 3 fixations per cluster and the true positives at 2 and 5 fixations per cluster.

"pop out" and some undergo considerable visual scrutinizing which is reflected by increased numbers of fixations per cluster. Furthermore, TPs required more fixations per cluster than TNs. Presumably this difference reflects a difference in information-processing load depending on whether the viewer makes a positive or negative decision. Chi square tests were performed to compare entire frequency distributions of numbers of fixations per cluster grouped into contingency tables (Hays, 1965, p. 595). The numbers of fixations per cluster ranged from one fixation per cluster to over 17 fixations per cluster. However, only 11 fixations-per-cluster categories were used in testing the frequency distributions by chi square because so little data existed beyond the 11 fixations-per-cluster category.

Using an alpha level of .01, chi square tests revealed that the TN frequency distribution of numbers of fixations per cluster differed from the other three decision-category frequency distributions ($X^2(10) > 23.21, p < .01$). The FN frequency distribution of numbers of fixations per cluster was similar to

Tab. 1: Means and modes of number of fixations per cluster for four decision categories in Experiment 1

Decision	Number of Fixations per Cluster		Mean Cluster Duration (ms.)	
	Mean	Mode	Exp. 1[a] Data	Kundel et al., 1978 Data
True Positive (TP)	5.2	2,5	950	960
True Negative (TN)	3.7	2	670	730
False Negative (FN)	4.4	3	800	950
False Positive (FP)	4.5	2	820	—

a. The mean fixation duration data from Exp. 1 was derived by multiplying the mean number of fixations per cluster by the mean fixation duration which was 183 ms. The Kundel et al. (1978) data were taken from Table 2, p. 180 and reflect total fixation dwell averages. No data were available on false positive decisions in Kundel et al.

the FP frequency distribution ($X^2(10) = 11.49, n.s.$), and the FP distribution was similar to the TP distribution ($X^2(10) = 21.65, n.s.$). But the FN frequency distribution was different from the TP frequency distribution ($X^2(10) = 25.11, p < .01$). The similarity between FN and FP frequency distributions of numbers of fixations per cluster is interpreted as indicating that it takes as much time to decide to reject a true nodule as false, as to accept a false nodule feature as part of an imagined nodule.

We assume that FN decisions are caused when anatomic scenery obscures or camouflages the nodule target. This interpretation fits our previous findings (Kundel et al., 1978) that showed that FNs required more visual scrutiny as reflected by differences between initial and total fixation dwell on nodule targets. Note that estimates of mean cluster duration in Table 1 for Experiment 1, which were obtained by multiplying mean number of fixations per cluster in each decision category by mean overall fixation duration (183 ms), are consistent with those obtained by Kundel et al.

Results of Experiment 2

In Experiment 2, we measured the number of fixations per cluster on image features that viewers indicated as being either "suspect" or "nodule containing." This was accomplished by first requiring the viewer to search the image for a nodule while his eye movements were being recorded (15 s) followed by questions designed to elicit the locations of suspicious objects on the image as well as suspected nodules. The suspicious objects presumably indicate locations that contain nodule-like features, but did not meet the viewer's criteria for nodule targets.

A total of 231 suspected nodule targets, defined by the viewer as being fixated during search and pointed out afterwards, were recorded. Almost 75% of these suspected nodule targets were resolved by the radiologists as not containing nodules, but rather normal features. However, 11 percent were containing nodules (FNs). The remaining 25% of suspect nodule targets were resolved by the radiologists as nodules. For this subset of suspected nodule targets, 48 percent were truly normal (FPs). The important question here is whether the non-indicated, but fixated, FN decisions differ in number of fixations per cluster from the TNs. If so, they can be played back to the viewer for re-evaluation and some decisions will change from FN to TP (Nodine & Kundel, 1987).

Tab. 2: Relationship between image objects classified according to degree of suspicion, decision and information-processing load

Contents of Fixation Zone:	Image Object Noted As:	Decision About Object:	IP Load: (Fix/Clust)	Decision Outcome:
	Suspect	Nodule	4.9	TP (Scrutinized)
Nodule	Suspect	Non-Nodule	4.8	FN (Scrutinized)
	Non-Suspect	None	4.5	FN (Default)
	Suspect	Nodule	4.7	FP (Scrutinized)
Normal	Suspect	Non-Nodule	4.6	TN (Scrutinized)
	Non-Suspect	None	3.9	TN (Default)

Table 2 shows the relationship between various combinations of image objects rated by degree of suspicion, decision, and information-processing load measured in terms of mean number of fixations per cluster. Table 2 indicates that, compared to a default TN, a scrutinized TN takes 0.7 of a fixation per cluster more, on average, to decide that a suspected object is truly not nodule containing. The same might be expected to hold for the situation in which the viewer suspects an object that is a true nodule, but decides that it is not. This is the case of the scrutinized FN which also shows an increase of 0.9 fixation per cluster. Even when the true nodule target is not recognized as a suspected nodule target as is the case for default FN, there is still a 0.6 fixation per cluster increase. One would expect the difference between default FNs and scrutinized FNs to be greater since a true nodule target was presumably missed in the latter case. However, even though it was missed, it may have been fixated. The data show that all of the suspected FNs (n =17) were fixated, whereas only 68 percent of the non- suspected FNs (n =70) were fixated.

Perhaps it is the nodules that were rated "invisible" that are not being fixated, since they made up 55 percent of all nodule targets. But the interesting point is that even though they were rated invisible, both types of FNs required more fixations per cluster than default TNs. This would suggest that there is something unique about the eye landing on a real abnormality that both attracts attention and suspicion. Maybe the truly abnormal objects raise suspicion because fragments of the abnormality are recognized, but the data are simply too sparce to unambigiously decide that it is a nodule target. Whatever the case, the fact that FNs required more fixations per cluster on average than most TNs, as shown in Figure 2, means that we can identify them using number of fixations per cluster as the eye-movement measure.

If we feed back to the radiologist the image locations of fixation clusters containing many fixations, determined by computing fixations per cluster threshold values based on maximizing the likelihood of suspected nodule targets which are known to drew more fixations per cluster, the radiologist will pick up some of the true nodules that were suspected but dismissed (scrutinized FNs) during initial viewing. This threshold is maximum when the log likelihood ratio of FN/TN is positive. Missed nodules made up 11 percent of the FN category. If half of the suspected nodule targets falling in the missed FN decision category were converted to TP decisions during feedback, this would significantly improve the diagnostic accuracy of nodule detection among radiologists since they are already performing at a relatively high level by ROC standards. A test of the use of visual feedback under these conditions is currently being investigated (Nodine & Kundel, 1987)

Fixation duration

In contrast to the cluster data, fewer differences among decision categories were obtained when frequency distributions of fixation durations were tested using 2 (decision categories) x 15 (fixation duration intervals of 40 ms) chi square contingency tables. Only the difference between TN and TP distributions and TN and FN distributions were significant ($p < .01$). These differences reflect a shift toward longer fixation durations for TP and FN frequency distributions compared to the TN frequency distribution. The overall average fixation duration was 183 ms. Figure 5 shows the distributions for all three decision categories. The fact that there is a difference between FN and TN suggests that fixation duration can also be used to predict missed true nodules on chest x-ray images.

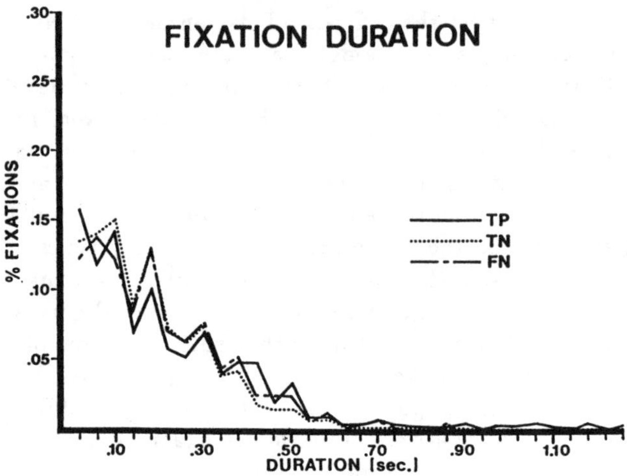

Fig. 5: The distributions of fixation durations for three types of decisions. The overall average fixation duration was 183 ms.

Conclusion

The comparison of the number of fixations per cluster with fixation duration indicates that the former is a more sensitive measure of information- processing load. This finding fits a theoretical interpretation that argues that increasing numbers of fixations clustering on objects of image scenery during search for a nodule target reflect visual scrutiny. Visual scrutiny implies information processing of image details designed to integrate suspected target features into a perceptual object that matches meaningful anatomical or pathological objects of chest imagery stored in the viewer's memory. Differences in the distributions of numbers of fixations clustering on target objects classified into true and false decision categories suggest that information processing is accomplished by directing a relatively large number of short-duration fixations to the suspected target rather than dwelling on it with a few long-duration fixations. Thus, the process of recognizing inconspicuous target objects in chest x-ray images seems to depend more on number of fixations per cluster than duration of individual fixations. The fixation still remains the natural unit of visual processing, but only a small portion of the total duration of a fixation is used to encode information; the bulk of the time being spent programing the next saccade which is either to acquire more local information or jump to a new image object. Because encoding time is limited and fixed (50 ms for reading tasks according to Rayner et al., 1981), number of fixations clustering on image objects may be a better predictor of information-processing load than duration of individual fixations for visual search tasks.

Acknowledgement

This research was supported in part by Grant No. CA 32870, National Cancer Institute, U.S.P.H.

References

Friedman, A., & Liebelt, L.S., *On the time course of viewing pictures with a view toward remembering*, in "D.F. Fisher, R.A. Monty, & J.W. Senders (Eds.), Eye movements, cognition and visual perception," Erlbaum, Hillsdale, N.J., 1981, pp. 137-155.

Jacobs, A.M., *Toward a model of eye movement control in visual search*, in "J.K. O'Regan & A. Lévy-Schoen (Eds.), Eye movements: From physiology to cognition," Elsevier, Amsterdam, 1987, pp. 275-284.

Just, M.A., & Carpenter, P.A., *A theory of reading: From eye fixations to comprehension*, Psychological Review **87** (1980), 329- 354.

Karsh, R., & Breitenbach, F.W., *Looking at looking: amorphous fixation measure*, in "R. Groner, C. Metz, D.F. Fisher, & R.A. Monty (Eds.), Eye movements and psychological functions: International views," Erlbaum, Hillsdale, N.J., 1983, pp. 53-64.

Kundel, H.L., Nodine, C.F., & Carmody, D.P., *Visual scanning, pattern recognition and decision making in pulmonary nodule detection*, Investigative Radiology **13** (1978), 175-181.

Loftus, G.R., *Eye fixations and recognition memory for pictures*, Cognitive Psychology **3** (1972), 525-551.

Loftus, G.R., *Tachistoscopic simulations of eye fixations on pictures*, Journal of Experimental Psychology: Human Learning and Memory **7** (1981), 369-376.

McConkie, G.W., Underwood, N.R., Zola, D., & Wolverton, G.S., *Some temporal characteristics of processes during reading*, Journal of Experimental Psychology: Human Perception and Performance **11** (1985), 168-186.

Nodine, C.F., & Kundel, H.L., *The cognitive side of visual search*, in "J.K. O'Regan & A. Lévy-Schoen (Eds.), Eye movements: From physiology to cognition," Elsevier, Amsterdam, 1987a, pp. 573- 582.

Nodine, C.F., & Kundel, H.L., *Using eye movements to study visual search and improve tumor detection*, Radiographics **7** (1987b), 1241-1250.

Rayner, K., Inhoff, A.H., Morrison, R.E., Slowiaczek, M.L., & Bertera, J.H., *Masking of foveal and parafoveal vision during eye fixations in reading*, Journal of Experimental Psychology: Human Perception and Performance **7** (1981), 167-179.

Schneider, W., & Schiffrin, R.M., *Controlled and automatic human information processing: Detection, search, and attention*, Psychological Review **84** (1977), 1-66.

Treisman, A.M., & Gelade, G., *A feature-integration theory of attention*, Cognitive Psychology **12** (1980), 97-136.

AUTHOR INDEX

SUBJECT INDEX

LIST OF CONTRIBUTORS

Prof. Dr. Wolfgang Becker
- see Jürgens

Rob Berg
- see van Gisbergen

Dr. Ir. Lo Bour
Department of
Clinical Neurophysiology, H2-214
Academic Medical Centre, AZUA
Meibergdreef 9
NL-1105 AZ, Amsterdam
The Netherlands

Dr. David Brogan
- see Findlay

Dr. Marc Brysbaert
Laboratory of
Experimental Psychology
University of Leuven
Tiensestraat 102
B-3000 Leuven
Belgium

Prof. Patricia A. Carpenter
- see Just

Dr. Pierre Courrieu
- see Pynte

Prof. Dr. Otto D. Creutzfeldt
Abteilung Neurobiologie
Max-Planck-Institut für
biophysikalische Chemie
P.O. Box 2841
D-3400 Göttingen
Federal Republic of Germany

Dr. Heiner Deubel
Lehrstuhl für Nachrichtentechnik
Technische Universität München
Arcisstr. 21
D-8000 München 2
Federal Republic of Germany

Dr. John M. Findlay
Department of Psychology
University of Durham
Science Laboratories
South Road
Durham, DH1 3LE
United Kingdom

Dr. Hessel Franssen
Afdeling Klinische Neurofysiologie
Academisch Ziekenhuis
Nicolaas Beetstraat 24
NL-3511 HG Utrecht
The Netherlands

Dr. Jan van Gisbergen
Department of
Medical Physics & Biophysics
University of Nijmegen
Geert Grooteplein Noord 21
NL-6525 EZ Nijmegen
The Netherlands

Prof. Dr. Rudolf Groner
Psychologisches Institut
Universität Bern
Laupenstr. 4
CH-3008 Bern
Switzerland

Prof. Dr. Dieter Heller
Psychologisches Institut
der Universität Fribourg
Route des Fougères
CH-1701 Fribourg
Switzerland

Dr. Arthur M. Jacobs
Groupe Regard, Laboratoire de
Psychologie Expérimentale
CNRS & Université René Descartes
28, rue Serpente
F-75006 Paris
France

Dr. Reinhart Jürgens
Sektion Neurophysiologie
Oberer Eselsberg
D-7900 Ulm
Federal Republic of Germany

Prof. Marcel Adam Just
Department of Psychology
Carnegie-Mellon University
Pittsburgh, PA 15213
USA

Prof. Alan Kennedy
Department of Psychology
University of Dundee
Dundee DD1 4HN
Scotland

Dr. Kazuo Koga
Department of Aerospace Psychology
The Research Institute of
Environmental Medicine
Nagoya University
Chikusa-ku, Nagoya 464
Japan

Dr. Anselm W. Kornhuber
- see Jürgens

Prof. Dr. Werner Krause
Friedrich-Schiller-Universität
Sektion Psychologie
Schillerstr. 8
GDR-6900 Jena
German Democratic Republic

Dr. Harald Kundel, M.D.
- see Nodine

Dr. Uta Lass
- see Lüer

Dr. Ariane Lévy-Schoen
- see Jacobs

Prof. Dr. Gerd Lüer
Institut für Psychologie
Georg-August-Universität Göttingen
Gosslerstr. 14
D-3400 Göttingen
Federal Republic of Germany

Prof. Dr. Tatsuro Makino
Department of
Educational Psychology
Waseda University
Nishiwaseda Shinjyuku-ku, Tokyo
Japan

Dr. George W. McConkie
Center for the Study of Reading
University of Illinois
51 Gerty Drive
Champaign, IL 61820
USA

Dr. Wayne S. Murray
- see Kennedy

Prof. Calvin F. Nodine, Ph. D.
Pendergrass Laboratory
Department of Radiology
University of Pennsylvania
School of Medicine
3 Medical Education Building
36th Hamilton Walk
Philadelphia, PA 19104-6086
USA

Dr. J. Kevin O'Regan
- see Vitu

James B. Polikoff
- see Nodine

Dr. Joel Pynte
Centre de Recherche en
Psychologie Cognitive
Université de Provence
29, Avenue Robert Schuman
F-13621 Aix-en-Provence
France

Katsuaki Sakata
Japan Color Research Institute
Nishiazabu Minato-ku, Tokyo
Japan

Prof. Dr. Roberto Schmid
Dipartimento di Informatica
e Sistemistica
Universita' di Pavia
Via Abbiategrasso 209
I-27100 Pavia
Italy

Dr. Josephine Shallo-Hoffmann
Universitäts-Augenklinik
Abteilung Strabologie &
Neurophthalmologie
Robert-Koch-Str. 40
D-3400 Göttingen
Federal Republic of Germany

Arend Smit
- see van Gisbergen

Dr. Ir. Dirk Frederik Stegeman
Afdeling Klinische Neurofysiologie
Instituut voor Neurologie
Reinier Postlaan 4
NL-6500 HB Nijmegen
The Netherlands

Nobuko Takahashi
Department of Psychology
Waseda University
Toyama Shinjyuku-ku, Tokyo
Japan

Lawrence L. Toto
- see Nodine

Dr. N. Roderic Underwood
Claremont Teachers' College
Claremont, Western Australia, 6010
Australia

Françoise Vitu
Groupe Regard
Laboratoire de Psychologie
Expérimentale, CNRS
Université René Descartes
EHESS, EPHE
28, rue Serpente
F-75006 Paris
France

Gary S. Wolverton
- see McConkie

Prof. Dr. Géry d'Ydewalle
- see Brysbaert

Dr. Daniela Zambarbieri
- see Schmid

Dr. David Zola
- see McConkie